Optical Play

SRLT

Northwestern University Press
Studies in Russian Literature and Theory

Optical Play

Glass, Vision, and Spectacle in Russian Culture

Julia Bekman Chadaga

NORTHWESTERN UNIVERSITY PRESS / EVANSTON, ILLINOIS

Northwestern University Press
www.nupress.northwestern.edu

Printed in the United States of America

10 9 8 7 6 5 4 3 2 1

Library of Congress Cataloging-in-Publication Data

Chadaga, Julia Bekman, author.
Optical play : glass, vision, and spectacle in Russian culture / Julia Bekman Chadaga.
pages cm
Includes bibliographical references and index.
ISBN 978-0-8101-3003-6 (cloth : alk. paper)—ISBN 978-0-8101-6788-9 (ebook)
1. Russian literature—History and criticism. 2. Glass in literature. 3. Vision in literature. 4. Glass—Social aspects—Russia. 5. Vision—Social aspects—Russia. 6. Glass construction—Social aspects—Russia. I. Title.
PG2975.C47 2014
891.70936—dc23
2014018889

♾ The paper used in this publication meets the minimum requirements of the American National Standard for Information Sciences—Permanence of Paper for Printed Library Materials, ANSI Z39.48–1992.

To my parents, Valéry and Larisa Bekman

Contents

Illustrations

Acknowledgments

This project has come a long way since its first glimmering in a strategy session with Vivek Chadaga in a Cambridge café; out of that conversation emerged a "glass matrix" and subsequently a paper for Julie Buckler's inspiring graduate seminar. Over the years, as that paper grew into a dissertation and then this book, I have benefited from the support and encouragement of many people and institutions. As I look back on my journey through Glassland, I am filled with gratitude toward all who have helped me in my quest and feel wonder-struck at their generosity.

I was able to conduct research for my project and do substantial amounts of writing and revision thanks to funding from the Abby and George O'Neill Research Travel Grant, a Graduate Society Term-Time Dissertation Fellowship, a Foreign Language and Area Studies award, and the Andrew W. Mellon Foundation–Humanities Center Interdisciplinary Dissertation Completion Fellowship. I received valuable materials and assistance from many institutions in Russia. In Moscow, I am grateful to the staff of the State Historical Museum, the State Literature Museum, the Russian State Library, the History Library, the State Museum of Ceramics (Kuskovo Estate), the Museum of Applied and Folk Art, and the Tsaritsyno Museum. In St. Petersburg, my thanks go to the staff of the Lomonosov Museum, the Museum of the History of St. Petersburg, the State Russian Museum, the State Hermitage (especially the department of Russian Culture), Oranienbaum, the Peter the Great Museum of Anthropology and Ethnography (Kunstkamera), the Palace-Museum of Peter I, and the Peterhof Museum.

The sense of sight is at the heart of this book, and so I am indebted to the museum staff members who helped me to obtain images and permission to use them: Mary B. Chervenak at the Corning Museum of Glass, Ol'ga Savvina and Evgeniia Petrova at the Russian Museum, Zhanna Etsina at the Hermitage, Natalia Zhukova at the State Historical Museum, Maria A. Yanes at the Kunstkamera, Tatiana Enikeeva at Kuskovo, and the staff of the House-Museum of Peter I in Vologda. I owe particular thanks to Liudmila Alekseeva Aksyonova at the Museum of the History of St. Petersburg, and Elena Aleksandrovna Ivanova at the Russian Museum. At the State Historical Museum in Moscow, Liudmila Aronovna Dement'eva, the head of the metal department, shared a number of valuable leads and showed me my first *zertsalo*, in whose physical existence I had not quite believed up until then; and Inna Ivanovna Sergeenko, head of the glass and ceramics department, gave me access to a treasure trove of glassware and provided illuminating information. I am grateful for the hospitality of those who provided housing and companionship during my travels in Russia: Nina Fyodorovna Lykova and Anna Dimitrievna Korshunova in Moscow, and Larisa Bondar and Yuri Kholkin in St. Petersburg; I also wish to thank Margarita Georgievna Nirman for her insightful cultural commentary.

The welcoming surroundings and rich collections of several libraries in the U.S. helped me to advance my research: Widener Library and Houghton Library at Harvard University; the Northwestern University Library; and the DeWitt Wallace Library at Macalester College, whose staff has provided invaluable assistance: the magic of interlibrary loan brought rare volumes within my reach, while Johan Oberg, Chris Schommer, and Elizabeth Hutchins helped immensely with capturing prized images and finding a home for them within my book.

I am thankful to the audiences at Amherst College, Yale University, Columbia University, and at conferences in San Francisco, Salt Lake City, Boston, and Middletown, Conn., who offered valuable comments on talks that I gave on various aspects of this project. Marcus Levitt provided wonderful feedback on my first conference paper and on my first publication. Isobel Armstrong and Oksana Bulgakowa were kind enough to meet with me and share their own perspectives on glass. I learned many things from fellow participants at the Objects of Affection conference at Princeton University in May 2012, including Krisztina Fehervary, Joan Neuberger, Kim Lane Scheppele, and Emma Widdis; and I am grateful to Serguei Oushakine for organizing the conference, a powerful way to affirm the cross-disciplinary potential of material culture studies that allowed me to clarify my thinking about how glass fits in.

My dissertation readers, Svetlana Boym, William Mills Todd III, and Julie A. Buckler, continue to be role models for me as scholars and mentors. All three were extraordinarily generous in sharing their ideas and offering substantive feedback; I am thankful for their encouragement and faith in the value of my project, which they championed during every stage of its development. Many friends, colleagues, and students had a part to play in the evolution of my book. I was fortunate to learn from stimulating conversations with Ellen Arnold, Edyta Bojanowka, David Brandenberger, Katia Dianina, Gitta Hammarberg, Tim Harte, Anna Katsnelson, Anastasia Kayiatos, Anna Krylova, Julia Livshin, Sasha Lyons, Ethan Ostrow, Sean Pollock,

Rachel Perlmeter, Polina Rikoun, Karen Rosenflanz, Svetlana Rukhelman, Beth Severy-Hoven, Cristina Vatulescu, and Jim von Geldern. Elizaveta Kundas provided valuable assistance in the U.S. and in Russia; Martha Davis and Judith Klasson were great sources of administrative and emotional support. Priscilla Meyer taught me about the thrill of literary detective work and nurtured my scholarly instincts in crucial ways. I am thankful to Louise Dickson and Matthew Thrasher for locating images; to Lazar Fleishman, Grigori Freidin, Natalia Melikova, and Janice Pilch for guiding me through the dark forest of copyright questions; and to Bill Butler for showing me the *zertsalo* in a different light.

Ernie Capello generously shared advice that proved essential for helping to move my book through the production process. My manuscript improved a great deal thanks to the feedback that I received from my anonymous readers, whose detailed responses to my work helped me to see the shape of my argument more clearly and to strengthen the book as a whole. At Northwestern University Press, Mike Levine and Gary Saul Morson provided steadfast support and useful suggestions throughout the revision process, Gianna Mosser was of great help with illustrations, and Anne Gendler shepherded me through the maze of copyediting with sensitivity and finesse; I am very thankful to them all.

I owe a special debt of gratitude to Julia Vaingurt, whom I am proud to call an intellectual fellow traveler, and whose eloquent critiques of hundreds of pages' worth of drafts from every stage of this project, as well as her brilliance, good humor, and kindness, sustained me through trying times and helped to improve this book in countless ways.

Some of the material in this book first appeared in *Russian Review* (January 2002); *Slavic Review* (Spring 2007); *Studies in Twentieth and Twenty-First Century Literature* (Summer 2010); and *Novoe Literaturnoe Obozrenie* (2013); and I would like to thank the editorial staff of each of these journals. Portions of chapter 6 have appeared in "From Lenin's Tomb to Avtovo Station: Illusion and Spectacle in Soviet Subterranean Space," in *Rites of Place: Public Commemoration in Russia and Eastern Europe*, edited by Julie Buckler and Emily Johnson (Northwestern University Press, 2013).

My work has benefited tremendously from the help and warm support of my family. My parents, Valéry and Larisa Bekman, gave me precious insights into the Russian language and Russian culture for which I am ever thankful; they have helped me to discover my intellectual passions and, leading by example, emboldened me to be an intrepid explorer in every aspect of life, from my childhood on Lomonosov Street and every step of the way since then. Svetlana Bekman has always been there as a thoughtful interlocutor and a trusted friend; her aptitude for everything from legal discourse to jewelry-making has encouraged me to be as multifaceted in my own life.

Mani and Sophia Chadaga have infused my life with a sense of play and wondrous defamiliarization, so important for scholarly inquiry and every other form of human flourishing. Vivek Chadaga, my most insightful reader, the best writer that I know, and the love of my life, challenged, cheered, and inspired me over the course of my work on this project; I am more grateful to him than words can say.

Note on Transliteration

I have followed the Library of Congress system for transliterating Russian in the endnotes and bibliography; in the text itself, I have also used this system, with the exception of some familiar names that are customarily known in an alternate transliteration, for example, Mayakovsky rather than Maiakovskii.

Optical Play

Introduction

> Our sovereign and his inner circle went beyond the sea, and he traveled through the foreign lands and visited Glassland. And in the foreign lands a maiden rules the Glass Kingdom; that maiden abused our sovereign; she put him in a hot frying pan, took him out of the frying pan and had him tossed into a dungeon. . . . That man is not our sovereign, but a foreigner; our sovereign, while among the foreigners, was sealed into a barrel and cast into the sea.
>
> —Folk legend cited by S. M. Solov'ev

ACCORDING TO POPULAR legend, Peter the Great met an untimely end in the perilous kingdom of Glassland. In ironic contradiction to the transparent name of that kingdom, the emperor, it seems, was hidden from sight in a dungeon, then sealed in a barrel and consigned to the depths of the sea. It was not Peter, but a foreigner masquerading as him (just as glass can masquerade as a more precious material, from amethyst to gold) who returned to rule over Russia. Peter should have never traveled abroad; and he certainly should have never, ever set foot in Glassland.

In this legend, glass becomes invested with several provocative attributes. It is a signifier of the foreign, the alien, the strange; it belongs to the fairy-tale realm, and more broadly, the domain of the imagination. The word *Stekgol'm* (Stockholm), enigmatic-sounding to the Russian ear, mutates into the more comprehensible *Stekol'nyi*, an adjective meaning "of glass." The foreign city-name acts as an incantation, and a city of glass emerges from a linguistic misapprehension. This invention then generates another: the city of Stekol'nyi is part of an entire "Glass Kingdom" (*Stekol'noe tsarstvo*)—which comes to stand for all that is hostile and menacing to Russia. The people among whom this legend arose were apparently predisposed to think of glass in such terms.

It is customary to consider glass as synonymous with clarity; yet the legend of Peter's demise makes Glassland a place where obscurity and darkness reign. Because of its transparency, we have also come to regard glass as a purely functional material—in other words, we do not really regard it at all. We simply look through it at whatever is on the other side. Yet glass is never merely functional; and in Russia, its uses are even more complex, as an example from more recent times shows. Urban dwellers are familiar with the way in which windows in subway cars turn into mirrors when the trains race through tunnels. As Elena Frolova reports, however, the window-mirrors in the Russian metro yield bizarre reflections, for reasons that have to do with an anxiety about foreignness, akin to the one that informed the legend of Peter in Glassland:

> You've probably noticed at one time or another the reflection of the passenger sitting next to you and thought: "What a freak of nature! How can he live with a face like that?" I don't mean to offend you, but you are, to put it mildly, no beauty yourself (I'm talking about your reflection). On the other hand, if there's nothing else to do during the ride, you can make funny faces and entertain yourself and the people around you.[1]

What is the source of these funhouse-mirror reflections? To create the panes of the windows in question, molten glass is stretched out between a series of rollers, then cooled and polished. This process inevitably leads to distortion, and thus, distorted reflections. Frolova observes that in the West they have come up with a way to combat such distortion, because "they don't appreciate our national form of amusement." The technique for producing perfectly smooth sheet glass involves floating the molten glass on a pool of molten tin.[2] While other countries have adopted this method, most factories in Russia—including the one where the metro windows are made—still use the old technique that yields distorted glass. On the bright side, Frolova concedes, "You'll never be bored riding the metro."

The windows in a metro car do not always serve as windows, but in the Russian case, even their mirror function is subverted. Instead of seeing a true likeness, the viewer finds himself changed, as if in a fairy tale, into something freakish and unrecognizable (just as Peter was swapped for a foreign impostor in Glassland). Frolova gently chides the backwardness of her compatriots, yet she takes pride in their imaginative reaction to their funhouse reality, enabled by a peculiar kind of glass. Thus the question of how glass transforms vision—literally and figuratively—is topical in Russia even today.

This study explores the uses and abuses of glass in the cultural history of modern Russia. As a material, glass is unique in the way that it has captivated people's imagination throughout its long history. In the modern world, glass has played a crucial role in the transformation of technology, art, and vision itself.[3] As a recent study on glass as a material at the intersection of art and science argues, glass production brought about "a technical revolution . . . capable of subverting the modes of perception of the outside world whether in daily life or in the area of philosophical and scientific reflection."[4]

Using selected case studies, I tell the story of how the appearance of glass objects in Russia over the course of several centuries following the Petrine reforms affected the lives of the human beings who interacted with them. My argument is that these objects transformed the ways in which their beholders saw as well as imagined; thus, in addition to its more apparent optical effect, glass had a profound influence on the workings of the mind's eye. I draw much of my evidence for these transformations from literary texts, because I believe that such texts serve not only to record the phenomena that their authors encounter in their day-to-day lives, but also to reflect upon the meaning of these phenomena and to suggest the implications of Russians' experience with glass for a broader consideration of this material's significance in the modern world.

Glass engages with the sense of sight; by changing how the *subject* of the gaze *sees* and how the *object* of the gaze *looks*, glass mediates the way we see through subtle, often invisible means: in Isobel Armstrong's formulation, glass is "always in between."[5] When we consider glass and its uses over the centuries, we see how our ways of seeing have changed.[6] Rather than attempt to provide an exhaustive survey of Russian seeing practices, I focus instead on several instructive case studies whose analysis yields wider implications for the study of visual and material culture in Russia; my hope is that this project will encourage fellow scholars to continue exploring the transformative effect that the things surrounding us have had in the past and continue to have in the present.

The issue of how Russians fashioned their self-identity while casting glances—now admiring, now antagonistic—toward the West is key for understanding the stories of Peter in Glassland and the Russian metro windows discussed above. These examples serve to introduce a central argument in my book about how glass simultaneously helped to both symbolize and realize modernity and the process of Westernization in Russia. I juxtapose Russian artifacts and texts with Western analogues in order to elucidate Russia's relationship toward the West as well as Russians' ambivalence about modernization. My focus is on specifically Russian cultural meanings; examples from other parts of the world serve to highlight what is unique about the Russian response to glass, but also to situate the Russian example within a broader context of human interaction with this material. Our response to sensory stimuli is to an extent universal, but at the same time, always culturally situated; both of these considerations shape my investigation of glass in Russia.

By locating Russia within the realm of glass discovery and innovation, my study serves as a corrective to histories of glass that claim to be comprehensive yet omit Russia from their map of the world. Thus, two recent studies, *Glass: From the First Mirror to Fiber Optics, the Story of the Substance That Changed the World* and *Glass: A World History*, do not take Russia into consideration. These omissions attest to a refusal, whether deliberate or simply automatic, to grant Russia those attributes of enlightenment, scientific innovation, and artistic brilliance that are associated with the development of glassmaking in a particular country. Exploring the prominent status of glass in Russian culture will therefore challenge the preconceptions that Western readers may have about Russia.

In this study I aim to excavate and explicate seldom-seen objects of beauty and significance that would otherwise be lost to scholars; beyond that, I trace the symbolic meanings assigned to glass in Russia from the post-Petrine period up to the present day. Building on Yury Lotman's idea about the textuality of artifacts, I propose that glass objects—"works of glass"—can be read as texts because they are part of the same sign system as the verbal documents that I analyze. Lotman defines culture as a form of interaction within a specific social group and posits that "any structure serving the sphere of social interaction is a language," that is, "a system of signs used according to rules known to members of the given collective." In the category of "signs" Lotman places words, visual images, and things—any form of "material expression that *has a meaning* and can therefore be used to *convey sense*. It follows that culture has, first, a communicative, and second, a symbolic nature."[7] Taking into account the experience of both the authors and the readers of the "works of glass" under consideration, my study examines glass from the dual perspective of production and consumption. In approaching glass as readable text, I am also inspired by Armstrong's insightful work on the transformations of the visible world and in the world of ideas engendered by the mass production of glass in nineteenth-century England. She combines a poetic imagination with scholarly rigor, reminds us that "texts disclose the invisible presence of an invisible layer of glass in innumerable ways,"[8] and shows glass itself as the eloquent text that it truly is.

This project seeks to broaden the boundaries of the Slavic field by exploring how material culture studies can help enrich the analysis of literature. Material culture studies is a subset of cultural studies; "material culture" may be thought of as culturally constituted relationships to objects; social relations as mediated through objects; and/or the material forms taken by culture (defined as a process through which human groups construct themselves and are socialized). Anthropologist Daniel Miller sees the task of material culture studies as a rescue effort, recuperating artifacts from fetishization and making them legible, understandable as embodiments of human values.[9]

We respond to material things with our senses, in contrast to processing abstract ideas with our intellect. Arguably, this former kind of response is more universal than the latter. Art historian Jules David Prown provocatively asserts that artifacts are material expressions of underlying cultural beliefs that are obscured or repressed in written documents and works of art, which are produced with the explicit intent to communicate.[10] Miller seems to argue rather for the duplicity of objects, which "often appear as more 'natural' than words, in that we come across them in the main as already existing things, unlike at least spoken language, which is produced in front of us. This quality of artefacts helps, as it were, to entrance us, to cause us to forget that they are indeed artefacts, embodiments of cultural codes, rather than simply the natural environment within which we live."[11] This line of reasoning can also serve as an argument in support of interpreting artifacts rather than taking them at face value—which is exactly what I seek to do with material objects depicted in literary texts.

My approach calls for analyzing texts that refer to particular objects and showing how the text and the object mutually illuminate one another. It is important to look at the elements of material reality in a work of literature because our relationships and self-definitions are always mediated by the objects that surround us. Glass is particularly relevant in this respect, because it mediates the way that we see. In reading verbal texts and artifacts side by side, I aim to shed new light on literary works whose authors deploy glass realia in telling ways. Literary critics conventionally regard the material world of a fictional text in terms that evoke the hierarchy of personage and stage property: just as in the theater, the actors have primary and the props only secondary importance, so too in fiction the material objects depicted—according to this assumption—only exist to fill in the space around the characters. I strive to undo this hierarchy in order to show that artifacts in literature can speak volumes.

This project began as a quest to solve a mystery about a parallel occurrence in eighteenth-century Russia: in the period when both the domestic glass industry and secular literature were starting to blossom, authors crafted the physical attributes of glass—such as its capacity to reflect as well as transmit light—into figurative language to describe the social transformations that they witnessed happening around them. This process, whereby the sensuous qualities of a substance are transformed into metaphors that are then applied to social phenomena, and which characterizes the Russian response to the presence of glass throughout the period under consideration, can be understood with reference to the concept of qualisigns, defined as the material attributes of things that can be perceived by the senses; this term was introduced by semiotician C. S. Peirce and developed in recent years by anthropologists exploring the signifying potential of material culture.

In her analysis of the emotional qualities with which people in

Soviet-bloc countries invested construction materials such as wood and plastic, Krisztina Fehervary shows how the concept of qualisigns sheds light on the way in which "sensory experience of the material world" generates meaning. Fehervary argues that iconicity, or resemblance, "characterizes the relationship between sensuous qualities of things and how we take them up in language to describe concepts, values or emotional states."[12] Focusing on one specific substance, olive oil, Anne Meneley calls for increased scholarly attention to "the material substrate of the symbolic"[13] and describes how such qualities as immiscibility, luminosity, and the capacity to cleanse, warm, seal and preserve, penetrate and permeate have served to imbue the material with symbolic meanings and immense value in both sacred and secular contexts: "Olive oil's persuasive qualisigns are the source of its longevity not only as a food, but as a source of spiritual succor."[14] Meneley notes that each of the physical qualities of olive oil "is potentially the material basis for a sign"; the potentiality is key, because different qualities are emphasized depending on the cultural context, and thus the meaning of this substance cannot be pinned down to something "universal [and] unchanging."

The qualisigns of glass include transparency and translucency; the capacity to refract and reflect light; fragility; coldness; chemical nonreactiveness; capacity to change the perceived size of an object; capacity to take multiple forms and imitate other materials; and acoustic and electrostatic qualities. All of these come into play in the analysis of various culturally significant glass objects in my study; over a period of time, reinforced by cultural texts and through social practice, the physical qualities of glass generate symbolic associations that then get assigned to the human actors using these objects. To cite a few examples that will be explored in subsequent chapters: the creation of ever-larger windows suggests a society increasingly oriented toward openness and honesty; the glass chambers of Tatlin's tower gesture at the "purity" of the political work carried on inside the building; the luster of the Crystal Bed conveys the magnificence of the empire that created it. In each case, some qualities of the object are foregrounded while others are elided, but those latter qualities haunt the object and threaten at any moment to disrupt the stable meaning that it is meant to convey. Thus, Lenin's display case is transparent, and provides the illusion of access to the embalmed, yet "more alive than all the living" leader, as well as evidence of his miraculous preservation; but the coffin is also fragile, inviting attempts to destroy it in order to symbolically lash out at what the object within represents.

Material culture studies fascinated me before I even knew that such a discipline existed. I have long sought to articulate to myself the connection between the linguistic realm and the material world. Possibly this has something to do with the violent rupture between signifier and signified that I experienced as an émigré who arrived in the United States in 1979 with a meager arsenal of English words (the Queen's English, as it turned out). In fact, those material remnants of our abandoned Soviet home that we managed to preserve—a carved wooden jewelry box, a tennis ball the color of smoke, an A-line *sarafan* in a florid pattern—made me conscious even then of the treasure trove of meaning that lies concealed, waiting to be discovered—a story waiting to be told—in the humblest of things.

The objects that I have just catalogued would find a home in the "lyrical museum" of Mikhail Epstein, theorist and practitioner of realogy (the science of things). By means of his writings as well as a museum that houses personal artifacts and their particular stories, Epstein seeks to bring to light the "endless variety and profound significance of things in human life, the wealth of their figurative and conceptual meaning, which can in no way be reduced to a utilitarian role. The whole of human life consists of things and is preserved in them, like so many geological layers, through which we can trace a succession of ages, tastes, attachments, fascinations."[15] Just as Epstein and his fellow thinkers try to preserve meaningful private artifacts from falling into obscurity, I am motivated to perform a similar rescue attempt with regard to objects that were once in the public domain, and seen by innumerable eyes. Even private artifacts, however, can be considered through the prism of the collective. We may have private relationships with our things, but when these things were made, their creation was informed by ideas prevalent in the culture at that time. One can think of them as material embodiments of the culture—sites where certain collectively held ideas crystallized.

Glass objects embody ideas that we can access to gain entry to the past, but it is just as important to consider their affective dimension. In her stimulating book *Vibrant Matter: A Political Ecology of Things*, Jane Bennett argues that bodies, whether animate or not, "affect other bodies, enhancing or weakening their power."[16] Bennett recalls serving on a jury and observing the persuasive power of a glass container known as a Gunpowder Residue Sampler:

> It was a small glass vial with an adhesive-covered metal lid. . . . This object/witness had been dabbed on the accused's hand hours after the shooting and now offered to the jury its microscopic evidence that the hand had either fired a gun or been within three feet of a gun firing. . . . This composite of glass, skin cells, glue, words, laws, metals, and human emotions had become an actant[,] that which, by virtue of its particular location in an assemblage and the fortuity of being in the right place at the right time, makes the difference, makes things happen.[17]

How does glass "make things happen"? In my view, the answer in large part has to do with the ways in which glass invites the human gaze by acting as a reflective surface or a transparent container, whether for objects or for light.

As a material that captures and manipulates light like no other, glass has contributed throughout history to the staging of spectacles whose aim was to discipline and indoctrinate. Michel Foucault's insights on the relationship between power and the gaze inspire my own approach.[18] I expand upon Richard Wortman's term "scenarios of power," which refers to performative mythmaking meant to consolidate autocratic power by appealing to "the symbolic sphere of ceremonies and imagery" in imperial Russia.[19] My focus, however, is not on processes that unfold in time, but on concrete objects that become part of the environment and that large groups of people are compelled to view—whether because these objects are always in their line of sight, or on the horizon, or part of an invented tradition in which they are obligated to participate. The objects themselves may be static, but the experience of seeing them is a potentially dynamic one in that it may bring about a transformation within the self.

Reflective glass plays a significant part in this book, but my interest in the collective gaze takes this project beyond the type of subjectivity typically associated with literary images of solitary mirror contemplation.[20] At the turn of the twentieth century, plate glass came into wider use in Russia and there emerged a kind of spectacular subjectivity, suggested by the image of multiple storefront reflections of passersby who simultaneously see themselves and others seeing them. Vladimir Mayakovsky, speaking for the Futurists at a public lecture in 1913, defined beauty as the frenetic street life of the urban crowd and enormous shop windows reflecting the images of tramways, trucks, and automobiles flying by.[21] The interaction of the shop windows and the urban crowds creates an environment of multiple reflection and aesthetic inspiration. Armstrong discusses this phenomenon in the context of nineteenth-century England: the human sensorium begins to respond to "the new production of mass-produced transparency in which one's body can be, glancingly, inadvertently, reflected back from the environment, belonging to the urban phantasmagoria outside one's control. For the first time in our culture, perhaps, the self can be a mirage returned from the surfaces of the city's landscape."[22] In the Russian literary tradition, such modernist works as Yury Olesha's *Envy* (1927) depict the psychological impact of this phenomenon.

Reflection is an obvious way in which glass mediates how we see the world, but even transparent glass alters perception. When advances in glassmaking technology allowed the manufacture of large shop windows, the commodities on display began to look radically different; consumer goods took on the aura of works of art. As Wolfgang Schivelbusch observes, "the uninterrupted, transparently sparkling surface acted rather like glass on a framed painting." A mid-nineteenth-century observer noted that "dull colours receive . . . an element of freshness, sparkle and refinement, because glass as a medium alters appearances and irritates the eye. . . . Putting paintings under glass makes them appear better than they really are. The protective glass confers upon good copies an additional element of deception. The plate glass of shop windows, too, has an 'improving' effect on some goods."[23] Glass bestows value on whatever it encases, by giving it a surface luster associated with more precious substances. My study asks: Why is glass a perpetually modern material? Why do so many futuristic visions include gleaming glass houses, and why did utopian thinkers want to live in such dwellings? Is it a matter of the democratic ideals associated with transparency—the destruction of the boundary between inside and outside, public and private, as championed by the advocates of architectural glass—or the desire to take on the luster that a glass case confers?

Studying the spectacular display function of glass can reveal much about the beliefs and anxieties of a society. In his *System of Objects*, Jean Baudrillard approaches glass as a material that fosters the denial of contact. The ambiguity of our appraisal of glass has to do with its capacity to take on contrasting functions: "it is at once proximity and distance, intimacy and the refusal of intimacy, communication and non-communication." We somehow cannot help but project a human value system upon this unassuming material because its functional uses create around it an aura of purity and reliability, "hygiene and prophylaxis"; in Baudrillard's view, these attributes make glass "truly the material of the future—a future, after all, that is to be one of disavowal of the body . . . in the name of a radiant and functional objectivity."[24] Yet Baudrillard's notion of the disavowal of the body is problematized by images in cultural texts that imbue glass with human, bodily attributes. This latter phenomenon may be a kind of wishful thinking, an attempt to draw a parallel between being human and such desirable qualities of glass as clarity, purity, and honesty.[25]

Glass is both utilitarian and mystical, and as such it speaks to the oscillation between these two poles in the human psyche. Utopian building projects are the most striking example of architecture that is designed to transform not only the outside world but mankind itself—architecture that works miracles. Inevitably, glass is involved in such projects; it is always already modern, but it also carries associations of ancient mystery and timeless magic. Glass signifies both the future just out of reach and, in the glass city from the Book of Revelation, the very end of history.[26]

At the opening ceremony of the Great Exhibition of 1851 in London, housed in the famous Crystal Palace, the archbishop of Canterbury delivered a speech invoking the glass city of the New Jerusalem. He bade his listeners to regard the Crystal Palace as "a heavenly palace," then cited a passage from the Book of Revelation: "And he carried me away in the Spirit to a mountain great and high, and showed me the Holy City, Jerusalem, coming down out of heaven from God. It shone with the glory of God, and its brilliance was like that of a very precious jewel, like jasper, clear as crystal. . . . The city was like pure glass. It did not need the sun or the moon to shine on it, for the glory of God gives it light, and the Lamb is its lamp."[27] The glass building that housed the exhibition was filled with plants and regarded by contemporaries as a gigantic winter garden (indeed, architect Joseph Paxton was a greenhouse designer); and at the time, gardens had strong associations with paradise. The building was also lit from within by numerous gas lanterns, which underscored the correspondences with the radiant glass city of New Jerusalem. Yet as Grigorii Revzin points out, while the archbishop's speech belonged to the genre of the sermon "where such associations are rhetorically appropriate," his audience took his words literally. "In 1851, Europe finally found out what heaven would look like. It is made of glass and steel, illuminated, and filled not with angels and righteous men, but with vast numbers of goods, merchants, and shoppers."[28]

From the advent of larger windows in the wake of the Petrine revolution in architecture to the Constructivist designs for glass houses, architecture is a central motif in my study. By virtue of its architectural applications, the ubiquity, and even the invisibility, of glass in our time make it a continuous source of wonder. In 2010, a viral video captured pop singer Justin Bieber walking through a revolving door and colliding with a pane of glass that he did not know was there. The scene played like a comical version of the verse opening of Nabokov's novel *Pale Fire* (whose plot line features a revolution that breaks out in a glass factory): "I was the shadow of the waxwing slain / By the false azure of the windowpane." In fact, the video clip and its Nabokovian antecedent embody the reason why glass is a perpetual object of fascination for human beings. This reason has to do with its role in the built environment. We build things in order to make our lives easier and happier, and sometimes we get good results, but at other times we only succeed in creating obstacles to that sought-after happiness; and glass in the built environment is a case study that testifies to this paradox.

My argument about how the presence and use of glass objects contributed to a transformation of vision in Russia and beyond draws upon evidence from texts that illustrate how this transformation is reflected in literature and how it influences the development of literature itself. Moreover, in tracing the functional and symbolic applications of glass in Russian culture, my study documents a transformation not only of vision (and attempts to create such a transformation) but also of the built environment—living conditions that arguably shape human beings in profound ways.

In his monumental work *Culture Two*, Vladimir Papernyi discusses larger manifestations of Stalinist culture through architecture, which for him typifies certain features of this culture, making them stand out in stark relief.[29] What makes architecture so telling as an illustration of broader cultural trends has to do with its scale and spectacular nature—it is always in view, and it reshapes the landscape—as well as with its function: as a space for dwelling, architecture "hits us where we live," to take the idiom literally.

For Walter Benjamin, the material components of architecture provide a way to access the ideas underpinning a particular moment in history. Benjamin writes on the phenomenon of Parisian arcades, most of which were built in the late 1830s, and whose beauty attracted visitors from abroad to their sparkling wares: "In their fittings art is brought in to the service of commerce."[30] He cites an *Illustrated Guide to Paris* that calls the arcade "a city, indeed, a world in miniature," apparently because the glass roof creates a sort of second firmament—in the same essay Benjamin characterizes the arcade as "both house and stars." One of Benjamin's most striking observations concerns the use of iron in the construction of arcades. Iron and glass have been called the modernist materials par excellence.[31] Benjamin draws an insightful connection between the use of iron in architecture and the material's earlier incarnation: the development of iron "accelerates in the course of the century. . . . The rail becomes the first prefabricated iron component, the forerunner of the girder. Iron is avoided in residential buildings and used in arcades, exhibition halls, stations—buildings serving transitory purposes."[32] In effect, Benjamin traces the association between modernity and speed (note his use of the word "accelerates" to underscore his point) back to the role that iron played in the construction of railways. The rail, the key structural element of a train track, evolves into the girder, the key structural element of a building, and the iron invests the building with a similar aura of acceleration in space and time.[33]

I would argue that glass presents an analogous case, whereby a technological innovation typical of modernity, in particular one that evokes the association of speed and transitoriness, can be linked to an architectural element. Mikhail Yampolsky draws a parallel between the transparency of film celluloid and that of utopian glass buildings at the turn of the twentieth century.[34] A contemporary example of the same principle is the use of glass in the information revolution. In the past several decades, the phenomenon of glass-based fiber optics has accelerated the pace of life in unprecedented ways.[35] The optical pathways along which light impulses travel can be seen as the most recent incarnation of the railway, with all its symbolic associations. In fact, buildings are being constructed already wired with fiber optical cables. Now the glass is on the inside: it has become another kind of structural element altogether.

In eighteenth-century Russian literature, one detects a phenomenon that can be called (with apologies to Marx) "glass consciousness." Throughout this study, I am interested in going back in time to moments when glass was considered precious and even magical; when people noticed its effect on the visible world. Even in the twentieth century, when the material was becoming ubiquitous, remarkable glass objects were still appearing for the first time. Written texts are records of the reception and experience of these objects; they also enrich our understanding of them.[36]

The span of time encompassed by my study is bracketed by the Petrine revolution in the eighteenth century and the Bolshevik Revolution (and the decades that followed) in the twentieth. I use "revolution" to refer to an ongoing process rather than a single discrete event; thus, "Petrine revolution" signifies the extensive reforms that Peter I instituted, the consequences of these reforms, and the events that followed in their wake. Looking at a broad span of time allows me to draw out meaningful patterns and show how cultural history repeats itself. Moreover, these two periods have much in common. Both revolutions ushered in transformations in consciousness—new ways of seeing; and thus it is fitting that in these time periods glass attracted particular interest: it is a material that, more than any other, engages with the sense of sight by reflecting, refracting, dazzling the eye, and serving as the omnipresent medium through which we access the visible world. Writers of the eighteenth century were obsessed with optics and vision—the legacy of the Baroque as well as the Enlightenment. The turn of the twentieth century saw a resurgence of the obsession.[37] From the Zor-Ved group to the Cine-Eye collective, many artists' organizations were interested in exploring the phenomenon of visual perception and in transforming the sense of sight in order to create better human beings. Technological advances and spiritual aspirations both played a major role in orienting Russian culture toward the sense of sight.[38]

With its emphasis on visual culture, my project is part of a larger movement in Slavic studies heralded by a number of recent publications, including the essay collection *Picturing Russia: Explorations in Visual Culture*. The editors of the volume note a consistent tendency among Russians "to turn to the visual in order to summon a new reality into being . . . to use the experience of viewing as an engine of historical or eschatological transformation,"[39] an idea that is fundamental for *Optical Play* as well. Central to my project is the artistic response to the phenomenological presence of glass: this presence influenced how artists perceived the creative process, the use of language, and their ways of seeing. Writers are sensitive to the stimuli of the phenomenal world and to the ideas in the air, and their work can serve as a barometer of public opinion of the time. I document the way that glass played on the imaginations of artists, but also of people from all walks of life.

Thus, I look not only at high art but at its more popular manifestations from songs to sayings; as I consider these texts as well as legal, journalistic, and other types of discourse, I draw attention to recurring motifs and rhetorical strategies.

HISTORICAL OVERVIEW

My study proper begins with glass in modern Russia, that is, Russia in the wake of the Petrine reforms that brought the country out of the medieval period. A brief look at the uses of glass in pre-eighteenth-century Russia, when this material was precious and rare, helps to underscore the dramatic role it would play in the culture in subsequent centuries.

Archeological evidence shows that glassmaking first developed on what is now Russian territory in the northwestern town of Old Ladoga in the second half of the eighth century.[40] The Mongol invasion put a temporary halt to the development of glassmaking in Russia;[41] small workshops "deep in the woods and in villages hidden away in oak groves" continued to function on the territory of Ukraine while Russia was under the Mongol yoke.[42]

The value of glass in pre-modern Russia is underscored by the fact that glass beads were an early form of money. These beads were known as *glazki* (with the accent on the second syllable). Even at such an early stage, the connection between glass and seeing is apparent: around the turn of the seventeenth century, the word *glaz* (which originally meant "shiny sphere" or "pebble") displaced *oko* as the signifier of the eye. The *glazki* beads, decorated with gold and silver foil, and dating to the eighth century, have been found in excavations at Old Ladoga; similar beads, including ones that were gold, yellow, blue, and green in color have also been found in Kiev.[43] The beads were frequently washed out by rains and ended up in the crumbling banks of large rivers. In 1114 the inhabitants of Ladoga informed the chronicler Nestor: "Around here, after a heavy rain, our children find *glazki*, big and small ones, with holes drilled through them, and others collect them near the Volkhov River when the tide washes them ashore."[44]

The beads known as *glazki* as well as tiny decorative beads (*biser*) were manufactured at a glass workshop that had been established in Old Ladoga as far back as the eighth century; according to Andrei Chernov, glassmakers from the Near East (brought in voluntarily or by force) plied their trade there. In addition to being the center of Russian glassmaking, Old Ladoga was a major trading post; the *glazki* made here were given to local hunters in exchange for furs,[45] which were then traded to Arabian merchants for silver coins. Chernov argues that these glass beads played a crucial role in the formation of the Russian state: "It is this silver that would pay for Riurik's mission, the construction on the 'upper river' of Novgorod, the transfer of the capital to Kiev, and the very birth of the unified Old Russian state." One of Chernov's cohorts conjectures that the *glazki* served as the currency of Ladoga for two centuries because these eye-beads recalled the left eye of the Scandinavian god Odin, who sacrificed it in exchange for wisdom.[46]

All kinds of vessels were fashioned from glass with functions from sacred to profane. Excavations of burial sites and settlements in Crimea and southern Ukraine have unearthed thick-walled spherical glass vessels, about the size of an apple, hermetically sealed and containing a saline liquid, dating to the eleventh through the thirteenth century. Scholars speculate that these were vessels containing tears, religious relics brought from the Holy Land.[47] The ancient chronicles show that glass containers were used in thirteenth-century Pskov and Novgorod to hold precious liquids such as myrrh.[48] Drinking vessels of light yellow and green glass called *sleznitsy* (from *sleza*, "teardrop") were widespread in the twelfth through fourteenth centuries. They were in the shape of funnels crudely soldered at the bottom, and when such a vessel was filled with liquid, the drinker could not put it down on the table but had to drain it at one go.[49]

Because glass was mostly imported from abroad and therefore an expensive luxury item in medieval Russia, windows at the time were made of such materials as bulls' bladders, fish eggsacks,[50] rags, or (for the privileged few) mica.[51] (See figure 1.) (In her novel *The Slynx* from 2000, set in a post-apocalyptic Moscow whose denizens have regressed to a primitive way of life, Tatiana Tolstaya includes numerous references to windows covered with animal bladders.) Glass windows only began to appear in the mid-seventeenth century, although most peasants continued to use other materials up to the middle of the nineteenth. During the construction of St. Petersburg in the early eighteenth century, even the homes of the well-to-do had windowpanes of mica, not glass.[52] Windows were of various shapes, sometimes round (produced by cutting off the base of a wide flat-bottomed blown glass vessel[53]) and other times in the form of the letter д; they were sealed off with iron bars and shutters on the outside.[54]

Mirrors in pre-eighteenth-century Russia were primarily small hand-held ones. A particularly lavish example was an implement of the tsar's grooming, consisting of a large fan of feathers, satin, or leather, with a mirror at the center.[55] Wall mirrors began to appear in the second half of the seventeenth century; they were hung only in interior rooms such as bedchambers, never in outer rooms used for receptions. These mirrors had frames of decoratively carved wood that was painted, gilded, or silvered, and frequently had pasted-on velvet and stamped leather embellishments. They were placed between windows or on blind walls and were always covered with taffeta, satin, or velvet curtains on rings, or were locked up in the manner of icon-

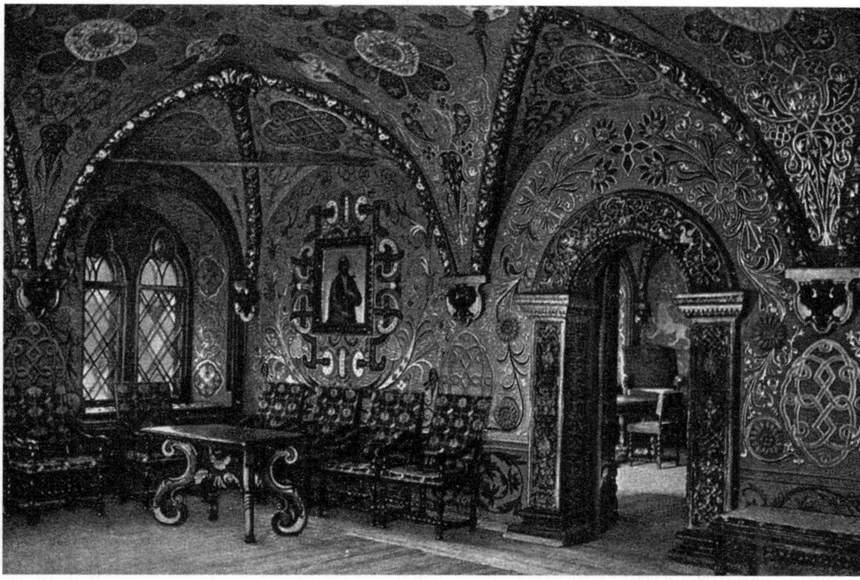

Figure 1. The Boyars' Room of the Terem Palace (built 1635–37) in the Kremlin, Moscow. The windows were originally glazed with mica. Private collection. Photo credit: CCI / The Art Archive at Art Resource, New York.

cases.[56] The prices for mirrors in Muscovy ranged from two kopecks to 100 rubles, with a median of 75 kopecks (four kopecks being equal to an average day's pay.)[57] Prince Vasily Golitsyn, "one of the wealthiest men in late Muscovy," owned 81 mirrors, for which he paid 679 rubles, an enormous sum at the time. The price of one of the mirrors—20 rubles—was equivalent to that of "six slaves."[58]

Glass in pre-modern Russia and the surrounding region was a popular material for adornment, of one's self and one's surroundings. Archeological digs on the territories of towns from Kiev to Kostroma have unearthed multicolored glass bracelets, bead necklaces, and rings dating to the tenth through the twelfth centuries.[59] Glass was used to decorate the interiors of churches: thus, in 1508 Grand Prince Vasily had the icons in the Church of Annunciation embellished with silver, gold, and glass beads;[60] and smalt mosaics were created for the St. Sofia cathedral in Kiev at about the same time as those of the St. Mark cathedral in Venice.[61]

The first Russian glass factory was built by Swedish artillery master Julius Koiet in 1639 in the village of Dukhanino near Moscow. This factory specialized exclusively in window glass and greenish apothecary vessels.[62] The factory could not keep up with the growing demand for glass from the court, let alone from other sectors of the population. Thus a second glass factory, this one belonging to the tsar, was established at Izmailovo near Moscow in 1668.[63] It is here that the history of modern Russian glassmaking begins.

Peter the Great actively supported the Russian glass industry. For example, he issued a decree in August 1709 in which he bequeathed to the Englishman William Lloyd a number of glass factories located in Moscow, near the village of Vorob'ev, for a period of ten years, tasking Lloyd with increasing glass production and teaching glassmaking techniques to a dozen Russian artisans.[64] Thanks to efforts such as these, Russian glass came into its own in the eighteenth century, when the country was emerging as an imperial power and a modern state. Glass artists produced objects glorifying the state as well as imitating nature. Mikhail Lomonosov, the father of Russian versification, was also a pioneer of glassmaking; his "Letter on the Usefulness of Glass," an expansive paean to the miraculously versatile (and poetically suggestive) material that is glass, implicitly celebrates the Russian literary language as an equally expressive medium that likewise bends to its master's will.

As Russian secular literature developed in the eighteenth century concurrently with the glass industry, the latter yielded optical devices after which literature sought to model itself. The function of the former suggested the function of the latter to writers looking for a way to define their endeavor. With its optical qualities evoking simultaneously the sparkle and grandeur of the Baroque, the clarity of Classicism, and, with objects from telescope lenses to windows and chandeliers, the discourse of the Enlightenment, glass provided a series of metaphors for eighteenth-century writers seeking to describe the character of the tumultuous times in which they lived.

Glass is thus mentioned in a multitude of eighteenth-century texts, but it also acts *as* a text to be read, from drinking vessels engraved with words and images alluding to imperial glory to the peculiar, prismatic Mirror of Law (*zertsalo*), which simultaneously demands and defies interpretation. The *zertsalo* symbolized jurisprudence and was employed as an emblem of surveillance—the sovereign's "all-seeing eye"—during all Russian legal proceedings. These objects appeared during the Petrine period and remained in use until the Bolshevik Revolution of 1917, when most were destroyed in a wave of iconoclasm. A complex of associations between the *zertsalo* and the emblem of the all-seeing eye illustrates the connection between seeing and power: the Petrine "mirror" ultimately was meant to be perceived as the eye of God.

As the nation's glass industry came of age alongside its literature in the nineteenth century, glass took on new meanings. Massive glass constructions played a role in the glorification of Russian imperial might through ceremony and spectacle. Eventually, large-scale glass production and the increasingly widespread use of windows allowed people to imagine a perfect future based on communal glass houses.

At the turn of the twentieth century, Russian artists rediscovered and revisited the eighteenth century to gain access to cultural memory and to shake off the fetters of Realism, which had reigned supreme in the previous century. The writerly gaze shifted from the tableau seen through the window (the leading metaphor for realist art) to the cracks on the window's surface; writers began to scrutinize language itself, reveling in its materiality even as they questioned its adequacy as a transparent container for meaning.[65] At the same time, in all spheres of cultural production, from writing to art, architecture, and film, glass took on a new importance. It became the modern construction material par excellence. Glass played key roles in technological developments, such as the search for a superior eye, from cameras to optical lenses. The material was instrumental in the creation of technologies of surveillance; in contrast to the *zertsalo*, these devices were far less spectacular and far more insidious.

Curiously, while modernists turned their attention to glass, what they prized most was its ability to become invisible. Kandinsky's paintings on glass (1912–17) were inspired by Russian icons and by Hinterglasmalerei, a style of folk art that had been in existence in Europe since late antiquity and flourished in southern Bavaria in the eighteenth century. In these works Kandinsky tries to present a pure play of color, with no canvas to mediate the viewing experience.[66] Because they were to be viewed from the reverse side, these paintings were done backward—the upper layers of paint were applied first. For Kandinsky, the glass medium thus transformed the creative process itself.

An analogue of sorts may be found in Marcel Duchamp's painting on glass, *The Bride Stripped Bare by Her Bachelors, Even* (1915–23). Apropos of his turn to a transparent canvas, Duchamp wrote: "If a painter leaves the canvas blank, he still exposes to the viewer something that is considered an object in itself. This is not true of glass; the blank parts, except in relation to the room and the viewer, are not dwelt upon." Calvin Tomkins explains that, because one could simultaneously look *at* and look *through* a painting on glass, the experience of looking became "ambiguous, open-ended, and unfixed"; this quality allowed Duchamp to take his exploration of movement to an entirely new level: whereas the artist had earlier tried to represent bodies in motion in such works as his *Nude Descending a Staircase*, now this interest "had been superseded by his concern with movement of another kind—with the transition from one mental or psychological state to another."[67] For artists, glass is an ideal material to respond to and articulate change—by its very nature, neither fluid nor solid entirely, it embodies the state of transition.

Already in the seventeenth century, the tension between looking-at and looking-through inherent in glass was a provocative one for writers, as in the case of George Herbert's poem "The Elixer" (1633): "A man that looks on glasse / On it may stay his eye; / Or if he pleaseth, through it passe, / And then the heav'ns espie." The way in which glass plays with our vision can evoke the possibility of moving between two planes of existence—the material and the spiritual, this world and the next. Therefore glass suggests the presence of another reality—and as an extension of this idea, to a number of thinkers over the last several centuries, glass has suggested utopia.

One such utopian thinker, the avant-garde poet Velimir Khlebnikov, made explicit the connection between glass and dynamism with his project for an easily transportable, feather-light glass architecture. In 1920 he imagined the house of the future as "a container of molded glass, a mobile dwelling-module" that can move from place to place with lightness and ease, fitting into empty metal frameworks to create cityscapes that resemble "glass and steel honeycombs." One of the dwellings that he proposes takes the form of an open book that consists of "stone walls set at an angle, and glass sheets of living modules arranged fanwise between these walls." This architectural merging of glass and text is appropriate for Khlebnikov's vision of an urban landscape inscribed with an "alphabet of iron consonants and vowels of glass."[68]

Khlebnikov was developing his ideas at a time when architectural projects worldwide called for extensive use of glass, which took on a significance that transcended its utilitarian value. Art critic Robert Hughes juxtaposes the age-old reverence for stained glass windows with modern architects' infatuation with glass as a construction material: "It was the face of the Crystal, the Pure Prism. . . . It suggested a responsive skin, like the sensitive membrane of the eye, whereas brick and stone were impervious, a crust against the world." Akin to stained glass, it was regarded by some with a nearly religious fervor. In 1914 Paul Scheerbart argued that replacing brick buildings with glass ones would bring about "a paradise on earth."[69] The idealization of glass architecture had a poignant significance in the years after the First World War; Hughes explains: "A world remade of glass would have evolved beyond throwing stones—or artillery shells. Glass architecture was pacifist architecture, the very image of exalted vulnerability which, given a new social contract, would remain forever intact."[70]

The sarcophagus built in 1924 to display the embalmed body of Lenin was an altogether different "glass house." In the days following Lenin's death, letters and telegrams to the Burial Commission called for the preservation, and continued visibility, of Lenin's body: "It is imperative that Il'ich physically remain with us and that he can be seen by the working masses . . . The body of Il'ich should not be consigned to the earth, but should be embalmed and placed in a central museum in order that the workers of future epochs will be able to see the leader of the proletariat."[71] (The anxiety about the leader's visibility again resonates with the legend of Peter in Glassland.) Soon after, Lenin's body was put on permanent display in a crystal coffin, a key component of the official attempt to create a cult, that is, a system of popular veneration, around Lenin.

This system of veneration was made possible by the physical properties of glass—the capacity of this material to manipulate light, which can be used to create a spectacle that holds sway over the emotions of large groups of people. Throughout this study I return to the spectacular potential of glass and show how both the tendentious capacity and the playfulness of this material have shaped Russian culture.

CHAPTER OUTLINE

My book identifies a number of ways in which glass functions, both materially and metaphorically: each chapter examines a particular function and shows its historical development as well as the evolution of the discourse around that function. Chapter 1, "Looking through Glass: The Transformation of Vision," explores the ways in which glass mediates how people see. In the form of the window, glass has historically transformed the psyche by changing what we can see of the outside world. "Transformation of vision" also refers to the effect that the presence of glass has on the imagination—the mind's eye. This chapter focuses on windows as a crucial site for examining how the Petrine reforms manifested themselves in the sphere of material culture. I analyze how windows shape perception in an eighteenth-century memoir as well as in several canonical nineteenth-century literary texts and address the attendant topics of the gaze, power, and powerlessness. I place this discussion in the context of the Petrine revolution in architecture: the transition from isolationism to an outward-looking perspective; in doing so I provide a new angle from which to consider Algarotti's characterization of St. Petersburg, promptly adopted by Russian thinkers, as a "window on Europe." In the twentieth century, the notions of voyeurism, surveillance, and collectivism combined as the avant-garde and then the Bolshevik revolutions ushered in new ways of seeing. Glass contributed to this phenomenon in the built environment and in the world of ideas.[72] The "satirical windows" of the Russian Telegraph Agency turned the display case for the commodity fetish into a site of political mobilization, and transformed vision in a very different way.

In chapter 2, "The Language of Glass: Making Rhetorical Objects," I show the correspondences between Mikhail Lomonosov's glassmaking and his literary work. While Lomonosov's "Letter on the Usefulness of Glass" praises the practical applications of this material, illustrating the multiple ways in which glass had transformed art, science, and everyday life by mid-century, this poem is also about the way that glass inspires writing. After situating Lomonosov's glassmaking in a historical context, I turn to Lomonosov's verse and document his battle with rivals in the Russian Academy of Sciences over his controversial use of glass.

Lomonosov's "Letter" serves as the central philosophical statement about glass in eighteenth-century Russia, spelling out the ways in which the physical qualities of this material generate symbolic meanings. In Lomonosov's time, the ability of glass to reflect and its potential to work on the conscience of the beholder gave rise to a powerful metaphor that came to be materialized in official iconography. The mirror became a symbol of jurisprudence, and this symbol was embodied in the *zertsalo*, which functioned as an object of surveillance, conduit of ideology, and sacred container. My discussion of the *zertsalo*, demonstrating how the scrutiny of an artifact can enrich literary analysis, serves as an example of the analytical practice that I employ throughout this book.

While the *zertsalo* was an artifact whose use was mandated in all government offices, glass values penetrated everyday life in Russia to an even more profound degree in the form of vision aids, from spectacles to telescopes. Here I develop the discussion of the transformation of vision begun in the previous chapter. In his play *The Trinket-Dealer* (1765), Vladimir Lukin adapts Robert Dodsley's comedy *The Toy Shop*, and adds a new element: the telescope and the lorgnette—glass eyes, in a sense—appear as stage props used for satirical effect. Lukin's version of Dodsley's play places a far greater emphasis on the optical. This emphasis suggests a preoccupation with issues of seeing and being seen—and the artificial means of doing so—among the newly Westernized Russian audience. I provide historical background on the way in which optical devices transformed vision; I then show how eyeglasses and lorgnettes functioned not only as devices to improve eyesight but also as a signifying costume over the span of several centuries. After examining Lukin's play, I focus on the modernist period as a time when writers were compelled to examine, with an intensity akin to that of their eighteenth-century counterparts, the effect of glass objects on the human psyche.[73]

Following up on the discussion of objects with a rhetorical value in chapter 2, I turn to the propagandistic potential of glass in chapter 3, "The Display of Power: Spectacular Glass in Imperial Russia." Glass has a capacity to imitate nature, and bears a striking resemblance to water and ice—elements with a special resonance in Russian cultural history that I address in this chapter. I begin with a description and analysis of a proto-glass house:

the palatial Ice House of Empress Anna—the first such structure ever built. The Ice House was both a dwelling and a spectacle; illuminated from within, this translucent edifice was created at the monarch's behest in order to mesmerize and discipline the Russian populace—and it did so with great success. This chapter then goes on to examine the spectacular potential of glass that stems from its inherent capacity to capture light. This potential allows glass to be crafted into an object that fascinates and holds sway over viewers' emotions. Throughout my study, I use "spectacular" to refer to objects made to be viewed and to impart a particular iconic impression; and I apply the term "ideological spectacle" to monumental glass objects created for rhetorical purposes.

Eighteenth-century glassware depicting symbols of autocracy demonstrates in miniature the spectacular potential of glass. This potential was harnessed more and more effectively in the nineteenth century, and colossal glass constructions were created that served to glorify Russian imperial might. A key example of such a construction was a crystal bed presented to the Persian shah in 1826; its massive scale and shimmering facets were designed to convey the splendor of the nation that had produced it.

In the next two chapters, I seek to answer the question of why glass appeared as a utopian building material for so many thinkers, in Russia and beyond. The idea of glass houses provoked controversy in the nineteenth century and in the first decades of the twentieth. More recently, the construction of glass skyscrapers in Moscow has elicited outcries in the press against the disturbing proliferation of reflections that such buildings generated.[74] In our day, it is important to consider why glass architecture continues to invite both awe and attack (in word and deed). As the glass industry grew and windows became more widespread, visionary thinkers began to imagine utopian glass palaces accessible to one and all. In chapter 4, "Glass Architecture: Glimpses of Utopia," I juxtapose Chernyshevsky's Crystal Palace with Dostoevsky's glass phobia using readings of literary texts by both authors. I place the analysis in the context of the material conditions of glass production as well as the worldwide interest in glass houses, and the ideals that they represented, from Fourier's phalansteries to Paxton's Crystal Palace.

Chapter 5, "The Glass House as Dream and Nightmare," focuses on the controversy around glass architecture as well as the creation and reception of such buildings in twentieth-century Russia. Living in glass houses promised physical well-being; at the same time, the transparency of those buildings was associated with moral purity, openness, and democracy, attributes that the inhabitants would take on as well. Thus the literal would magically become the figurative.

Glass architecture was at the heart of the utopian aspirations and dystopian fears in twentieth-century Russia. I present two opposing views on the notion of a glass utopia: Khlebnikov's enthusiastic embrace versus Zamyatin's rejection of the idea. At the turn of the twentieth century, Zamyatin set his anti-utopia in a world where not only the buildings, but also the sidewalks, the furniture, and virtually everything else is made of glass. With his transparent world in which every citizen is subjected to the all-seeing eye of the state, Zamyatin uncannily predicts the society of surveillance that would rise in the Soviet Union in decades to come; moreover, he shows how our physical surroundings can condition the way we think and imagine, especially when we do not notice them. At the same time, Zamyatin chooses a material whose apparent stability conceals a fragility that threatens the very existence of the oppressive state. In his film project *The Glass House*, Eisenstein devised a skyscraper with glass walls as a space within which to carry out his ideological critique of the Western bourgeois way of life. However, the anxieties about surveillance that emerge from his project echo those found in Zamyatin's anti-utopia, and make it seem as if his attack is aimed at a target much closer to home.

Chapter 6, "Light in Captivity: The Glass Object as Ideological Spectacle," demonstrates how the Soviet state strove to legitimize its existence and glorify its achievements by harnessing the spectacular potential of glass, and how writers such as Olesha and Platonov challenged this strategy. The chapter narrates how electric lightbulbs appeared on the scene in Soviet Russia and contributed to the sanctified image of Lenin (the association of his name with lightbulbs, or "Lenin's little lamps"), thus taking on a significance unlike that in any other country. Turning to the gigantic red stars on the Kremlin towers, I argue that "Lenin's little lamp" is on the same continuum as the Kremlin stars as an attempt by the Soviet state to lay claim to the domain of light, an idea that I explore with reference to Jean Starobinski's concept of the "solar myth of the revolution." Today, Lenin's body remains on display in a glass case designed to evoke associations with saintly relics and Sleeping Beauty. My study describes how this object came into being, the ideas and hopes that informed its creation, and the public and private response recorded in the press, literature, and letters. Placing Lenin's body in a glass case rendered him, and the symbolic order he represented, both powerful and vulnerable. The glass spire of Moscow State University and the Avtovo metro station in St. Petersburg serve as further illustrations of the ideological uses of glass in Stalinist Russia. Close readings of literary works and press accounts provide evidence for my argument about the propagandistic potential of captive light.

In the conclusion, I address the religious uses and corporeal associations of glass in order to further illuminate the question, central to my study, of how spectacular glass served as a means to play upon people's hearts and minds. Before summing up, I propose ways to understand the relationship between glass and Logos in the work of Osip Mandelstam—a writer notable for his poetics of thingness—and consider some enigmatic passages in his poetry in the light of this relationship.

Does materiality itself have a unique status in Russian thought? Epstein raises this provocative suggestion when he highlights the enduring concerns in Russian culture regarding the traditional opposition between matter and spirit. Arguing that Russians embraced Western materialism because of a native philosophical tradition, a "long-standing preoccupation . . . with material objects as phenomenal codes of being," Epstein finds the roots of this concern in such Russian belief systems as the emphasis on corporeality in Russian Orthodoxy and tradition of "dual-faith" (*dvoeverie*), "whereby the cult of Mother-Earth and the cult of the Heavenly Father continually interacted to produce a unique mentality of 'idealistic materialism.'" This tradition informs a range of beliefs, from the revolutionary materialism of Herzen and Chernyshevsky to Nikolai Fedorov's doctrine of resurrection.[75] In foregrounding the preoccupation that Russian culture has with a material whose transparency, which at times seems to efface its materiality, has inspired idealistic associations for centuries, my project provides a way to think through the hypothesis that Epstein offers.

Epstein's novel *Cries in the New Wilderness: From the Files of the Moscow Institute of Atheism*[76] takes the form of a document describing the beliefs and practices of banned religious sects that led a secret existence during the Soviet period. These sects are fictional creations, but their tenets are based on actual ideas that were in the air in Russia in the 1970s and 1980s.[77] One of the sects profiled in the novel is a glass-obsessed doomsday cult known variously as the *steklovidtsy* (glass-seers), *steklodely* (glassworkers), and *stekol'shchiki* (glaziers). They are a secret brotherhood, at once a professional union and mystical society, with origins reaching back for thousands of years—their beliefs having been propagated in Russia by Count Shuvalov, the addressee of Lomonosov's "Letter on the Usefulness of Glass"—and thus analogous to the Masons; yet unlike the Masons, the Glaziers are virtually unknown, because their basic guiding principle is that of invisibility.

Inspired by the image of the New Jerusalem in the Book of Revelation, the Glaziers predict that at the end of time, the earth shall turn to glass and become a transparent vessel for divine light. They believe that transparency is itself divine, and thus they strive to purify and transform the world, and themselves, in God's image. They see glass architecture in mystical terms: "Whereas through stone the earth sends its weight up to heaven, through glass heaven lends its transparency to earth. . . . Glass, which is smelted from sand, from a component of the earth, celestializes it, as it were, from within."[78] The Glaziers seek to make not only their surroundings but also themselves transparent; for them, glass becomes a model for being in the world:

> A transparent human being is one who has attenuated his earthly existence to such a delicate state that it begins to transmit light . . . You do not even notice such a human being, but in his light you see yourself, you see more deeply into yourself. The highest status in this impenetrable world is that of invisibility. The invisible one is he who does not prevent others from being seen. . . . A man becomes a void in the Universe—and then he fills it, as air fills a glistening bubble. A glassblower blows void into solid matter to thin it out until it shines. Let everyone become the glassblower of his own "I"![79]

Extending the analogy between glass and self, the Glaziers carry vitreous amulets (watches, eyeglasses, lenses) not only as tools but as secret signs, self-definitions, in a perfect illustration of how glass is both utilitarian and symbolic: "Sometimes they use these things, but, even more important, they constantly study their magical property: to be without concealing being."[80]

The Glaziers have a privileged place in Epstein's "comedy of ideas": they are the last of four doomsday sects, and the penultimate sect to be discussed; last of all is the "literary sect" known as the Pushkinians, who have built an elaborate religious system around the poet. Tellingly, Epstein—the founder of the "lyrical museum"—juxtaposes the Russian national poet and the poetic material of glass. Epstein is attentive to the plurality of voices in his culture, and deftly picks out the recurring motifs. It is not surprising, then, that he introduces us to the Glaziers; indeed, parallels between glass, language, and consciousness, as well as a general preoccupation with the material, are manifested at various discursive levels within Russian culture. I would like to let the voices of the Glaziers serve as an overture to my own project.

Chapter One

Looking through Glass: The Transformation of Vision

> [Following his journey to the Russian capital, Algarotti wrote]: "St. Petersburg is a great big window on Europe" . . . When we say 'St. Petersburg is a window on Europe,' we are quoting not Algarotti himself, but Pushkin. But Pushkin translated this expression not from the language of the original but from the French. The French translation did not contain the augmentative suffix. For Algarotti this expression had a somewhat different meaning than for Pushkin, because in Italy the term 'big window'—with the augmentative suffix!—is also used to refer to a window through which you can step out onto a balcony or a loggia. That is, it is an exit into an exterior space. Whereas among us it has become merely a window, which has given rise to jokes to the effect that normal people use the door, but we're always trying to climb in through the window.
>
> —Mikhail Tallai, Russian Genealogical Society

TRADITIONAL RUSSIAN CULTURE viewed the window as the border between the world of one's home and the hostile external world; as such, this aperture was considered one of the most dangerous places in the house. People believed that demonic forces (*nechistaia sila*, literally "unclean power") could gain access to the home through the window and cause harm to the residents and their loved ones. This belief gave rise to numerous omens: for example, a bird flying into a window signified someone's imminent demise; a woodpecker knocking on a window frame presaged death or misfortune. A positive counterpart to these feared intrusions was the sunbeam, the only element from outside whose entry through the window Russians welcomed. One old riddle reified solar energy as a "golden log" poking into one's window (*iz okna v okno zolotoe brevno*), while another presented sunlight juxtaposed with solar rays extending into the home as "a lady in the yard with her sleeves in the hut [*barynia vo dvore, a rukava v izbe*]." To prevent anything "foreign" from getting inside the home, Russians drew crosses with chalk or coal on the upper part of the window and sprinkled holy water on the frame.[1]

These beliefs reveal a set of anxieties about border-crossing and the foreign that are also observable in a multitude of Russian superstitions and sayings regarding mirrors.[2] Thus, these glass expanses that appeared in Russian homes carried with them a powerful symbolic charge alongside with their pragmatic light-giving function. To stand or sit next to a window was to become a border guard of sorts in the microcosm of one's own home.

Another reason that windows have a particular resonance in the Russian context is that their function evokes the conflict between openness and isolationism that is at the heart of modern Russian identity. The eighteenth century saw a Petrine revolution in architecture: windows became larger as Russia became more open to Western influences. In 1739 Count Francesco Algarotti famously dubbed St. Petersburg, the capital that Peter built ex nihilo, a "window through which Russia looks at Europe." Algarotti had in mind a large window through which one can step out onto a balcony; subsequently, as Algarotti's phrase was absorbed back into Russia and served to shape the nation's self-identity, this specific definition gave way to the broader meaning of openness and, perhaps, wistful surveillance of a lovely and inaccessible view.

WINDOW GLASS: FRAMING THE WORLD AND SHAPING THE INTERIOR

The symbolic significance of glass can be fruitfully examined as part of the larger phenomenon whereby building materials take on meanings distinct from their utilitarian designations. The construction of St. Petersburg serves as a vivid case study of just such a process. In the consolidation of state power though secularization, symbols with previously religious significance became associated with the state.[3] In the case of Peter the Great, attributes that were once Apostle Peter's became those of the emperor. Feofan Propokovich, referring to the emperor Peter in a speech, cited the Gospel's etymologically based association of Peter with "the rock" upon which the future was to be built. The emerging myth of Petersburg reinforced this symbolism through the opposition of *wooden* Russia versus *stone* Petersburg, established by a total ban in 1714 on the erection of stone buildings anywhere in Russia except in the new capital.[4]

Peter has always been associated with the stone out of which his city was built. Yet an equally important material in this respect is glass, for the new, European-style architecture in St. Petersburg called for much greater lighting of interiors, therefore much larger windows, than had been the norm in seventeenth-century Russia. In his biography of Lomonosov, P. P. Pekarskii notes that "many country- and even city-dwellers in [the mid-eighteenth century] considered simple glass windowpanes to be a luxury and used mica and animal bladders instead."[5] This state of affairs was changing, however, and architecture in Peter's newly constructed capital set the tone. Tiny mica windows and stained glass in leaden sashes receded into the past. The first palaces built in Petersburg featured hallways brightened by rows of evenly spaced windows.[6] William Craft Brumfield notes this innovation in describing the Kikin Chambers (*palaty*), which served as the initial site for the Kunstkamera; he calls attention to the "large window frames, whose expanse of glass provides a telling contrast to pre-Petrine dwellings, which seem to have been designed to exclude a view of the exterior world."[7] Peter's famous Domik (little house), the new capital's first dwelling, featured log walls painted to resemble brick and large windows composed of numerous panes of glass, a radical departure from Russian architectural conventions of the time.[8] The architecture of the Petrine period was characterized by structures that let more light and air into buildings, as well as by expanded interior spaces, thinner walls, and lighter constructions. By the second half of the eighteenth century, windowpanes as large as five meters long and three meters wide began to be produced.[9] Daylight entered palaces and then more modest homes, while the improved construction of lamps as well as extensive use of wall mirrors and optical capacities of faceted glass in chandeliers gradually led to brighter interiors.[10] (Glass contributed to brighter exteriors, too: glass panes for lanterns were cast in bronze molds and then polished; the first lanterns began to appear on the streets of Moscow in 1730.)[11]

In their attempt to dematerialize the solidity of walls and create an overwhelming, ostentatious ambiance, Baroque architects painstakingly arranged mirrors in order to best reflect the room's numerous light fixtures, which were themselves made of glass.[12] In upper-class interiors, mirrors and windows alternated with one another, creating the illusion of expanded space; this effect can be seen, for example, in the Italian House at the Kuskovo estate near Moscow and the Catherine Palace.[13] At the court of Empress Elizabeth, the grand hall that was used for her beloved masquerades was described by a visitor as having twelve large windows in a row "corresponding to the same number of mirrors of a truly enormous size."[14] (See figure 2.) (Here I would like to note how radical this proliferation of mirrors

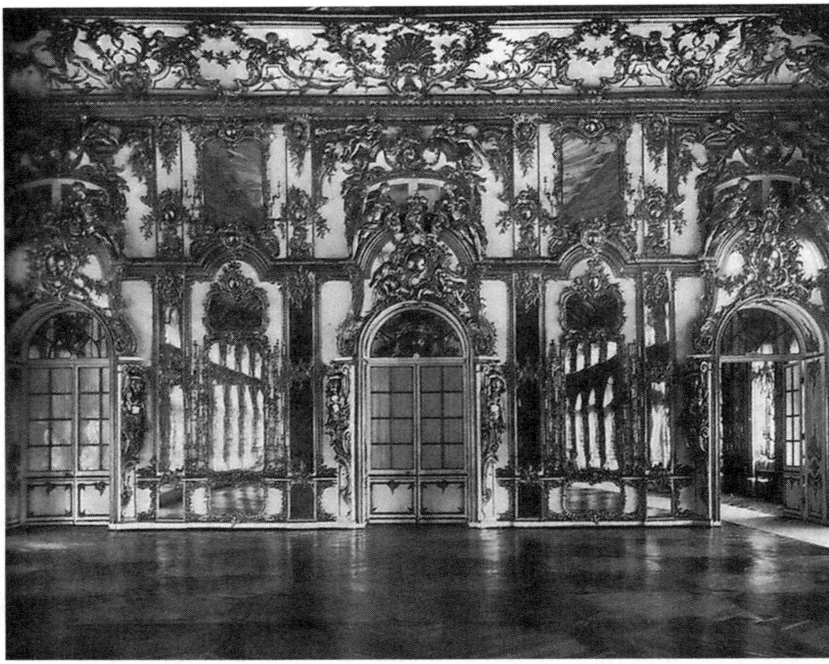

Figure 2. Interior of the Catherine Palace in Tsarskoe Selo, designed by Francesco Bartolomeo Rastrelli, 1752–56.

was in a country where such objects had been virtually taboo not long before; this is a topic that I will discuss in detail in chapter 2.)

At the turn of the nineteenth century, Karamzin provided a sketch showing how profoundly the urban landscape had changed, and how the internal landscape had changed with it:

> Our age might be called the age of *laying bare* [*otkrovennosti*] in the physical and moral sense: just take a look at our charming beauties! . . . There once was a time when people hid in dark homes and beneath the shield of tall fences. Nowadays everywhere there are bright homes and big windows facing the street: go ahead and peek in! We want to live, act, and think in transparent glass.[15]

Karamzin's evocation of transparency is fitting in a work entitled "My Confession" (1802), whose narrator unapologetically reveals his amoral way of life to one and all. This passage brings up another important aspect of the Petrine architectural innovation: not only did windows let light inside dwellings, but they allowed the dwellers to look out, and potentially, outsiders to look in. The introduction of more and larger windows ushered in a new psychological state (this would, of course, affect primarily those who could dwell in buildings affected by the changes, although the position of outsider-looking-in was potentially open to anyone) based on a changed relationship to interiors as well as a greater interaction with and awareness of the world outside—a widening of one's outlook (*krugozor*).

In her *Memoirs* written in 1767, Princess Natal'ia Borisovna Dolgorukaia describes herself at age sixteen, observing from a window as history marches past in all its ceremonial garb. The first such procession, taking place in 1730, is the funeral march for Peter II that moves past the Sheremetev house in Moscow. First come archpriests and archimandrites, followed by medals and coats of arms borne aloft; finally Dolgorukaia's fiancé Ivan in a mourning cape passes by:

> They had to carry the Emperor's body past our house, where I sat by the window, gazing at the woeful ceremony. . . . When [Ivan] came up even with our windows, he looked over with weeping eyes, his countenance saying: "Whom are we burying! It is the last, last time that I shall see him!" I felt so faint that I fell against the window; I was too weak to sit up.[16]

Soon afterward, another procession makes its way past Dolgorukaia, who this time finds a window in a palace anteroom from which to watch Empress Anna's accession ceremony:

> I sat in an anteroom in the palace and saw the whole ceremony. It went by the windows where I was sitting, and now for the last time I saw my fiancé commanding the Guards: he was a Major and he sat on a horse saluting [the Empress]. Imagine how I felt viewing that spectacle.[17]

Each of the window passages above also contained a reference to Anna that was cut from the 1810 and 1840 editions of the *Memoirs*. In the former case, Anna's right to the crown is questioned, while the latter paints a monstrous portrait of the empress: "she was truly terrible to look at, with a repulsive face, and she was so large that when she walked among her cavaliers she was a head taller than all of them, as well as extremely fat." Dolgorukaia's view from on high paradoxically allowed her to look down upon the most sovereign figure in the land while observing the procession of autocratic power that signified her imminent undoing, whose trajectory she was helpless to stop. Re-creating through writing a gaze through a window, Dolgorukaia wrote from a doubly cloistered perspective: a position of power and powerlessness.

The official procession viewed from a window reappears once more, in a transformed state, in Dolgorukaia's *Memoirs*. The Dolgorukii family is banished to their remote estate in Penza. They stop to rest in a village belonging to Dolgorukaia's mother-in-law. They have been there for less than a month when soldiers of the new regime invade their home; the family is ordered to pack, and they are subsequently transported under heavy guard to an even more remote Siberian town. Dolgorukaia sees danger approaching through a window:

> In the distance I could make out a large number of men and horses coming toward us at great speed. . . . We could see immediately that we were in for more trouble, that ill-feeling for us was growing rather than declining. You can imagine the state I was in then. I collapsed down on a chair, and when I came to, the manor was full of soldiers.[18]

Dolgorukaia spoke of collapsing against the window at the culmination of her description of the funeral; here, she loses consciousness at an analogous point in the narrative, again as if the sight is too overwhelming. The window allows her to see out, but it also suggests protection and a border that is not supposed to be breached; her loss of consciousness allows her to elide the violation of her family home by the soldiers, who are already inside when she comes to. Previously, Dolgorukaia watched official processions through a window; the approach of Anna's soldiers is a variation on the procession motif.

As Lewis Mumford observes, windows presented the world in a frame, and by virtue of this function, glass came to both symbolize and facilitate "the double process of naturalism and abstraction which had begun to characterize the thought of Europe. . . . [Glass] made it possible to see certain elements of reality more clearly: and it focussed attention on a sharply defined field—namely, that which was bounded by the frame."[19] Windows and paintings both present an image within a frame; Dolgorukaia's depiction of her window views may have been informed by the visual art of the time. For example, an engraving of 1709 depicting Peter the Great's triumphant entry into Poltava avoided the use of perspective and situated the whole of the procession on one page. Wortman observes: "The effect is to take the entry procession out of the ordinary and give it a sense of otherness."[20] The engraver Ivan Sokolov was instructed to follow the example set by this work in his depiction of Elizabeth's triumphant entrance into Moscow, which shows the entire procession arranged in seemingly endless rows snaking back and forth across a single page. Visual art was a part of Dolgorukaia's cultural vocabulary: hence in the midst of describing the hardships of her exile journey, she digresses to praise the beauty of her husband's riding horses: "Were I an artist, I would not have hesitated to paint their portraits."[21] In her memoir, Dolgorukaia uses windows to frame and thereby to control and alleviate the distressing events that she is narrating.

The final window image in the *Memoirs* appears when the exiled family is journeying down a river on the way to Berezov; when the weather is calm, Dolgorukaia sits by the window in her cabin and either weeps or washes handkerchiefs. She also finds another way to amuse herself: "Sometimes I would buy a sturgeon and tie him on a line so that he could swim along beside me, a slave as I was."[22] This time Dolgorukaia is in an even more liminal space—drifting between water and dry land. And this time she controls what she sees out of the window by creating her own spectacle, complete with her own "captive"—a fish, a creature that is heavily weighted with Christian symbolism and, to a mind so inclined, embodies the hope of rebirth.

The way in which Dolgorukaia stages the turning points of her life around windows echoes the strategic use of these glass portals by writers and artists in other times and places; thus, in post-Renaissance paintings the motif of the window serves as a boundary separating "places of contemplation, of detached introspection, of protective domesticity, and later of romantic longing from the world's hustle and bustle, its sensual lures, its impermanence, its lack of order and control."[23] Windows introduce a paradoxical dynamic into our relationship with visible reality, which we can access with our gaze but are helpless to control. Glass thus makes us mindful of the connection between seeing and power. On the one hand, looking is a kind of possession that grants power over the object of the gaze.[24] On the other hand, the glass pane wavers between visibility and invisibility; when it cannot be seen, it gives the illusion of direct access to the object beheld, but that illusion can be dashed in a moment, showing that the power dynamic is more complex than it may seem. Several key Russian texts from the nineteenth century elucidate this connection by staging encounters between the male and female protagonists around windows. When authors working in the period of nascent Realism deployed windows in their texts, they were mindful of both the materiality and the symbolism of these objects; they drew upon a wealth of associations stemming from the anxiety around border-crossing as reflected in the symbolic status of windows peculiar to Russia.[25]

In what follows, I shall focus on three examples: the way in which a window mediates Liza's relationship with Hermann in Pushkin's short story "The Queen of Spades" (1833); Bazarov pressing his forehead against a windowpane in Turgenev's *Fathers and Sons* (1862); and the heroine of Tolstoy's *Anna Karenina* (1873–77) rubbing her book knife against a train window as she thinks about Vronsky, while her affair with him is already taking shape. In each case, male-female relationships are at stake (with the attendant power dynamics), and there is something perverse about each of them—a transgression is involved, and the window plays a crucial role in the scenario.

In "The Queen of Spades," we initially see the encounter from Liza's point of view: one day, "Lizaveta Ivanovna, while sitting at the window and doing some needlepoint, happened to glance outside and saw a young engineer who was standing still and directing his gaze toward her window."[26] Hermann has come in search of treasure, which he hopes to obtain by compelling the Countess to share her secret winning card combination, but Liza does not know this; she merely sees a mysterious stranger looking intensely in her direction. She lowers her head and occupies herself with her work, until she is called away; here she again happens to look out the window and sees the same officer, which seems "fairly strange" to her.

Subsequently, the story gives us Hermann's view of the same encounter: haunted by dreams of winning big at the card table, he finds himself helplessly drawn to the house where the Countess dwells. "He stopped and began looking at the windows. In one of them he saw a little head with dark hair, bent down over what was probably a book or some handiwork. The little head raised itself up a bit. Hermann saw a fresh little face and dark eyes. This moment decided his fate."[27] What is striking about the wording in this passage is the fragmentation of the woman whom Hermann sees. This is the decisive moment when Hermann decides to launch his intrigue; the fragmented way in which the window presents Liza to him enables him to think of her in instrumental terms rather than as a real person whom he might hurt.

The window serves as a frame presenting both characters to one another in the most desirable light: Liza soon begins to think of Hermann as a personage from the novels (most likely non-Russian ones) that she reads[28]—he appears to her framed within a literary text, as it were; and his passionate letters to her, whose text Hermann copies from a "German novel," serve to strengthen her delusion and make it that much easier for Hermann to exploit her. The windows that frame Liza and Hermann then become analogous to the pages of the foreign novels that shape their worldview. Moreover, their romance remains text-based throughout—they exchange letters; Liza, for her part, tosses her letters to Hermann out of the same window that framed their first encounter. The motif of card-playing that is prevalent in the story further underscores the way in which a window objectifies the one who is beheld within its frame: note how the human figure is framed inside the "face cards" as if the king, queen, and jack were themselves looking out of a window.[29] And indeed, the device of replacing the animate with the inanimate is a key to understanding Pushkin's story.

In Turgenev's novel *Fathers and Sons*, a window once again mediates the interaction between the two would-be lovers (who likewise do not end up together). This time, a moment of contact between one of them and the window is filled with enigmatic significance. The two window episodes occur in Odintsova's room on sequential days. In the first episode, it is late in the evening; Bazarov predicts that as soon as the clock strikes ten, "you will throw me out." Odintsova protests that she will do no such thing, and then asks Bazarov to open the window because the room feels stuffy. "Bazarov stood up and pushed on the window. It instantly flew open with a bang . . . He did not expect that it would open so easily; besides, his hands were shaking."[30] The sudden violent action of the window is notable: in this way, the customarily transparent and thus self-effacing object now calls attention to itself, and begins to seem animate, as if it possesses a will of its own. This window that noisily flies open gestures at the power of the pent-up passion within Bazarov and the imminent release of out-of-control sensuality within Odintsova as well.[31] The mechanics of the window play an important role in this scene, but so does the material of which it is made. Bazarov effectively transfers his agitation to the static window, while in a subsequent scene, he attempts to take on that same window's physical properties of coldness and containment.

After their initial conversation ends inconclusively, Odintsova invites Bazarov back to her room on the following day to continue where they left off. She compels Bazarov to admit to his infatuation with her, a confession that is agonizing for him; standing with his back to her, he admits that he loves her "'stupidly, madly . . . See what you have achieved.' Odintsova stretched out her arms, and Bazarov pressed his forehead against the glass on the window. He could not breathe; his whole body trembled visibly."[32] The body language here is telling: while Odintsova reaches out to Bazarov, he presses his forehead (the seat of his rational faculty, now overrun by irrational passion) against the window as if trying to numb himself. The fact that the window is a barrier between wild nature and constructed civilization, as well as a key component in the scientific attempt to comprehend and control the elements, can help us to decipher the image of Bazarov leaning against the windowpane. In the novel, glass is linked to western Europe through its association with the positivist scientists whose ideas inspire Bazarov. He is accustomed to dissecting frogs—the central trope in the novel for his uncompromising empiricism and determination to master the natural world—by pressing them against transparent glass slides and observing them through microscope lenses; and now he is seeking to master himself by means of glass.

Window-touching is also a crucial, and cryptic, element in an early scene in *Anna Karenina*. Once again, the window is linked with a problematic love affair; this time, the male side of the equation is both "out there," in the world beyond the window, and simultaneously inhabiting Anna's consciousness, becoming inextricably linked with the literary text (once again, of non-Russian origin) that she reads (recalling the intersection of reading and ill-advised falling in love in Pushkin's text). Anna is riding in a train compartment, holding a book knife (*razreznoi nozhik*) and an English novel, trying to concentrate on her reading, but she is distracted by the snow that blankets her window (*sneg, bivshii v levoe okno i nalipavshii na steklo*). She finds it unpleasant to read, "that is, to observe the reflections of the lives of other people. She yearned to live too much herself."[33] The use of the word "reflections" here to refer to the literary depictions of human beings is appropriate in light of the window's proximity: the window, rendered opaque by snow, is capable of generating literal reflections, and when Anna sees her image in the window, she can easily imagine herself as the heroine of a literary text.

As Amy Mandelker points out, the framing function of the window echoes that of the novel that Anna holds; moreover, both apertures offer only the illusion of escape: "the narratives she reads are so many windows onto so many worlds; yet none of them offers a genuine outlet for her desires that thus become repressed and frustrated."[34] Central to this scene is the material essence of a window, which offers an appealing vista while precluding true escape: hence, Tolstoy draws attention repeatedly to the presence of the snow-covered window; by covering it with snow, he makes the invisible glass visible and its shielding/imprisoning function explicit.

Anna puts down her book and begins thinking about her recent acquaintance with Vronsky, scoffing at the idea that there could be anything significant between herself and "this boyish officer [*ofitser-mal'chishka*]"; she ends up caressing the window with her knife, then pressing "its smooth and cold surface" to her cheek—an action that evokes a feeling of inexplicable joy.[35] In physical terms, there is a transfer of cold from the snow-covered window to the knife and then to Anna's cheek. The window is a barrier, hinting at the lines that respectable citizens dare not cross in Anna's society. The barrier in this case is the prohibition against adultery (a social as well as a biblical taboo); the image of the window that is usually transparent, but now rendered visible by snow, foregrounds the prohibition that now stands out in stark relief in Anna's mind.

Why does Anna feel joy after touching her cheek with the "smooth and cold" knife? This scene can be read as a moment of (illusory) liberation brought about by contact with the cold knife (in other words, she achieves the "cooling off" that Bazarov fails to attain when he presses his brow to the windowpane). The transparent window is rendered in this scene as white as the page of a book, and thus presents to Anna's gaze the notion of herself and Vronsky as the protagonists of a brand-new novel, whose author she can become and whose outcome she can thus determine; this fantasy of escape and control is made possible by the physical qualities of the windowpane, which captivates the eye and fires the imagination with its capacity to convey metaphorical meaning.

As Mandelker argues, the English novel serves "as a generator of mimetic initiation: Anna no sooner reads of an event that she longs to inscribe it in her own life." Moreover, Mandelker sees Anna's use of the knife as an attempted escape into the textual reality that "seduces" her: "Anna places the knife against the window glass—the membrane that separates the world from the vision of the world, the frame that imprisons experience. The knife directed against the text purchases Anna's only possible entry into the pictured world."[36] The critic's use of the word "inscribe" helps us to make further sense of Anna's knife-play with the page-like window; by using the knife in an imaginative rather than utilitarian way, not to cut the pages of a new novel, but to press it to the window as if preparing to carve words in the surface, Anna enacts that fantasy of inscription to which Mandelker alludes. Anna's failure to leave a mark is poignant in light of her desire for agency that is palpable in this scene.

The woman at the window is a popular motif in art, traditionally seen as an emblem of woman's lack of agency in society: thus she is relegated to viewing instead of doing.[37] Yet the situation may be more complex, and the woman at the window, more active than she might seem. At times windows also serve as surfaces for inscription. According to legend, Catherine II wrote her *Instruction* in the lavish "agate rooms" in the palace at Tsarskoe Selo. Not far from these rooms was the modestly appointed bedchamber upon whose window a date—May 21, 1786—had been engraved with a diamond, possibly by the empress herself. The meaning of the date remains a mystery.[38]

The image fits almost too neatly into the paradigm of Peter I as builder and Catherine II as writer. If Catherine was indeed the author of that inscription, in any event a nicely transgressive gesture, was it done in daytime, in a moment of contemplation of the world outside, or at night, when the empress would have seen her own image in the glass? Princess Dolgorukaia narrates the decisive events and crises of her early life as seen through and happening around windows. In Catherine's bedroom, on the other hand, the event is encrypted into a date that does not reveal its referent; in fact the event may have been the act of inscription itself. Historian M. I. Pyliaev notes that a certain general made off with the glass when the windowpanes in the room were replaced;[39] nothing more is known of the fate of this curious eighteenth-century document.

Window-writing was an established practice by the time that Catherine made her mark. References to windows inscribed with words appear in the poems of Edmund Spenser and George Herbert; such inscriptions could be performed with the use of diamond rings designed specifically for this purpose. Two centuries before Catherine's enigmatic inscription, Princess Elizabeth, held under house arrest at Woodstock Manor, used a diamond to engrave in her window: "Much suspected by me / Nothing proved can be. Quoth Elizabeth, Prisoner."[40] Closer to our time, the dissident Soviet writer Vasily Aksyonov liked to show visitors the inscription on a windowpane in his high-rise Moscow apartment: "This house was built by prisoners."[41] Windows, then, can serve as writing surfaces for captives of various kinds who are seeking transcendence.

Windows offer not only vistas, but also reflections, and at times a superimposition of various visual planes. John Donne's poem "A Valediction: Of My Name, in the Window" (1633) suggests that the reflection of one's image is itself a kind of inscription. Donne's narrator, who is taking leave of his mistress, informs her that has inscribed his name in her window as a memento of his love; paradoxically, he states that this act of inscription has not weakened, but rather strengthened the glass: "My name engrav'd herein, / Doth contribute my firmness to this glasse, / Which, ever since that charm, hath been / As hard, as that which grav'd it, was; / Thine eye will give it price enough, to mock / The diamonds of either rock." What motivated the poet to become a graffiti artist was apparently the desire to merge with his beloved in a peculiar way—for his name "to become part of his lover's reflection—to be written, as it were, across her face."[42] The poet takes the opportunity to merge with glass himself in proclaiming that he shares the material's transparency—a sign of his sincerity: "'Tis much that Glass should be / As all confessing, and through-shine as I, / 'Tis more, that it shewes thee to thee, / And clear reflects thee to thine eye. / But all such rules, loves magic can undo, / Here you see me, and I am you." In a later stanza, Donne's narrator urges his addressee to consider the inscribed letters in corporeal terms as the very bones of his body: "think this ragged bony name to be / My ruinous anatomy"—again evoking the confluence of body and glass.

To write on the surface of a window through which one habitually looks is to alter one's visible reality and to apply one's personal stamp to the outside world. Another way to do this is by turning a clear windowpane into a picture—a stained glass window. Such windows were not produced in Kievan Rus for reasons ranging from the local climate to the spatial organization within Orthodox cathedrals, which differed from that found in western Europe. Moreover, as Tatiana Volobaeva explains, Orthodox tradition prohibited painting icons on glass "owing to the brittleness and fragility of the material, and consequently of the image depicted thereupon" and the belief that the depicted sacred being somehow dwelled in the painted surface itself.

Yet glass, true to its transgressive nature, began to appear in Russian Orthodox churches in the nineteenth century. Volobaeva has traced over

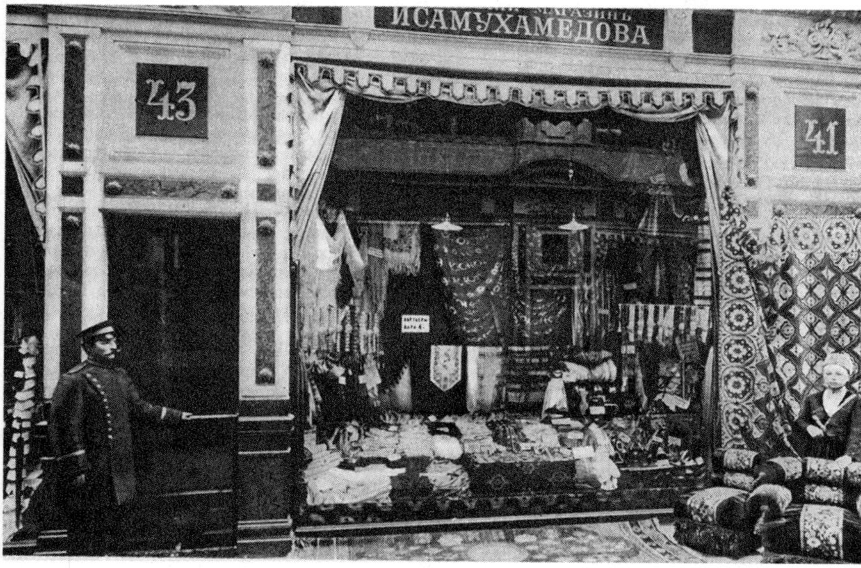

Figure 3. Early twentieth-century shop window. Reproduced from Ia. N. Rivosh, *Vremia i veshchi: Ocherki po istorii material'noi kul'tury v Rossii nachala XX veka*. Moscow: Iskusstvo, 1990.

thirty references in written sources to Orthodox churches in St. Petersburg alone that were decorated with stained glass windows in the period between the 1820s and the 1910s. This change was connected with a broader transformation within Russian religious culture starting in the eighteenth century, when icons began to be perceived in aesthetic as well as spiritual terms, "not only as an object of religious worship, but increasingly as the finely wrought creation of an artist or an artisan." Stained glass windows began to appear in Russia not only in ecclesiastical buildings, but also in private homes whose well-to-do residents wished to transform their view of the outside world, transfiguring a commonplace reality into "a fantastic world of beauty."[43]

The shop window, which made its Russian debut in the mid-nineteenth century, likewise helped to create a fantasy realm. (See figure 3.) Shop windows are eloquent spectacles; they speak to the haves and have-nots, and they help to construct that binary opposition. They epitomize privilege yet beckon with promises of equal access to visual pleasure and possession:

> A pane of glass, not more than 1.5 centimeters thick, divides the shop from the pavement. On one side, the climate-controlled interior welcomes those who can buy; on the other, the intemperate street is where those who cannot

> buy may look without paying . . . [Shop windows] are relatively democratic . . . yet what display windows point at and push us towards, is financially inaccessible to many people much of the time . . . [Window-dressers] walk a fine line between cultivating exclusivity and letting the rest of us down so softly that we feel uplifted.[44]

Shop windows were a necessary accoutrement of the department stores that appeared in Russia's major cities and "directly challenged the previous conventions of the urban market."[45] The pane of glass signified the elimination of the face-to-face interaction, the personal engagement intrinsic to haggling over prices, and the spontaneity of the earlier marketplace. The fact that the Russian word for "shop window," *vitrina*, is a borrowing from the French can be traced back to the fact that a French merchant opened Russia's first department store.[46] For a long period of time, the main department stores in Moscow were operated by foreigners, and hence, an aura of foreignness hovered around these shops, their wares, and their display windows. In Vladimir Lukin's play *The Trinket Dealer* from the preceding century, the speeches of the dandified Russian gentry are replete with French borrowings, and Lukin decries this foreign invasion, which manifests itself as an influx of words and commodities.[47]

As a scene in Gogol's story "The Overcoat" demonstrates, the association between shop windows and "the French" had already become automatic by 1842, the date when the story was written. The poor clerk Akaky Akakievich, clad in his new overcoat, gazes "with curiosity" at an illuminated shop window that contains "a picture of some sort of beautiful woman who was kicking off her shoe, thereby laying bare her entire foot, one that was not at all bad-looking; meanwhile, behind her back some sort of man with sideburns and a handsome goatee was sticking his head through the doors leading to the adjacent room." After taking in the spectacle, Akaky shakes his head and smiles, and then goes on his way, while the narrator wonders whether that smile had been a response to "an altogether unfamiliar thing about which, nevertheless, everyone retains a certain sense," and speculates that Akaky, "akin to many other clerks," must have thought something along the following lines: "Oh, the French! What can you say, if they get a hankering for that sort of thing, then you can be sure . . ."[48]

The woman in the shop window is an object of desire—"an unfamiliar thing" for the celibate clerk, but something that instinctively stirs him: he has already come to view his overcoat as his "life companion," so he is predisposed to think of commodities in erotic terms, which is exactly the sentiment that the window display is designed to evoke. Moreover, the bearded man depicted in the display serves to model adult male desire for the sexually immature Akaky. Elizabeth Outka formulates the way in which shop windows came to serve as sites of identity formation in the nineteenth century: they "offered the consumer different views of possible selves, obtainable for a price. The displays always suggested that the viewer was lacking, producing a never-ending loop of desire, buying, and dissatisfaction."[49] As in the case of the windows in Pushkin and Tolstoy, the frame of the shop window functions analogously to the page of a novel and creates a kind of identification scenario, this time between Akaky and the man peering at the woman; here the text underscores the relationship between gaze and possession.

The combination of the erotic and the mercantile in "The Overcoat" resonates strongly with the first encounter between Hermann and Liza in "The Queen of Spades." Hermann decides that the pretty (and fragmented) girl in the window will lead him to the treasure he seeks, and conflates the figure of Liza with the notion of wealth; from that moment on, he is doomed. Gogol's poor clerk, whose new overcoat-bride means everything to him, sees a pretty (and fragmented) girl in a shop window, a spectacle that stirs a new kind of desire—and from that moment on, he too is doomed. Akin to the window scenes in Pushkin, Turgenev, and Tolstoy, the shop window scene in "The Overcoat" is another nexus of glass and desire, and the desire again has illicit overtones (Akaky ogles the image of a woman disrobing; moreover, there is already a man in the picture, which makes Akaky's gaze even more voyeuristic); indeed, his interaction with this image sets off a chain reaction of catastrophic events for the poor clerk, so the woman in the shop window display functions as a kind of femme fatale. The shop window glass again represents a barrier, and its invisibility complicates the viewer's relationship with that which is beyond the glass: the desirable commodity is simultaneously untouchable and within reach.

POST-REVOLUTIONARY WINDOWS: TRANSPARENCY AND FRAGILITY

In 1928, Aleksandr Rodchenko began taking experimental photographs showing the play of light on glass surfaces. That year, he proclaimed: "We are taught to look in a routine, inculcated manner. We must discover the visible world. We must revolutionize our visual thinking."[50] The Bolshevik Revolution precipitated a transformation of vision, and glass contributed to this phenomenon in the material environment and in the world of ideas. It was appropriate that the new Soviet state was eager to establish, quite literally, an autonomous way of seeing:

> Even before the end of the Civil War, during a time of hunger and devastation, the State Optical Institute was founded in December 1918 on Lenin's

> initiative. . . . Domestic production of optical glass was established in the Soviet Union in the beginning of the 1920s, making the import of such glass unnecessary.[51]

During the War Communism years (1919–21), the display function of shop windows was appropriated by the Bolsheviks and given a Marxist twist: the commodity fetish gave way—only to return with a vengeance with the advent of the New Economic Policy (NEP)—to political propaganda in the form of the "windows" (*okna*) of ROSTA, the Russian Telegraph Agency, which served to inform and indoctrinate the masses from September 1919 until January 1922. As Stephen White recounts, during the Civil War "the printing industry was in a poor state and reproduction in color was almost impossible, so [ROSTA] decided to organize special 'windows' in all its sections containing color drawings on themes of the day" and to mass-produce them using human labor. The first such window, addressing the subject of Denikin and the fall of the Hungarian Soviet Republic, and labeled "Rosta Satire Window No. 1," appeared in the window of a shop formerly known as Abrikosov and Sons, a purveyor of sweets.[52]

Numerous "windows" followed in its wake; they consisted of colorful posters displayed in Moscow and later Petrograd and other towns. Positive heroes—workers and soldiers—in bright scarlet hues vied with enemies of the Bolsheviks (kulaks, the bourgeoisie, Social Revolutionaries, White Army generals, Entente powers) depicted as grotesque caricatures.[53] These windows provided the latest news and information, propagandized and explicated the decrees and resolutions issued by Soviet power, and exposed and ridiculed its enemies.[54] Thus the commercial function of the windows was displaced by a new ideological function; now it was a political imperative that was on display. Mayakovsky was one of the artists who worked on the ROSTA windows—he produced about one third of the total output;[55] later, he channeled his talents into ads for commodities that had reasserted their role in the shop windows of the NEP.

The phenomenon of the tsarist shop windows transformed into revolutionary "windows of satire" should be viewed in light of the connection between glass and theatricality. While the shop windows were given brand-new roles as conduits of propaganda, their beholders would not immediately forget their previous power to stage a scene of desire and fulfillment by means of expenditure. In 1909, a British journalist writing in the *Daily Mail* described shop windows, each of which "formed a sort of proscenium for a deep-set scene with a painted background in colours delicately harmonizing with the articles occupying what may be termed the centre of the stage." This description sheds light on the nature of Akaky's experience as he gazes at the risqué window display; as Outka points, out, such windows compelled viewers to "imagine performing within the atmosphere and even playing with a new identity suggested on this stage."[56] The theatricality of shop windows is likewise a helpful framework within which to analyze the repurposed shop windows of ROSTA, in that the period of War Communism was one in which identity became crucial to survival and the taking-on of a new identity was a prevalent social strategy.[57] In this light, it makes sense that shop windows, already accustomed to serving as stages for potential new identities, were appropriated as theaters in which the struggle between the forces of revolution and counter-revolution was played out in graphic images, accompanied by helpful captions.

In Fedor Gladkov's novel *Cement*, the unsettling depiction of the shop windows that serve as harbingers of the NEP may be linked with the author's memory of the ROSTA windows and the very different purpose that they served. A description of the lavish expanses of glass of the shop windows follows after recurring images of glass shattering in combat scenes set during the period of War Communism; hence the intact shop windows, when they appear, seem that much more obviously a negation of the revolutionary cause. On the other hand, the restoration of the broken factory windows constitutes a key leitmotif in the novel, and is depicted as an unambiguously positive phenomenon. The distinction between two kinds of window—*okno* and *vitrina*—is crucial to Gladkov's novel.[58]

The display function is certainly not alien to ideological applications in the Soviet context: as we shall see in chapter 6, the Lenin sarcophagus is a perfect illustration of the display function put to the service of the state. What is important to note is that the presence of the posters transformed the shop window into a glass-covered opening onto reality (as a window is meant to function); at the same time, these "windows" were also known as *okna satiry* ("windows of satire"), a combination that complicates the idea of a window providing a wholly objective view. The fact that the posters themselves came to be identified with "windows" is curious as well, implying that the cartoonish, ideologically motivated pictures were to be taken as an image of the real world. These annotated images appeared not only in shop windows but also in other well-traveled places, for example, in the form of street posters; when artists were faced with paper shortages, they stenciled the posters directly onto walls, fences, and sidewalks[59] (and later inside clubs, military units, and agitation centers).[60] The resulting images, however, were still known as *okna*—"windows." Thus the notion of the patently propagandistic image standing in for an objective view of reality extended beyond the shop window, and projected itself onto every possible urban space.

Moreover, the designation of "windows" for these images is notable because Soviet citizens were being encouraged to literally *peer into windows*—setting the tone of mutual surveillance for decades to come. A vivid

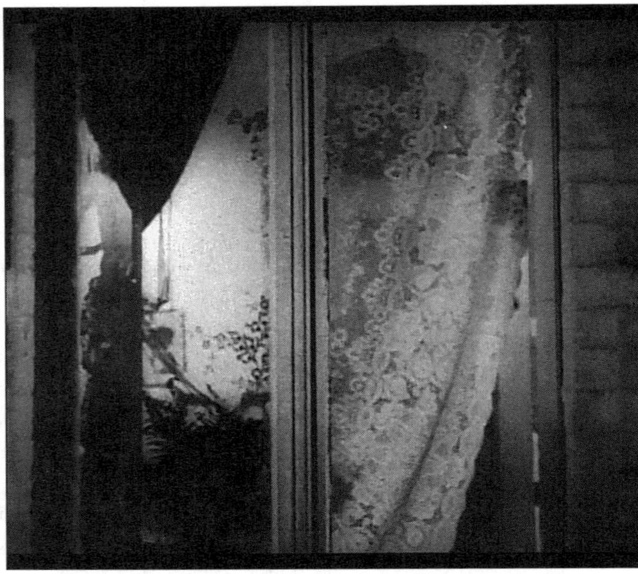

Figure 4. The camera eye peers into a sleeping woman's window. Dziga Vertov, *Man with a Movie Camera*, 1929.

illustration of this imperative appears in the tracking shot at the beginning of Dziga Vertov's documentary film *Man with a Movie Camera* (1929) when the gaze of the camera-eye carries us past the threshold of a lace-curtained window into the bedroom of a fitfully sleeping woman, who proceeds to wake up, throw off her covers, and pull on stockings and a bra without a hint of modesty. (See figure 4.) The message seems clear: private ownership and private space have been abolished in the land of the Soviets; in the film's narrative, this revolution in the realm of possession and desire is accomplished via the invasion of a glass barrier by a glass-based technology.

The Russian words for "window" (*okno*, formed from a Slavic root) and "shop window" (*vitrina*, a French borrowing) are distinct from one another. Thus, the Bolsheviks' transformation of *vitriny* into *okna* was a vivid demonstration of the profound change that the revolution promised to bring to every facet of Russian life, from the economic domain to language itself. While the connection between the eye and the window exists in English,[61] it is even more apparent in Russian. The word *okno* is etymologically related to the Old Slavonic word for eye, *oko* (still in use in high-style speech and writing). In addition, the word *zenitsa* (most commonly used in conjunction with the archaic *oko* in the idiom, "to protect as the apple of one's eye [*ze-*

nitsa oka]") means both "pupil of the eye" and "window." According to Dal', *zenitsa* signifies the pupil as well as "*gliadel'tse, zerkal'tse, chelovechek glaza*" ("little mirror, tiny being of the eye") and derives from the Vologda dialect *zenko*, which means "windowpane"—a formulation that envisions the eyes as the windows of the face.[62]

A rhyming Russian saying, "*chto v vitrine, to i v magazine*" ("what's in the shop window is what's in the store") turns on a fanciful metaphor whereby a person is likened to a shop, human qualities are presented in terms of consumer goods, and "what you see [in the display window] is what you get"; compare the lexical duo *oko/okno*, which presents the house as a face with eyes. While the etymology of the English word "window" signifies an opening in the home to let in air,[63] emphasing the function of the aperture, the Russian *okno* derives from *oko*, underscoring the eye-ness of the window, and thus, implying the animacy of the house rather than focusing on what the window lets in. In both the proverb and the etymology of *okno*, we note a tendency to blur the distinction between animate and inanimate entities that is not found in the analogous English phrasing.[64] This willingness to see the spark of life within the inanimate, deep-seated in the language, may have some bearing on the particular reception of glass in Russian culture. Because of its playful optical qualities, glass has suggested the qualities of a living entity to observers in Russia and beyond. This phenomenon can be glimpsed, for example, in the anthropomorphic depiction of glass architecture discussed in chapter 5 as well as the personification of material that appears in Lomonosov's "Letter on the Usefulness of Glass," to which we will turn in the next chapter.

Chapter Two

The Language of Glass: Making Rhetorical Objects

> Thanks to mirrors, rooms were transformed beyond recognition . . . A slight shift in perspective would turn the room into a kind of illusory space in which the world of the home and the outside world became mixed in the most fantastic way; the space was refracted, doubled, seemed to become multidimensional, its boundaries were virtually erased . . . The figures of visitors, multiplied by intersecting reflections, would glide along in different directions inside the fairy-tale realm beyond the looking glass [*zazerkal'e*]. A mirror placed at the end of the suite of rooms in its turn created the impression that the house extended into infinity.
>
> —P. Baiburova on the décor of mid-eighteenth-century Russian country houses

GLASS PLAYS A part in culture that is often overlooked, perhaps because of the transparent nature of the material and its manifold uses in modern life. Yet there was a time when glass seemed a wondrous substance. Its transparency makes it tend toward invisibility, yet invisibility suggests the presence of magic, as does the protean quality of glass that has led to its present-day ubiquity. Glass is a creation of culture whose basic substance is shaped into myriad forms to suit the idiom of that culture, with the potential to magnify, reflect, embody, or distort the world. In that way, it is like literary language. The kinship of glass and language drives Mikhail Lomonosov's poetic celebration of the material, his "Letter on the Usefulness of Glass" (1752).

The quality of usefulness can apply not only to literal utility but to the figurative sphere as well. Lotman provides examples of objects, including a loaf of bread and a sword, with practical, utilitarian functions as well as symbolic ones. A sword may be broken, displayed in a museum, or used to kill a man: "In all of these ways, it can be used an object, but when it is fastened to one's belt or attached to the hip and held in place by a sling, the sword symbolizes a free man; it is a 'signifier of freedom.'" A miniature sword intended to be worn at parades functions not as a weapon but as "virtually a depiction of a weapon." Thus, an object such as a sword may exist in culture—which is "always the sphere of symbolism"[1]—in any incarnation, from an actual weapon suitable for battle, to a symbol quite detached from its intended function.

I hope to demonstrate that in eighteenth-century Russian culture, glass moves from its utilitarian aspect toward a symbolic and signifying function, and back again. Inasmuch as glass is valued for its optical qualities, its sparkle, play of light, and capacity to reflect the outside world, it resonates with the eighteenth-century vogue for spectacle and display. The use of glass to substitute for precious stones evokes another aspect of Russian culture during the eighteenth century: the imitation of Western forms, from dress to literature, on the one hand, as well as a general trend toward artifice and artificiality. Lomonosov's experiments with glass enter into the then-current discourse of the Enlightenment; while architectural trends from larger windows to ever more elaborate chandeliers join that discourse in a more figurative manner. In a number of ways, the eighteenth century in Russia can be considered an Age of Glass.

Spectacular glass offered numerous expressive possibilities to artisans in Russia. In interiors, designers of light fixtures could take advantage of one of the main decorative qualities of glass—the capacity for reflection and refraction. Candles lit in chandeliers and girandoles decorated with crystal pendants (called "leaves," "teardrops," "stars," "icicles," "raindrops," etc.) created a magical play of light.[2] (See figure 5.) Glass can appeal to the emotions through its visual and its acoustic properties: striking the wall of a crystal vessel produces a gentle ring.[3] Little wonder, then, that in the first quarter of the eighteenth century, glass was used to make musical instruments. In 1724 in the Peterhof palace complex a musical fountain was constructed in which falling water set crystal bells in motion, producing a range of tones. One of these bells survives to this day in the State Russian Museum. It is made of high-quality clear, colorless glass and engraved with the image of a double-headed eagle, Peter the Great's monogram, and an inscription in German naming the place, time, and makers of the bell.[4]

Scholars trace the birth of Russian decorative glass (*khudozhestvennoe steklo*) to the Izmailovskii imperial factory in Moscow, founded in 1668. It was here that Russian glassmakers learned their craft from Ukrainian and western European colleagues. The Izmailovskii factory manufactured apothecary glass for the tsar and wares for the general market. It specialized in "amusing" (*poteshnoe*) glassware: vessels in the form of animals,

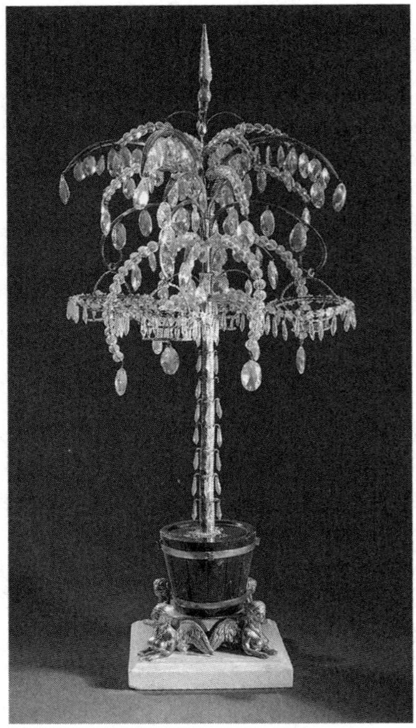

Figure 5. Girandole in the form of a palm tree in a tub. Potemkin Glass Factory. Russia, late eighteenth century. Crystal, bronze, and black marble, height 94 cm. The State Hermitage Museum, St. Petersburg. Photograph by Vladimir Terebenin, Leonard Kheifets, and Yuri Molodkovets. Copyright © The State Hermitage Museum.

fruit such as apples, as well as objects of unusual size and shape, including a clear wineglass two meters in size,[5] "a tall amusing goblet," and "a church-chandelier [*panikadila*] with figures." These objects were designed to appeal to the aesthetic of the emperor and his court.[6] Glass factories were initially state-controlled, but as the demand for glass began to exceed its production,[7] factory ownership fell increasingly into private hands; this pattern follows the typical sequence of privatization for other forms of mass production during the Petrine period.[8] The center of Russian glass production moved from Moscow to the Iamburg and Zhabin factories near St. Petersburg shortly after that city became the new capital.[9] The craft of Russian glassmaking developed at a remarkable pace thanks to the influx of foreign masters and the ardent support of the state.[10] By the time the crystal fountain at Peterhof had been built, the "apprentice phase" of Russian glassmaking was over. Now Russian artisans skilled in every aspect of the trade were able to pass on their expertise to subsequent generations.[11]

LOMONOSOV'S LETTER: WRITING ON GLASS

Mikhail Lomonosov is best known as the creator of majestic odes that glorified Russian monarchy and imperial splendor through words, as the site of Peterhof had done through visual means. Yet he also occupies a unique place in the history of world literature as one who simultaneously transformed both his nation's literary language[12] and its glass industry. Here I would like to take a closer look at the meanings behind Lomonosov's turn to glassmaking, and to consider the correspondences between versification and vitrification.

In Russia, Lomonosov is credited as being the first to take a scientific approach to glassmaking.[13] Indeed, his pioneering work on colored glass, which led to a rediscovery in Russia of the lost art of glass mosaics,[14] and then a revitalization of the glass industry as a whole, originated in laboratory experiments in which he sought to understand the nature of color. In 1748, shortly after Lomonosov received a professorship in chemistry, he had the Academy build for him a chemical laboratory on Vasilievskii Island in St. Petersburg. Here he undertook to devise a "Theory of Color," and soon realized that colored glass was essential for his experiments. Such glass was unavailable in Russia at the time. Whether out of patriotism or thrift, Lomonosov chose not to seek help from western European masters who possessed the secret recipes he needed. Instead, he conducted close to 3,000 experiments in which he added various minerals to molten glass until he arrived at his own rich palette of colors.[15] Along the way, he rediscovered the recipe for gold ruby glass (of a brilliant red color achieved through the addition of just the right amount of gold to the molten glass mixture), a secret that alchemist Johann Kunckel had taken to his grave in the previous century.[16]

By this time, glassmaking had taken hold of Lomonosov. He petitioned the Senate in 1752, asking for support in establishing a glass factory "for the benefit and glory of the Russian empire," where he would manufacture beads as well as numerous household items "that are currently not made in Russia, but imported from abroad in vast quantities, at a cost of many thousands [of rubles]." Lomonosov argued further that the items he would produce at his factory would find a market not only in Russia, but in other countries as well. Finally, he claimed that it would be cheaper to produce glass at his factory than to order it from abroad, since Russia has abundant sources of precisely those materials (wood, sand, potash) that are crucial for glassmaking.[17] His request met with success. At the new factory at Ust'-Ruditsa, Lomonosov produced clear glass for optical devices and opaque glass for mosaics[18] and such vessels as drinking glasses, candy dishes, ink pots, and snuffboxes;[19] larger-scale items including glass tabletops made to mimic precious and semiprecious stones such as striped and spotted jasper; glass cuff-links, buttons, pendants, fragrance holders, and letter-writing sets.[20] In the wake of Lomonosov's discoveries, colored glassware of various colors, particularly deep cobalt blue, displaced colorless glass in popularity in the second half of the eighteenth century. Russian factories vied with one another to develop the broadest range of colors. In the second half of the century, glass came into broader use in interiors, as seen in palace floors, portrait frames, and tables inlaid with Lomonosov's mosaics.[21]

Lomonosov's "Letter on the Usefulness of Glass" ("Pis'mo o Pol'ze Stekla"), sent to his patron Ivan Shuvalov in 1752 and published in 1753, sings the praises of glass in a seemingly exhaustive list of its virtues. Lomonosov wrote the poem in anticipation of having to petition the empress about opening his factory,[22] yet this pragmatic dimension does not begin to account for the enthusiasm and sheer sweep of Lomonosov's work. As we shall see, in celebrating glass, Lomonosov exults in the shape-shifting potential of a material that speaks to the poet's concerns about personal power and self-identity.

Lomonosov opens by launching a preemptive strike against those who would attack his interest in glass—introducing the theme of (self)-protection that will become a recurring one in the poem. He asserts that glass is no less useful or beautiful than natural stone:

> Those people are mistaken, Shuvalov,
> Who consider Glass to be lower than the Minerals
> Whose shining rays entice the eye:
> There is no less usefulness in it, and no less beauty.[23]

Lomonosov then defines the task of the poem: before his addressee Shuvalov, "in ecstasy" he sings the praises "not of precious stones, nor of gold, but of Glass." A mythological narrative follows describing the volcanic origins of glass. As Mount Etna erupts, day turns to "terrifying night" and the world fears its imminent demise. Then the apocalyptic tableau gives way to a peaceful sunlit scene: a "dear child, beautiful Glass" (*Liubeznoe ditia, prekrasnoe steklo*) has been born from a geological catastrophe.

Now Lomonosov turns to the manifold ways in which "mortals" have striven to follow nature in the creation of glass, and indeed, how they have surpassed her achievements.[24] It now appears that the metamorphosis of day into night on the eve of the birth of Glass was a harbinger of the material's talent for self-transformation, as Lomonosov's list of its manifestations makes clear. Lomonosov begins by praising the clarity of wine and beer glasses; then, so as not to dwell too long on the joys of inebriation (in fact, Lomonosov's rivals liked nothing more than to promote his reputation as a drunkard)[25] he offers transparency as a model of sincerity: "he who can be seen through is surely no sycophant." Likewise (the poet is unable to keep from returning to the subject of drink) a clear glass will not conceal any "admixture" placed therein, presumably by some malefactor. From liquor Lomonosov moves to life-saving medicines, which can be safely prepared and stored only in nonreactive glass vessels: "we owe our health and lives in part to Glass!"[26]

After this hyperbolic claim, Lomonosov once again shifts to the strategy of contrast, showing us the virtues of glass by telling us what it is not. This time he addresses the art of ceramics, which, at first glance, appears to have allowed the Chinese to dispense with glass altogether; yet glazing is what allows a ceramic vessel to hold water, and furthermore turns an ordinary pot into a work of art. Thus the poem demonstrates yet again the merged beauty and usefulness of glass. In mosaics, the attributes of beauty and utility fuse even more: these colorful bits of glass preserve the beauty and nobility of human faces for all time, protecting the precious human likeness from the ravages of age.[27] The motif of protection continues with the next use of glass: windows, which let sunlight in while we stay warm inside, and greenhouses, which let flowers thrive even in winter.

The mention of hothouse flowers turns the poet's mind to the "beauties" who use them to play dress-up. Now "the fair sex" becomes Lomonosov's addressee, and women's self-adornment, his topic. Yet Lomonosov does not condemn women's vanity; on the contrary, he drinks in the vision of their beautification rituals with the ardor of a Robert Herrick contemplating his beloved clad in silk. Glass plays a crucial role in such rituals: mirrors enable women's artifice and even double their beauty: "you are twice as comely when you use Glass"; and glass beads adorn society ladies and peasant girls ("rural nymphs") alike.[28]

The discussion of glass beads provokes Lomonosov to address the cruelty and greed of his fellow man, exemplified by settlers who swindled and slaughtered the Native American peoples. According to Lomonosov, we might think the Native Americans to be "simpletons" for accepting glass beads in exchange for precious metal; but in fact they are "more sensible than we" for choosing the one in favor of the other. Lomonosov lists the atrocities, from mining under inhuman conditions to warfare, perpetrated for the sake of silver and gold; by contrast, glass would never drive anyone to such extremes.[29] As if anticipating an attack on the perceived cheapness of glass, Lomonosov subjects that very quality to a curious revision into a morally commendable feature.

The poet thus makes the reader shift his point of view; and accordingly, the focus of the poem now shifts to optical glass. The digressions in the poem serve to make us aware of the way in which optics alter or divert the gaze. Lomonosov calls the capacity of glass to restore eyesight a "divine gift," which creates the opportunity for another digression, part of Lomonosov's polemic with the Orthodox Church: using lenses to capture the heavens' fire, we "imitate Prometheus harmlessly" (another way in which glass enables imitation) yet "the science of Prometheus" invites the wrath of ignorant proponents of religious obscurantism striving to block scientific progress. Lomonosov shows how intrinsic glass was to the discoveries of those he champions, from Copernicus to Newton, who, "having learned the laws of rays refracted in Glass," sought to tell the truth about the world. The telescope shows the full glory of God's creation, as does the microscope. It is the transformation of vision enabled by glass, in fact, that liberates our minds and allows us to travel from one state to another: "Probing infinite space with our reason, we pass from thought to thought, from one world to another [*Iz mysli khodim v mysl', iz sveta v svet inoi*]."[30]

Lomonosov then declares that a year would not suffice if he were to enumerate *all* the virtues of glass, and therefore, he is going to leave off praising the material and move from talk to action. Yet, carried away by the momentum of his own words, Lomonosov acknowledges that he cannot refrain from mentioning just one more marvelous feature of the material, one that helps to control nature by reproducing its effects, and keeps fear at bay. In fact, control of nature, imitation, and freedom from fear are all recurring themes in the poem; what seems therefore a spontaneous addition, another bead on a string, actually helps to sum up Lomonosov's argument rather neatly. Thus, the "Letter" informs us that glass spheres serving as electrical generators can duplicate the effects of lightning, which learned men can study and thereby eliminate the fear of lightning; and glass lightning rods divert disaster from our homes. Lomonosov reports that "marvelous news" is circulating around the world "that, knowing the rules discovered by Glass, we can turn thunder away from our homes."[31] Here Lomonosov's use of the instrumental case creates an ambiguity: the phrase "*pravila, izyskanny Steklom*" can be read as "rules discovered *by means of* Glass" or as "rules discovered *by* Glass." Following the latter reading (which is supported by the next reference to glass, four lines later, an obvious personification: "then Glass shall assure us of the truth [*togda o istine Steklo uverit nas*]"), we see that Lomonosov again personifies Glass, and this time even grants it agency—it is the substance itself that "discovers" the rules of nature; human beings merely need to learn what these rules are.

If we trace the argument of the poem, we see that Lomonosov does not have to choose between beauty and utility; the attributes of glass are such that he can conflate the two. Yet ultimately science, as a force for social, collective good, takes the upper hand over personal gain (from the enjoyment of wine to the pleasure of self-adornment). This peculiar poem might appear less so if seen in the context of a genre of "scientific poetry" that thrived in the sixteenth century. A collection of such poems was compiled by François Ouden as *Poëmata didascialica* (*Edifying Poems*), published in Europe in the late seventeenth and early eighteenth century, and by the mid-eighteenth century came to the attention of Lomonosov (he twice cites the work in his private papers). The poems, some in epistolary form addressed to leading scholars of the day, were written in Latin by French, Italian, and German authors and addressed such topics as chess, silkworms, tea, barometers, clockwork mechanisms, gunpowder, fire, gold, magnets, comets, earthquakes, rainbows, and northern lights.[32] Lomonosov may well have taken his cue from this compilation to use verse to introduce and popularize not only scientific discoveries but also science itself.

In 1746 Count M. I. Vorontsov bought ancient Roman mosaics to Russia; Lomonosov saw them the following year. From the notes of Lomonosov's fellow academician Jacob Stählin, we learn that these mosaics spurred the poet to copy and then surpass the originals.[33] What appealed to Lomonosov about mosaics was that, unlike painting, their colors would not fade over time.[34] He makes this very point in his "Address on the Usefulness of Chemistry" ("Slovo o pol'ze khimii") (written a year before the "Letter on the Usefulness of Glass"), where he praises science for providing "the means to make long-lasting works of art":

> Chemistry, seeing that her fragile creations [*neznhye sostavy*] fade and go to ruin from drastic atmospheric changes and the rays of the sun, used the mightiest instrument of her art—fire—combining hard minerals with glass at a high temperature, and created substances [*materii*] that excel in brightness and purity, and that resist the moisture of the atmosphere and the burning of the sun to such an extent that after many centuries they have not lost the least part of their beauty, which is attested by mosaics from a thousand years ago found in Greek and Italian cathedrals.[35]

The Italian mosaics were made from natural semiprecious stones, but Lomonosov set out to create a similar effect by artificial means.[36]

A notable feature of the "Letter" is the emergence of the poetic "I," not as pronounced as in lyrical poetry, but playing a more active role than in other, more typical odes.[37] Lines such as the following demonstrate Lomonosov's image of himself as a scientist: "Nowadays Europe has focused all its thoughts on this subject, and has already established suitable technologies. I, following in her footsteps, descend from Mt. Parnassus, and for a time I shall apply all my labor to Glass." An anecdote from 1757 further elucidates this self-image. When the French engraver Etienne Fessard created a portrait of Lomonosov, showing his subject in the act of composing the ode "To His Imperial Highness" at his desk, with two ships at sea and a flash of lightning seen in the window to his right, Lomonosov objected to the way in which he was represented ("as a court composer of odes," Bezborodov speculates) and invited the Academy artist Vortman to fix the "errors" in the portrait. The new version replaced the stormy sea in the background—too "poetic" an image—with the Ust'-Ruditskaia glass factory complete with smokestack, and pleased Lomonosov as the earlier portrait had not.[38] The contrast between the two images is between writing odes that praised the monarch and doing pioneering scientific work; hence for the background of his portrait, Lomonosov preferred his glass factory as opposed to a lightning storm—a demonstration of nature's might rather than that of his own mastery thereof; the former image would empower Lomonosov himself and take him out of the position of subservience. This issue of power, especially in light of the poet's humble origins and desire to transcend them and "re-create" himself, is an important prism through which we can view Lomonosov's broad-ranging artistic and scientific endeavors, in which he had so much at stake.

It might be too simple to conclude that for Lomonosov, his scientific activity took precedence over his literary work: he was performing experiments and creating new forms in the literary laboratory as well. Indeed, the two spheres of activity were so inseparable for Lomonsov that he cited his odes in his scientific papers. For example, in his "Address on Atmospheric Phenomena Originating from Electrical Power" (1753), Lomonosov notes the way in which his theory about northern lights differs from "[Benjamin] Franklin's conjecture" and adds: "Moreover, my ode on northern lights, composed in 1743, and published in 1748 in the *Rhetoric*, contains my long-standing opinion that northern lights may be generated by the movement of the ether."[39] As Morozov notes, for Lomonosov both poetry and science were "ways of attaining knowledge of the objectively existing world in all its beauty and grandeur."[40] Hence Lomonosov's celebration of glass, which plays such a crucial role in letting human beings come to know the perceptible world. We recall the genesis of Lomonosov's interest in mosaics: art emerging from science. The emergence of the "I" in Lomonosov's "Letter" is in part a reflection of the poet's understanding of his role as innovator and creator of Russian culture.

Glass in Lomonosov's poem undergoes numerous transformations; it seems to have an unlimited potential for self-reinvention. In a similar vein, Lomonosov celebrates the pliability of the Russian language in his *Russian Grammar*. He juxtaposes it against other European languages and argues that it can take on the functions and attributes of each:

> The Holy Roman Emperor Charles V has said that one should use Spanish for speaking with God, French—with friends, German—with enemies, Italian—with the female sex. But if he had been acquainted with Russian, then he

> surely would have added that it is a suitable language for speaking with all of them. For he would have found in it the splendor of Spanish, the liveliness of French, the solidity of German, the tenderness of Italian, and moreover the richness and powerful brevity in depiction of Greek and Latin. . . . My years of work on the Russian language have thoroughly convinced me of this.

Lomonosov believed that such flexibility made Russian an all-purpose language well suited to various contexts, from literature to science.[41]

In his *Rhetoric* of 1748, Lomonosov assigns precise semantic characteristics to particular letters of the alphabet: "The hard *с*, *ф*, *х*, *ц*, *ч*, *ш*, and fusible [*plavkoe*] р have a sonorous and swift pronunciation, and therefore they may be used to best represent forceful, great, loud, terrifying and majestic things and events. As for the soft ж, з, and fusible в, л, м, н, they have a delicate pronunciation and are therefore suitable for the depiction of delicate and soft things and events."[42] What is striking here is Lomonosov's emphasis on the materiality of the signifier; the use of the adjective *plavkoe* for certain letters even suggests the glassmaking register itself. For Lomonosov, glass and language both appear as wondrous substances with a capacity to be crafted into forms both useful and beautiful.

Among Lomonosov's ancestors were famous master carvers from Kholmogory, who turned ivory (usually from walrus or mammoth tusks) into delicate lace, then lined it with lilac, green, and red foil,[43] utterly transforming the original material, as glassmakers transform humble sand into something dazzling and translucent. Lomonosov grew up among these artists of metamorphosis, and his "Letter" testifies to a view of glass as a material with an even richer potential. Roland Barthes's essay on plastic provides a way to understand the evocation of wonder in Lomonosov's "Letter." For Barthes, this material's ability to transform unpromising matter into something precious evokes alchemy; he equates plastic with "the very idea of its infinite transformation." This capacity of plastic arouses "a perpetual amazement [that] is a pleasurable one, since the scope of the transformations gives man the measure of his power . . . an artificial Matter, more bountiful than all the natural deposits, is about to replace [Nature], and to determine the very invention of forms."[44] We might think of Lomonosov's "pleasurable amazement" in the "Letter" as a pleasure that is doubled, stemming as it does from the ability to craft new forms from an infinitely pliable substance, and an equally obliging language.[45] Glassmaking offered to Lomonosov the rationalism of science and the magic of alchemy.

Lomonosov created an impressive spectrum of colored glasses at the Ust'-Ruditskaia factory. From his laboratory journal we learn, for example, that mercury yielded "pale purple," iron—yellow, and gold—ruby-colored glass. The addition of copper resulted in glass in numerous shades of green:

"an excellent grass-green color resembling genuine emerald"; "green, close to the color of aquamarine"; "a beautiful beryl color"; "an excellent blue-green color (that of a scallion)"; and "semi-transparent, like the leaf of a stinging nettle."[46] Notable here is the frequency with which Lomonosov seeks correspondences between the products of nature and his own synthetic creations.

In a 1754 letter Lomonosov writes of the three-year period in which he conducted experiments on the nature of color, leading to his discovery of homemade colored glass:

> After nearly three thousand trials . . . I not only had a vast amount of material for a true theory of color, but I had also begun to work on the production of mosaics. I presented a little sample [*obrazchik*] of my work, namely, an icon [*obraz*] of the Mother of God, to the Empress in celebration of her name-day in 1751.[47]

Through linguistic play that turns on the correspondence between *obrazchik* and *obraz*, Lomonosov imbues glass with sacred associations. In his "Letter on the Usefulness of Glass," in a passage celebrating the greatness of God as Creator, Lomonosov praises His generosity in sending "His beloved son" down to Earth (an allusion to a scriptural passage from Luke 9:35); the image of the "beloved son" recalls the epithets "worthy offspring" and "dear child" that Lomonosov applied to Glass, new-born into the world, at the start of the poem—a "child" with its own mythological lineage.

As he sought to master the art of mosaics, Lomonosov did not wish to limit himself to tiny icons; he liked to think big. At the end of his life, Lomonosov devoted himself to a grandiose project to build a massive mosaic-lined mausoleum for Peter the Great. Soviet scholars argue that Lomonosov was moved by patriotism to undertake this project. But we might look at it instead as Lomonosov's attempt to pay tribute to a fellow artist of metamorphosis. His plan was to use mosaic from his own factory to decorate the mausoleum (to be housed in the St. Paul Cathedral of the Peter and Paul Fortress) with twelve tableaus depicting heroic moments in the emperor's life. Each scene would be accompanied by an appropriate biblical image. (This project had a literary analogue: Lomonosov also set out to write a "heroic epic poem," *Peter the Great*, consisting of twenty-four songs and embracing all the events of the tsar's reign.)[48] Lomonosov only lived to complete one of these heroic images—the *Battle of Poltava*.[49] Members of his workshop nearly finished another tableau, but eventually abandoned it and the project as a whole.[50]

It seems to have been a praiseworthy endeavor. Yet controversy plagued Lomonosov from the start. His rival, the poet Trediakovsky, made an oblique attack on Lomonosov's artistic medium in his article "On Mosaics," published in *The Industrious Bee* in 1759. Trediakovsky argues that contemporary mosaic artists favor marble and semiprecious stones over glass and enamel (*steklo i finift'*), which they consider "materials too cheap and base to use."[51] It was not long before Lomonosov became the target of official ridicule among his colleagues at the Academy. According to Stählin, "All the artists and experts enjoyed a good laugh at this folly and pitied the church if it should end up having to be inlaid with glass." Stählin disdainfully adds that it was only "through intrigues" that Lomonosov managed to receive a commission and a monetary advance from the Senate in 1761 "to carry out his brilliant plan."[52]

What can account for the hostility that Lomonosov's project inspired? I would suggest that the answer has to do with Trediakovsky's characterization of glass as a "cheap and base" material. This might appear to clash with the prestigious status of glass that glass enjoyed in eighteenth-century Russia;[53] yet what seems to have provoked these countervailing associations was the capacity of glass to imitate other, more expensive substances. Already in the mid-eighteenth century, glass was known for its capacity to take on the guise of other materials—recall, for example, that the output from Lomonosov's factory included imitation jasper and precious stones; in the nineteenth century, the capacity of glass to simulate other materials came to the forefront in domestic glass production. Thus, at an industrial exhibition in 1858 in St. Petersburg, the imperial glass factory was represented by, among other things, two turquoise-colored vases "in the Byzantine style," a greenish cup with veins "in imitation of jasper," and glassware painted with copies of Raphael and Fragonard. The Bakhmet'ev factory exhibited vases of opalescent and frosted white glass "resembling alabaster and marble."[54] The attacks against Lomonosov were driven in part by negative views of the capacity that glass has to masquerade as other materials. Self-consciousness about being an imitator—of "Western" forms that are by implication superior—is a recurring motif in Russian culture and may help to account for mixed feelings about the copycat capacity of glass: an unsettling connection between imitation and imposture begins to suggest itself.

The imitative capacity of glass, then, gave rise to peculiar anxieties about authenticity, and provoked accusations of "baseness," especially to those already unkindly predisposed toward Lomonosov, such as Trediakovsky and Stählin. The latter (who in fact conspired with fellow academicians to have Lomonosov expelled from the Academy in 1763) carried over this association of glass with inauthentic imitation to Lomonosov himself. In his papers he referred to the poet-inventor as a "savage" and an "uninvited guest in the world of art."[55]

The fact that the famously lowborn Lomonosov had launched his career by claiming to be the son of a priest (to gain admission to the Slavo-Greco-Latin Academy in 1731) may have also spurred his enemies to tar

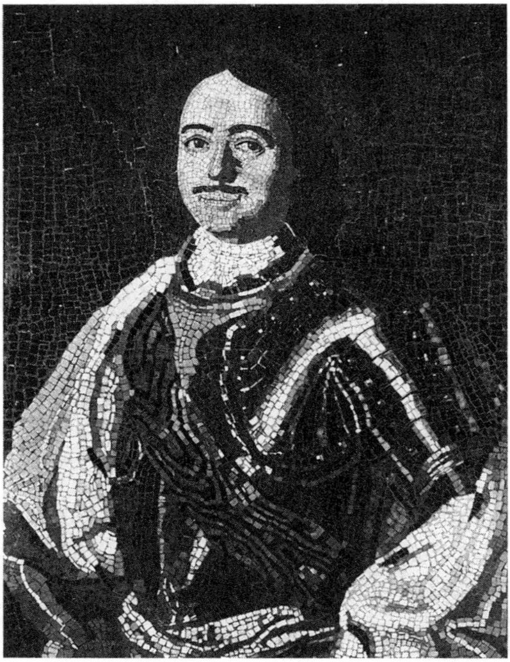

Figure 6. *Portrait of Peter I*, Mikhail Lomonosov, 1754, Russia. Smalt; mosaic. 89 × 69 cm. The State Hermitage, St. Petersburg. Photograph by Vladimir Terebenin, Leonard Kheifets, and Yuri Molodkovets. Copyright © The State Hermitage Museum.

him with the brush of inauthenticity. By accusing Lomonsov of being an impostor, not a genuine artist, his rival drew upon the negative connotations of glass, the material that held such profound meaning for Lomonosov and was inextricably associated with him. Lomonosov's heartfelt defense of the virtues of glass against more traditionally valued materials can then be seen as, in part, a self-referential move. The multiple metamorphoses of glass so nimbly demonstrated in Lomonosov's "Letter" are analogous to moments of human self-reinvention.

Lomonosov strove to immortalize Peter the Great by capturing his image in mosaics (see figure 6), and this was an apt material in light of the fact that glassmaking blossomed in Russia precisely in the Petrine period. Another object bearing the vitreous name of *zertsalo* (mirror) originated in Peter's legal reforms and came to serve as a peculiar monument to the monarch for centuries to come. This object epitomizes the way in which the physical properties of glass gave rise to figurative language and didactic associations. The optical phenomenon of reflection inherent to glass inspires the creation of mirrors. Then, this quality of reflection enters verbal art as a metaphor, generating the popular notion of the book as mirror. And then—only in Russia!—does this metaphor take on material form once again and is called a mirror, but this mirror is unlike any accoutrement of interior design that the reader is likely to have ever seen.

THE *ZERTSALO* AS MIRROR OF LAW AND ALL-SEEING EYE

In Nikolai Gogol's "Tale of How Ivan Ivanovich Quarreled with Ivan Nikiforovich" (1835), the chatty narrator tears himself away from the quarrel in question to describe the courthouse where the fate of the two friends is to be decided.

> The building is divided into two parts: in one there is the court, in the other, the jail. In the first part, there are two clean, whitewashed rooms: one is the outer room for petitioners; in the other is a desk adorned with ink stains. On the desk stands a *zertsalo*. There are four oak chairs with high backs; along the walls, ironbound chests in which the slanderous lawsuits of the district are piled up. On one of these chests, a polished boot was standing at the moment.[56]

What is the reader to make of the *zertsalo*—the term is an archaic form of *zerkalo*, "mirror"—that stands at the head of this Gogolian catalogue? This is a story whose very title thematizes the mirroring that will take place in it (as in, for example, the description of the two Ivans: one has a head "like a radish, tail downwards"; the other, "like a radish, tail upwards"). What exactly then is the *zertsalo* that has pride of place in this ambivalent description of a court of law? One sign of ambivalence is the series of bifurcations in this passage: the courthouse is divided into two halves; the court half is further split in two. (This splitting also mirrors the irreparable chasm that has opened up between the previously inseparable Ivans.) The clean, whitewashed rooms present a facade of unstained virtue that is thrown into question by the splotches of ink on the official desk; and the *zertsalo* is drawn into an uneasy association with those stains, for it, too, rests on the surface of the desk. Finally, the *zertsalo* atop the official desk rhymes visually with the shiny solitary boot atop the iron-bound chest filled with slanderous lawsuits. The "mirror" and the boot are monuments of sorts—but to what?

There are certain works of literature that we think we know so well, we feel confident in saying that no detail has escaped us, no nuance has slipped below our line of sight. Yet such details do exist, placed in the text according to the author's intricate design; in missing them, we miss an entire dimension of textual, and contextual, richness. For such details are often references to components of material culture, the furnishings of what once was everyday reality, but now seems irretrievably remote. These fragments of material reality can serve as a key to textual poetics.

One such object is the *zertsalo*, or, as English translation sometimes has it, the Mirror of Law. The *zertsalo* is an emblem of eighteenth-century Russia's bizarre marriage of Baroque and Classicist sensibility; yet this artifact survived through the nineteenth and into the twentieth century. It is situated between the realms of law and literature; the utilitarian and the aesthetic; the secular and the sacred. The *zertsalo* is a metaphor made concrete; it is *literally* a mnemonic device; and as a text-bearing artifact (with Peter I as author), it offers itself to a variety of readings. A spectacular object, it invites the gaze; a symbol of surveillance, it transforms the subject of the gaze into the object of it and plays a key role in a perpetually replicated scenario of power.[57] It is a conduit of ideology coded as iconography.

Here I would like to introduce and explicate the *zertsalo*. My goal is twofold: to rescue from obscurity an important object that deserves further elucidation; and to show how literary analysis can benefit from the examination of concrete objects. I have looked to well-known works of imaginative literature for references to my object of study, not only because these are canonical texts in which the *zertsalo* has been, up to now, hiding in plain sight, but also because authors of such works do more than document reality: they deploy realia to create meaning and effect, and it is instructive to see how they have chosen to describe, juxtapose, and otherwise make use of an artifact that itself required of its perceiver a formidable leap of the imagination.

The artifact known as the *zertsalo* came into being during the Petrine period. It took the form of a three-sided prism, and was designed to stand on the desk of every government official during legal proceedings as a symbol of law and order as well as a reminder of the sovereign's unblinking vigilance.[58] These were ornate, sizable objects meant to catch the eye. Judging by the *zertsala* on display and in storage in Moscow, St. Petersburg, and Vologda, they ranged in size from small and elegant (roughly a foot tall) to enormous and unwieldy (several feet in height), the majority tending toward the latter.

The *zertsalo* consisted of three planes joined together at the edges, with the figure of a double-headed eagle typically attached at the top. Each side of the prism displayed, usually behind glass, the text of a Petrine decree: on the observance of civil rights (April 17, 1722); proper conduct and honest service in the courts (January 21, 1724); and the importance of knowing and obeying government statutes (January 22, 1724). These decrees are considered to have been the three cornerstones of Russian law, at least until the judicial reforms of 1864.

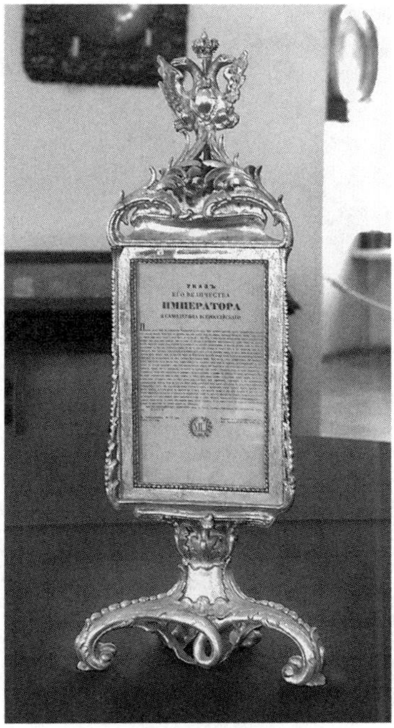

Figure 7. *Zertsalo*, sculpted by Mikhail Pavlov, 1762. Gilded wood and glass. Copyright © Museum of Anthropology and Ethnography (Kunstkamera) of the Russian Academy of Sciences. Lomonosov Museum, Kunstkamera.

Zertsala were made of carved, gilded wood, and occasionally metal.[59] A typical *zertsalo* was a large prism with rectangular sides. An exception is the spectacular oval *zertsalo* of gilded cast bronze, originally kept in the Synod and dating from 1775, currently on display at the St. Petersburg Historical Museum. Its rounded frame is adorned with plant-like forms, garlands, and official seals; a double-headed eagle sits at each of the three corners at the base, while the regal orb gets pride of place at the top. Another exception is a bronze *zertsalo* with oval sides dating from the 1760s–1770s that once belonged to the Senate, now kept at the State Russian Museum in St. Petersburg. It is decorated with sinuous leaves and three seated allegorical female figures. The decrees themselves are engraved in nielloed script on each side.[60] (See figures 7 and 8.) In the same museum, a second, larger model (approximately 2.5 feet tall) stands at the center of an official desk draped in red cloth in a reconstruction of the room that witnessed the sentencing of the Decembrists in 1826. Perhaps appropriately, this *zertsalo* is more severe, a rectangular prism crowned with a double-headed eagle that itself wears a crown and clutches the orb and scepter in its claws.

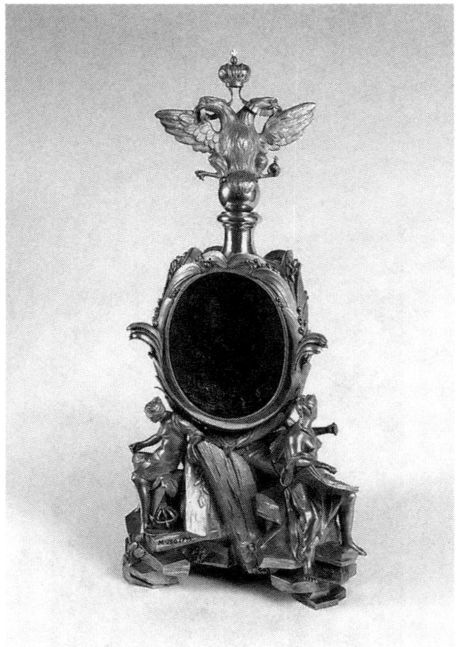

Figure 8. *Zertsalo*, 1760s–1770s. Bronze, steel, gilding. Copyright © 2013, State Russian Museum, St. Petersburg.

The name *zertsalo* apparently derives from the figurative language of the earliest decree displayed upon it, "On the observance of civil rights," in which Peter reminds his addressees to heed the laws, and orders a (literal) mnemonic device to be constructed for the officials:

> And therefore this decree shall be printed, entered into the Regulation, and published; likewise the Senate shall have a board on a pedestal with the above-mentioned printed decree pasted thereupon; and always in all places of official business, from the Senate down to the lowliest office, it must be present on every desk, *like a mirror before the eyes of the officials*. And as a penalty for neglecting to display this decree, a hundred rubles [shall be donated] to the military hospital.[61]

The decree contains the instructions for its own reproduction and dissemination. The rhetorical move at the end from the figurative to the pragmatic is characteristic of the hands-on emperor, whose interest in symbols had practical aims.[62] A well-known example of this interest is his commissioning of Daniel de La Feville's *Symbola et Emblemata* to be printed in Russia in 1705.[63] The fact that Peter would ask his officials to regard a "board on a pedestal" with a legal text attached as a "mirror" attests to his belief in the autonomy of the sign, or at least in his own ability to make one thing signify another, a power extending from the literal to the symbolic sphere. The *zertsalo* typifies the important role of allegory[64] in Russia during the eighteenth century, an epoch of transition that frequently saw the overlap of the Baroque and the Classicist sensibility.

It is not known when the "board on a pedestal" with a pasted-on decree became a prism with decrees displayed behind glass, nor when its figurative meaning—that is, a document serving "as a mirror" for one's conscience—became its name. What is clear is that, as early as February 1723, Peter envisioned the initial "mirror" decree as the seed crystal for a three-sided emblem of law.[65] The texts of both of the decrees from 1724 include a note in the emperor's hand indicating that these were to be added to what was then known as "the standing decree." It is tempting to speculate that Peter himself, in his incarnation as the artisan-tsar, built the prototype for the *zertsalo* with his own hands.[66]

Zertsala were still in use far into the nineteenth century. A law from November 20, 1864, during the reign of Alexander II, specifies that a *zertsalo* must be present at every court session. They continued to be manufactured until the Bolshevik Revolution in 1917; subsequently most of these lavish, overbearing symbols of autocracy[67] fell prey to a wave of iconoclasm. A small number of *zertsala* survive in Russian museums—a few on display, most tucked away in dusty storerooms.

Mirrors, Material and Metaphorical

In this section I shall discuss how the *zertsalo* came to acquire its name by sketching some important meanings associated with the mirror as everyday object and as metaphor. The term *zertsalo* was used to distinguish the Mirror of Law; the use of the Old Slavonic form signified that this object was something loftier than a mere physical mirror.[68] This term refers to a uniquely Russian artifact that came into being during a time of widespread adoption of European models yet, strikingly, had no European analogues. To be more precise, one can think of it as the progeny of didactic literature (the medieval genre of "mirror" books) and religious regalia, particularly such sacred vessels as the monstrance.

Decorative glass has a remarkable capacity for mimesis: for examples from the eighteenth century, one need only think of chandeliers decorated with crystal pendants in the shape of leaves, icicles, and stars,[69] or of the

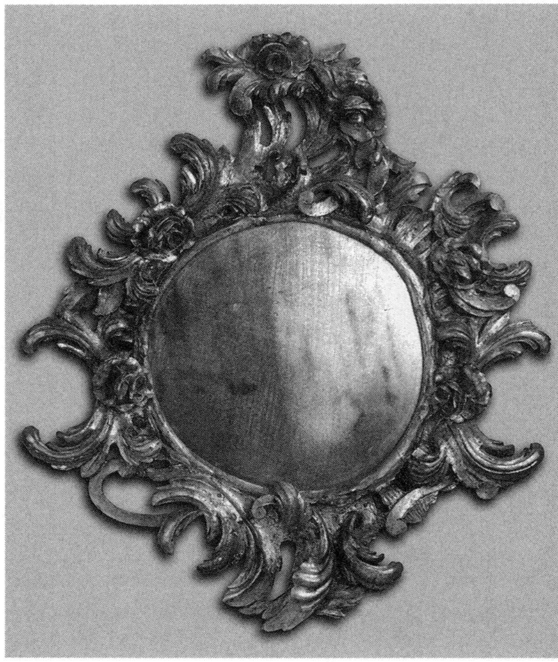

Figure 9. Mirror in a frame decorated with carved roses and acanthus leaves, 1750–1760s, Russia. Wood and glass; carved and gilded. 76 × 66 cm. The State Hermitage Museum, St. Petersburg. Photograph by Vladimir Terebenin, Leonard Kheifets, and Yuri Molodkovets. Copyright © The State Hermitage Museum.

mosaics that Lomonosov created in order to re-create historical events and personages. Optical glass too has the potential to create copies of the world—a potential that invited controversy, as seen, for example, in the medieval taboo against mirrors. In Russia, the mirror was just beginning to find wide use during the Petrine reforms, defying the long-standing church prohibition. Prior to this time, mirrors usually had to remain covered; gazing into mirrors was to be kept at an absolute minimum; on rare occasions, large imported mirrors were hung high on walls, so as to reflect neither people nor large spaces.[70] During his travels in Europe, Peter the Great took note of the prevailing Baroque aesthetic—the spatial expansion and play of light enabled by mirrors—and brought this influence home with him. Petrine mirrors differed from those of the previous century: they enjoyed increasingly widespread use,[71] were kept uncovered, and tended to be much larger, with lavish frames.[72] (See figure 9.) As the epigraph to this chapter shows, mirrors transformed upper-class interiors to such an extent that the residents could come to believe that they dwelled in a fantastic realm with no spatial limits.

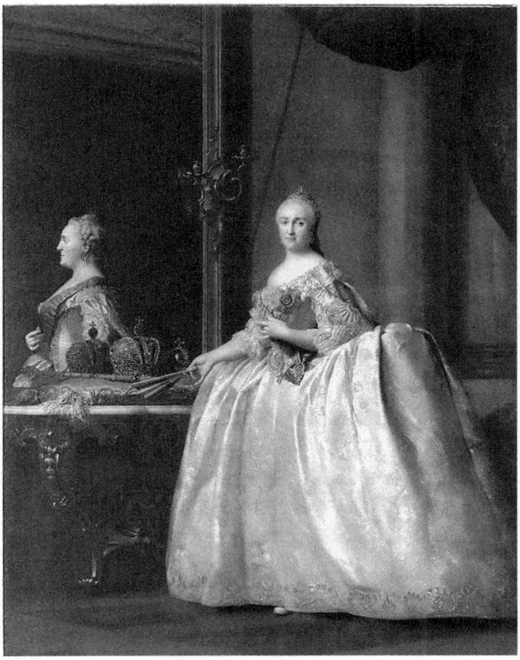

Figure 10. *Portrait of Catherine II in front of a Mirror*, Virgilius Erichsen (Ericksen), between 1762 and 1764, Denmark. Oil on canvas. 262.5 × 201.5 cm. The State Hermitage Museum, St. Petersburg. Photograph by Vladimir Terebenin, Leonard Kheifets, and Yuri Molodkovets. Copyright © The State Hermitage Museum.

A portrait of Catherine II from the mid-eighteenth century illustrates the potential for playful symbolism that mirrors took on at this time. (See figure 10.) The portrait shows the empress in a gala dress standing in front of a large mirror that takes up a fourth of the painterly space; she wears the order of Saint Andrew and a small crown on her head, and with a fan in her hand she gestures to the imperial regalia that is doubled, as is the empress herself, in the reflective glass. In the mirror Catherine faces a direction that can be read as "west"; like the double-headed eagle (whose body forms the background for the figure of Saint Andrew), she is oriented in two directions simultaneously. Yet that westward orientation is thrown into doubt by its location in the unreal, illusory space of the mirror.

The word "mirror" itself signified more than the looking glass of everyday use. On the figurative level, the mirror served as a marker for didactic publications, as seen in the proliferation throughout Europe of books of an edifying character with the word "mirror" in the title (for example, the

German *Mirror for Princes*).[73] Many such works reached eighteenth-century Russia in translation. They were soon joined by native versions;[74] the best known of these is *The True Mirror of Youth*, a compilation by different authors whose publication was ordered by Peter's decree in 1717. It addressed itself to the young nobility and set forth the standards for proper behavior in a new Russia that was becoming increasingly oriented toward the West. In contrast to the commonplace association of mirrors with superficiality and vanity, the mirror here was made to connote the rules of propriety and thus a concern with one's inner condition.[75]

The metaphor of the book-as-mirror has roots reaching back to the New Testament. In his Epistle to the Corinthians (1 Corinthians 13:12), Paul expresses the idea that the visible world available to human senses is but a pale reflection of the glory of God's kingdom; while currently, we see that glory "as if in a glass, darkly" (mirrors were indeed quite obscure before the advances in glassmaking made by the artisans of Murano), in the next world, we shall see it clearly, as it truly is: "face to face." In another passage (James 1:23–24), a parallel is drawn between contemplating one's reflection in a mirror and heeding the word of God. On the basis of a Neoplatonic treatment of the mirror analogy stemming from these two passages, Scripture came to be regarded as a mirror reflecting divine truth.[76] Augustine likens Scripture to a mirror in that it shows man both the perfection he can attain and the imperfection of his current state, so as to facilitate his spiritual makeover.[77]

From the twelfth to the sixteenth century, the "speculum genre" gained broad acceptance and gradually underwent secularization, as indicated by titles such as *A Mirror for Magistrates* and *The Mirour of Good Manners*.[78] The didactic function of a "mirror" publication could also be more subtly manifested in a form such as a genealogy of rulers or an encyclopedic collection of information about a subject such as natural history; the encyclopedia was thus seen as a mirror whose reflection captured the entire world.[79] In eighteenth-century Russia, the dominant association was with the trend toward edification and enlightenment. For example, an astronomical chart published in Russia in 1717 that addressed itself to "industrious youths and persons of any age who desire to understand the movement of the heavens and the Earth according to the treatise of Copernicus" was titled *The New Celestial Mirror*—in other words, this publication purported to capture and reflect the starry skies for readers eager to learn about them.

The figurative function of mirrors extended to the visual medium as well, as evidenced by such works as the popular print, *A Sinner's Mirror* (*Zertsalo greshnago*), dating from the second half of the eighteenth century. This didactic print illustrates the vanity of all human affairs. At the center, a knight and lady playfully banter while poised on the edge of an open grave. They are flanked by Death with a scythe on one side and a demon on the other.[80] In the Russian translation of *Symbola et Emblemata*, mirrors are presented in the guise of allegory. A mirror appears with such captions as "It spares no faults," "I tell the truth," and, in a tableau in which a heart is burned by the sun's rays reflected off a catoptric lens, "I burn but I am not consumed." The latter image curiously juxtaposes the iconography of the Bible with that of the modern empirical quest, and suggests that science and mysticism were in equal measure a part of the mirror's aura and not very far apart in the Baroque imagination.[81]

The *zertsalo* constituted a hybrid of the physical and figurative aspects of the eighteenth-century mirror. It was a spectacular object meant to bring about a moral transformation in the one who gazed into it. But the *zertsalo* had still another function: it was intended to invite contemplation, but also to suggest surveillance; it was not only the object of the gaze, but, in a sense, the source of it.

The Glass Eye

To monitor the judges was of paramount importance to Peter, who remained suspicious of their potential to undermine his authority by either disobeying the laws already in place or, on the other hand, using the existing laws to usurp his power.[82] On January 27, 1722, Peter created the official post of the procurator-general, whose duty was to keep a vigilant eye on the conduct of Senate officials and report any wrongdoing. As seen from the text of the decree "On the post of the procurator-general," Peter was interested in the idea of remote surveillance: "The procurator-general is duty-bound to preside in the Senate and keep a sharp lookout . . . This official stands for the sovereign's very eye."[83]

In this connection, let us note a prevalent motif in the iconography of eighteenth-century Russia—the "all-seeing eye," in its most basic form an eye inside a triangle,[84] a symbol of divinity that came to accompany depictions of the emperor starting in Petrine times. It graces the cover of the first Russian book of geography alongside other symbols of knowledge and power. An engraving shows the image of Peter carried by cherubs up toward a triangle with rays emanating from it and the word "God" inscribed within.[85] Another engraving, from 1712 by Alexei Zubov, shows Peter in armor and regalia beneath another such radiant inscription.[86] Zhivov and Uspenskii point out that a Russian viewer conditioned by the visual language of icons would take this inscription as referring to the tsar.

The use of the all-seeing eye in depictions of military triumph was another way in which the emperor was invested with divine power. The symbol appears on a wineglass made in 1770 that celebrates the victory

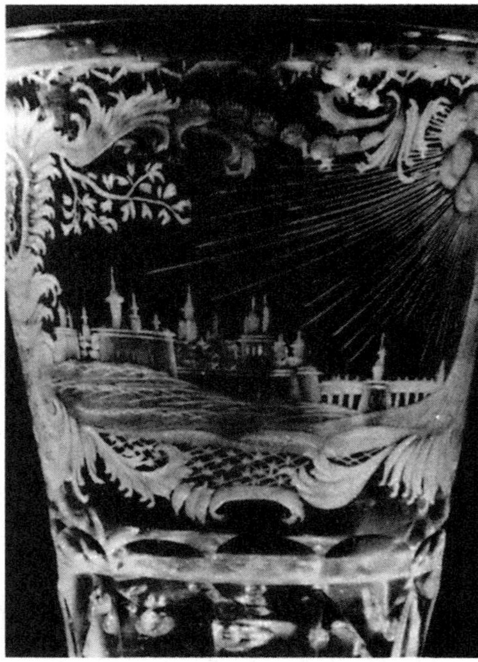

Figure 11. Wineglass, 1770, made to commemorate the victory of the Russian navy over Turkish forces. State Museum of Ceramics, Moscow.

of the Russian fleet over Turkish forces: the all-seeing eye peers from the clouds, signifying the heavens' approval.[87] (See figures 11, 11a, and 11b.) The transparency of the glass superimposes the face of the empress and the all-seeing eye. In an allegorical scene engraved on a glass goblet from 1720, the goddess Themis stands on a cliff amid waves with a sword in one hand and the scales of justice in the other, while the all-seeing eye hovers over her. The cliff represents Russia, against which enemy ships dash themselves while the goddess of justice rules in Russia's favor. The design on the goblet reproduces that of an illumination used to usher in the New Year and celebrate Russia's military might. On the eve of the display, engravings of the image were distributed to foreign diplomats, and Peter himself took the time to explain the allegory to them.[88] There appears to be a link between the all-seeing eye, Peter's passion for surveillance, and the shape the *zertsalo* would eventually take: the triangle could have inspired its ultimate prismatic form. As scholars have shown, throughout the eighteenth century the tsar was often conflated with divinity.[89] Thus the all-seeing *zertsalo* in its ideal incarnation would have conveyed the idea that the eye of the sovereign and the eye of God were one and the same.

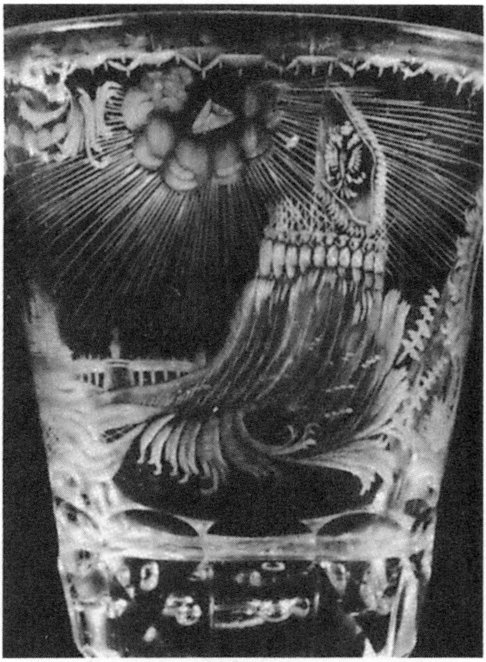

Figure 11a. Detail.

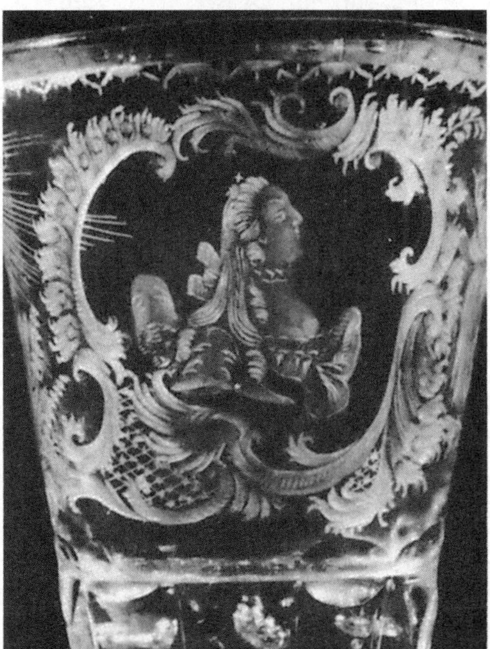

Figure 11b. Detail.

In eighteenth-century Russian law, the realms of the secular and the sacred intersected.[90] The *zertsalo* itself was imbued with a mystical, ceremonial quality.[91] That it had no European analogues is striking in light of the widespread emulation of Western models typical of this period. (The decrees themselves were part of Peter's overall attempt to create legislation according to the European model, with particular reference to Swedish law.)[92] It may be helpful to look not to the trappings of officialdom but rather to religious regalia to find objects resembling this artifact in form and function. One such object is the monstrance or ostensorium, a vessel displaying the Blessed Sacrament or saintly relics in a glass cylinder, used in prayer services and processions. The glass served to protect the sacred objects while letting the faithful feast their eyes on them at close range. An edict issued by the Fourth Council of the Lateran (convened by Pope Innocent III in 1215) stipulated that relics could not be exhibited without protection; subsequently, reliquaries began to be designed in the form of glass cylinders, and these vessels ended up as display cases for the Host as well: "These glass cylinders were . . . designed to hold long objects—a finger, arm or leg, which made them less suitable for the Host. And yet the traditional cylinder continued its existence from the fourteenth to the sixteenth century in the monstrance, even when this was built exclusively to contain the Eucharist."[93] In 1711 Alexander Menshikov acquired a silver monstrance made in Revel (now Tallinn) in 1474 and presented it to Peter I; it is currently housed at the Kunstkamera. On display at the Hermitage is a ciborium (*darokhranitel'nitsa*) of nielloed and gilded silver, made in Moscow in 1782, whose tiered construction is likewise evocative of a *zertsalo*. On their grand tour of Europe, Peter and his emissaries saw numerous Baroque splendors, including church interiors. Could the design of the *zertsalo* have come about as a result the "conversion to new norms of imagery" of Peter's ambassadors to the European capitals?[94]

The fact that a *mirror* was used to represent legality suggests the importance of glass in generating symbolic meaning in eighteenth-century Russia. In this period, glass was also an ideal material to carry allegory and ideology into enclosed, even intimate spaces:[95] thus, images appearing on the transparencies used in illuminations to celebrate imperial glory reappeared on transparent drinking glasses.[96] The *zertsalo*, a metaphorical mirror, was an imposing presence, looming before the eyes of government officials in silent testimony to the state's usurpation of sacred power. In his funeral oration for Peter, Feofan Propokovich, praising the tsar as a lawgiver, called him Russia's Moses. In fact, during the Petrine period the written law had come to be ignored as a matter of course. Numerous decrees were created that were either contradictory or impossible to fulfill. In this situation of utter legal chaos, Peter saw it necessary to issue decrees that ordered the strict observance of laws, which should have gone without saying. The *zertsalo*, perhaps an all too appropriate monument to the Petrine legacy in the legal realm, resembles a mock-evocation of the biblical Tablets of Law.[97]

The texts of the decrees displayed in the *zertsalo* are notable not only for pragmatic, procedural aspects, but also for elements that do not seem to belong in an official document at all, such as figurative language and narrative digressions. Each decree sets out to prevent certain transgressions and spells out the dire consequences facing the transgressor. The severity of the punishments may well have something to do with the notion, explicitly stated in the second decree, of the divine status of the court (*sud' bozhii est'*).[98]

The figurative language in the first decree suggests that eighteenth-century Russian law was a domain ruled by allegory and symbol. It was fitting that the figurative language of this decree would go on to generate the *zertsalo*, a figurative mirror. This decree gave the *zertsalo* its name: the simile "like a mirror" (*iako zerkalo*) was eventually transformed into the signifier of the text-bearing object itself. The shift from the figurative to the literal was, however, accompanied by a corresponding linguistic shift from the low (*zerkalo*) to the lofty (*zertsalo*). Thus, one could argue that the figurative aspect never went away: it just became subsumed under the ц of *zertsalo*. Also, as the single decree evolved into the three-sided prism and gained a symbolic name, the move forward, toward presumably a more enlightened time in which the rule of law would be absolute, was also, in a sense, a move backward from the Russian form to the Old Slavonicism. It was this Slavonic form that retained a memory of the original transcendent meaning of the *zertsalo*.

Reading the Mirror: The *Zertsalo* in Catherine's Time

Documentation of the *zertsalo* in paintings and engravings is elusive, perhaps because visual artists deemed it unworthy of representation.[99] In the eighteenth century, the law clerk was regarded as a shyster, a shifty Frol Skobeev figure, and the domain of judges was seen as ruled by bribery and *in*justice.[100] In addition, there was the *zertsalo* itself—a symbol deprived of its intended meaning (its presence did not appear to stem the tide of corruption in the courts) and surrounded instead with an aura of shame. On the other hand, well-known literary works contain many references to the *zertsalo*. Vasilii Kapnist's satire *Chicanery* (*Iabeda*, 1798) is a rich source of such references. Serving as a condemnation of legal abuses that range from rampant bribe-taking to outright incompetence, the play joins the tradition continued by writers such as Sukhovo-Kobylin and Gogol (who provides his own mirror reference in the epigraph to *The Inspector General*: "Don't blame the mirror for your own crooked mug").

In a scene from the play that was cut by the censor, the corrupt officials carouse, drinking, gambling, and plotting judicial mischief. The aptly-named judge Krivosudov declares that all laws can be combined and manipulated in one way or another: "*Zakony vse otchasti kleiatsia*"; disgruntled servant Anna mutters under her breath as she gathers the cards that have fallen on the floor: "*Stanem zhe i my kleit' mast' k masti*." The latter is such an obvious allusion to the wording of the first decree displayed on the *zertsalo* (in which Peter accuses officials of playing with the laws "as if they were cards, matching the suits to one another") that the crooked judge looks around in fear:

KRIVOSUDOV ("CROOKED JUDGE"): Shouldn't there be a *zertsalo* here? I don't see one.
BUL'BUL'KIN ("DRUNKARD"): Someone's hidden it away—good riddance.
ATUYEV ("HUNTING ADDICT"): Can't stand to look at it.
KHVATAIKO ("GRABBER"): It's been looking at *us* since time immemorial.
ANNA: I'll bet it's had its fill of looking at you all.[101]

This exchange underscores the fact that the *zertsalo*, as an all-seeing eye, was not only meant to be the object of the gaze (that of the officials) but the source of it as well (that of the sovereign): "*na nas ves' vek smotrelo*." The *zertsalo* clearly was a symbol of surveillance. To look at it was to meet another's glance, as is evident in several lines in *Chicanery* that survived the censor. The character Dobrov ("Good Guy") exclaims: "Peer into the Mirror of Law [*v Zertsalo vzglian' sudov*]: you'll see Peter's holy features there, bidding you to serve in the name of truth."[102]

The *zertsalo* thus projects the vigilant gaze of the emperor. The officials' irreverence toward the *zertsalo* might even begin to seem justified in this light; theirs is a sort of *ressentiment* born of paranoia and powerlessness. Before the ax descends, they can at least share a Bakhtinian chuckle or two as they poke fun at their inanimate oppressor. In a censored passage, Dobrov complains that crooked judges play with the *zertsalo* "as if it were a pinwheel."[103] Perhaps it was inevitable that in the Age of Trifles, officials' idle hands would turn the "Mirror of Law" into a plaything.[104] Yet what else could one do with this embodiment of paradox, a mirror that wasn't a mirror, that "reflected" not the face of the beholder but the "holy features" of the emperor himself?

The metaphor of the theater as a mirror that became widespread in the criticism as well as the literary production at the end of the eighteenth century sheds light on the prominent role played by the *zertsalo* in *Chicanery*. Both Krylov ("Theater is a school for morals, a mirror for passions, a trial for delusions")[105] and Plavil'shchikov ("Comedy tears the mask off the vice, so that whoever sees himself in the amusing mirror of moral edification will laugh at himself during the performance, and the impression he takes away will provoke an inner trial")[106] characterized the didactic function of the theater by joining the motif of comedy as mirror with the motif of the trial. Contemporaries perceived *Chicanery*, with its juridical theme, as a mirror of Russian mores.[107]

A number of literary texts by Gogol, Tolstoy, and Dostoevsky make use of the *zertsalo*, illuminating both its intended meaning and the ways in which it was perceived in actuality. Gogol's work in particular conveys a note of irreverence toward the *zertsalo* that had received its full expression in *Chicanery*.[108] Why did the *zertsalo* not always inspire proper conduct or even respect? Was it, in the final analysis, a touch grotesque in its forcible juxtaposition of sculptural flourishes and serious intent? The conflicting treatment of the *zertsalo* was likely due to a disjuncture between the real (ridiculed) and the ideal (respected). The *zertsalo* exemplified the folly of trying to embody *any* ideal in gilded wood and glass. The scorn toward the *zertsalo* may have been directed at the object itself as unworthy of representing the transcendent idea of law—or, more troublingly, toward what it represented.[109] Moreover, the allegorical meaning of the mirror in eighteenth-century Russia was ultimately unstable, wavering between gravity and whimsy.[110]

If we juxtapose the response to the *zertsalo* with the treatment of other imperial emblems, we are not likely to find the same degree of ambivalence. What set the *zertsalo* apart was its three-dimensional thingness—one could characterize it as an emblem in the round. Like the Tablets of Law, the *zertsalo* demanded to be read; covered with text on every side, it laid claim to absolute legibility. Yet its very form precluded a straightforward "official" reading; instead, the *zertsalo* gave off mixed signals. That may have made the *zertsalo* vexing to officials, but appealing to the literary imagination as a text-bearing artifact and the symbol of a polyvalent (and impossible) ideal.

In his "Letter on the Usefulness of Glass," Lomonosov basks in the ability to play God—or at least a miniature version thereof—that the material grants to him. As literary texts attest, the *zertsalo* took on a sacred status and conferred that sanctity upon the monarch whose "holy features" it was meant to reflect. Together, these examples demonstrate how material artifacts allow for the transfer of sacred power to non-divine human beings. Mirrors are artifacts that lend themselves to symbolic applications particularly well because of the optical properties of glass, their key component.

Let us recall that the Mirror of Law served as an emblem of surveillance—the imagined source of the sovereign's gaze. Glass, as a material and a metaphor, is inextricably linked with issues of power and the gaze.

A revolution in architecture that introduced more expansive windows into interior spaces radically changed the way in which people saw themselves and the world around them. At the same time, as optical technologies developed, glass vision aids became more widespread, and literary texts documented a growing anxiety provoked by the bespectacled gaze. In the preceding chapter we began to explore the transformative effect of looking through glass by considering the proliferation of windows; let us now turn to eyeglasses, which had a similarly profound effect on Russians' way of seeing.

Why do everyday objects, such as eyeglasses, merit scholarly scrutiny? Lotman argues that things shape the behavior of the people who use them (as an example, he cites how differently women began to walk and otherwise carry themselves once they began to wear trousers), and then live on as links to a history of the human gesture that would otherwise be lost forever:

> Things imperiously dictate our gestures, style of behavior, and ultimately our psychological state . . . Long ago objects were crafted by hand, their form was worked out over the course of decades, and sometimes centuries. [This process] inevitably turned a thing into the *history of the thing*, into the memory of the gestures associated with it.[111]

When Alexander Pushkin attended the Imperial Lycée at Tsarskoe Selo, he and his fellow students were not allowed to wear glasses, because it was considered rude to look through them at elders.[112] The act of gazing at someone through one's glasses was seen as an impudent gesture, on a par with staring fixedly into a person's face. Starting in the eighteenth century, etiquette in Russia went so far as to forbid a person to look through his glasses at a superior in age or in rank.[113] During the reign of Alexander I, glasses were so strongly associated with political nonconformism that they were all but banned at court (at the same time, the emperor himself was quite fond of lorgnettes, and always kept one concealed on his person).[114] Lotman describes the behavior of I. V. Gudovich, the commander-in-chief of Moscow at the turn of the nineteenth century, who was a great enemy of eyeglasses and was prone to tear them off a young man's face with the words, "You don't need to be scrutinizing me like that [*Nechego vam zdes' tak pristal'no razgliadyvat'*]!"[115] As Lotman's example suggests, there was something disquieting to the eighteenth-century Russian mind about being regarded through glasses, by a look focused and defined by artificial lenses into a studying, analytical gaze.

The following reminiscence by Goethe, cited by his contemporary Johann Peter Eckermann, provides a parallel instance of spectacle-phobia outside Russia and gives insight into the unease felt by the object of glassy scrutiny:

> Whenever a stranger steps up to me with spectacles on his nose, a discordant feeling comes over me, which I cannot master. It annoys me so much that on the very threshold it takes away a great part of my benevolence . . . It always seems to me as if I am to serve strangers as an object for strict examination, and as if with their armed glances they would penetrate my most secret thoughts, and spy out every wrinkle of my old face. But whilst they thus endeavour to make my acquaintance, they destroy all fair equality between us, as they prevent me from compensating myself by making theirs. For what do I gain from a man into whose eyes I cannot look when he is speaking, and the mirror of whose soul is veiled to me by a pair of glasses which dazzle me?[116]

Goethe's alarm at being contemplated through eyeglasses thus seems connected to the perception of being diminished, as if targeted by a withering ray that emanates from those magic spectacles; the gaze under which he squirms is always already superior, hostile, and even "armed"; most telling, perhaps, is Goethe's candid reference to "every wrinkle on [his] old face" being laid bare to the onlooker, as if the process of aging were a scandal to be concealed above all others. The spectacle-wearer, on the contrary, is "veiled" and thus protected from such intrusive "examination."

The notion that optical glass fostered an indecent kind of looking is underscored by the social role played in eighteenth-century Russia by the telescope (and for women, the lorgnette):[117] Lotman locates these vision aids among the props of the Russian dandy, who typically would, instead of watching the stage in the theater, train his enhanced vision upon loges occupied by the opposite sex. It was in the eighteenth century that eyeglasses became a fashionable requisite. A comparison with the social function of spectacles in eighteenth-century France reveals how these objects enabled the migration of Western forms of behavior to Russia: according to Pierre Marly, a scissor-shaped lorgnette was worn "with affectation and impertinence" by the dandies known as the *Incroyables* (who feigned having weak eyesight just to wear them) during the Directory of 1795–99: "The attraction they offered women was that they gave them the chance to show off the flattering curves of their naked arms as they peered, while in men they accentuated the impertinent attitude which was so in vogue at the time."[118] In Russia, telescopes and lorgnettes were referred to as "insolent optical devices" (*derzkaia optika*—the latter word was introduced into the Russian language by Lomonosov).[119] A character in Vladimir Lukin's play *The Trinket Dealer* (1765) illustrates an aspect of this: he speaks of donning his glasses at the theater so as not to hear the actors. Thus, the complex of glasses/telescope/lorgnette not only participates in what Lotman calls the theatricalization of everyday behavior, but it serves as a cloak of invisibility, shielding the eyes to lend the viewer the illusion of withdrawing from society.

OPTICAL GLASS IN THE AGE OF TRIFLES AND BEYOND

Lukin's one-act comedy *Shchepetil'nik* (*The Trinket Dealer*) concerns two kinds of "spectacles": vision aids that transform how one sees and is seen, and theatrical displays that compel others to look, appropriate for a period in which, in Lotman's account, everyday life became highly theatrical as members of the Russian nobility strove to refashion themselves as Westerners.[120]

Lukin's play is structured around a series of encounters between persons and things. Each such confrontation of customer and commodity culminates in the witty shop owner proffering a moral lesson grounded in materialism, a lesson that the recipient, for the most part, rejects. The shop owner's point about his age being an "age of trifles" is well taken; what is interesting for our purposes is that a number of the articles he offers for sale are notable for their optical properties. In fact, the very first person-thing encounter, which derives its humor from a simple working man's misperception, occurs in scene 3 when the laborer Miron mistakes a spyglass (*zritel'naia trubka*) for a musical instrument: "In our town people play these sorts of pipes, but here they use 'em to look at somethin' while screwing up one eye."[121] The prototype for Lukin's play, Robert Dodsley's *The Toy Shop* (1735),[122] does not contain an analogous scene—the spyglass is Lukin's own contribution. Miron's inability to identify this object shows that such optical devices were still relatively rare in mid-eighteenth-century Russia. The production of optical glass in Russia began in the eighteenth century in special workshops based at the Academy of Sciences, founded by Peter the Great. In 1737, master lens-crafter Ivan Beliaev created optical devices including microscopes, convex lenses to be used in telescopes, and eyeglasses made to order for professors and members of the Academy. He also built a variety of instruments calling for the use of finely crafted glass, including microscopes, barometers, and thermometers, used in an expedition to Kamchatka that departed from St. Petersburg in December of that year.[123] At mid-century, Lomonosov himself did pioneering work on optical lenses: he created and perfected an array of instruments including a microscope, a periscope, a multi-lens apparatus used to generate burning rays, and a universal barometer; and he invented a large single-mirror telescope that was the first in the world to allow people to see in the dark.[124]

In scene 7 of Lukin's play, the first customer, a "flighty woman" (*vertoprashka*) named Marem'iana requests to see a mirror. The shop owner responds by describing a special mirror made of "the best glass in the world" (Dodsley's original has "the finest in all England") that strips away pretenses and shows pretenders for who they are; it paradoxically reflects not the polished outside of a gallant or a coquette, but rather the false and corrupt inner self (this is in keeping with the didactic associations of mirrors discussed above). Interestingly, in the analogous scene in Dodsley's play, the prospective customer decides against this purchase: "Lord, I'm afraid to look in it, methinks, lest it should show me more of my Faults than I care to see."[125] Lukin's characters, however, have no such qualms; this line is elided in his version.

In subsequent scenes, the shop owner continues to use optical instruments for moralizing purposes. A certain Pritvorov (Mr. Pretense) asks the price of the spyglass. In response, the shop owner uses the instrument's optical functions as a metaphor for the moral failings of Pritvorov and his ilk: making one's own sins seem smaller than they really are while seeing the flaws of others as disproportionately large, and, conversely, deemphasizing others' achievements while exaggerating one's own.

In scene 17, the aged Starosvetov (Mr. Old World) asks to see some porcelain snuffboxes with depictions of "passionate love" in miniature. The shop owner suggests that Starosvetov first buy a pair of eyeglasses, which "grant new vision [*novoe zrenie*] to elderly people" (Lukin, *Shchepetil'nik*, 116). Starosvetov protests that he has no need of them, and refusing to accept his own advanced years, he argues: "it's indecent to look through glasses at my age [*neprilichno smotret' v ochki v moikh letakh*]."[126] (This line, emphasizing the "indecency" of the bespectacled gaze, is likewise not found in the English original.) Yet he cannot resist inquiring about their cost. The shop owner again launches into a tirade against the world of surfaces by enumerating the rare "virtues" of the glasses: they make the wearer see the empty head beneath the fancy wig, and will even allow one to distinguish good materials from cheap substitutes ("no one will mistake gravel for gold, nor a bast mat for a carpet"). The latter juxtaposition can be read as Lukin's dig at Russians posing as foreigners whose perceived superiority they seek in vain to emulate.

When the final customer, the scribbler Samokhvalov (Mr. Self-Praise) (most likely modeled on Lukin's contemporary Sumarokov), requests a pair of glasses, the shop owner finds a pair "made especially" for him. These special spectacles will cover his *ears* and allow him to criticize his fellow writers without having to hear their work, which Samokhvalov already knows is of poor quality. In this case, the glasses are given a new set of attributes, one that has little to do with their original optical function. Instead, the shop owner foregrounds the social role of the glasses as signifying costume, or "spectacle"—as Samokhvalov himself says, "I'll go to comedies, put on the glasses, and look at the theater while not listening to a word of what the actors are chattering about."[127] Here the glasses become a sort of mask for the wearer to shield himself from participation in social life while reserving for himself the empowered position of spectator. While these imaginary spectacles are worn over the ears, Lukin's play suggests by analogy that ordinary eyeglasses likewise function as a shield, obscuring the very "mirrors of the soul" that are the eyes.

The Trinket Dealer presents the character of Samokhvalov as a figure of ridicule for being a writer of mere trifles (*bezdeliushek*). The trinket dealer, a self-admitted purveyor of trifles, peddles many an optical device that somehow, in a hypostasized demonstration of its actual powers, shows in a true light the foibles of human nature to would-be customers. In the eighteenth century, Russian secular literature was developing concurrently with the glass industry; the latter yielded optical devices after which literature sought to model itself (the etiquette manual *True Mirror of Youth* is a well-known example). The function of the former suggested the function of the latter to writers looking for a way to define their endeavor. With literature placed in this role of an optical lens, Lukin and his contemporaries may well have aspired to create a "true mirror" instead of a forgettable "trifle." This helps to explain the prominence of optical devices in Lukin's play.

The very act of seeing is thematized in the first scene of Lukin's play through the repeated use of the word "eye" (*glaz*). One of the ways in which Lukin departs from Dodsley's original is by adding two sets of characters, each a pair of outsiders who provide a commentary, and thus an estranged *point of view*, on the central transactions. One set of outsiders is the pair of workers, whose befuddlement at the expensive bric-a-brac is another means to ridicule those who value such trifles so highly; the other set is the moralizing Major Chistoserdov (Pure Heart) and his eager-to-be-enlightened nephew. The play opens with a speech by Chistoserdov in which he praises his nephew for taking the proper approach to comedies, treating them "not as amusement for the eyes [*poveseleniem dlia glaz*] but as beneficial to the heart and mind." This is a meta-textual instruction to the audience on how to properly watch and derive benefit from Lukin's own comedy; the nephew here serves as their stand-in. The instruction also foreshadows the way the shopkeeper shall treat his wares—while the customers seek them out as "amusement for the eyes," he attempts to transform them into moral lessons "beneficial to the heart and mind."

Later in the same scene, Chistoserdov continues to instruct his nephew: "everyone's eyes are turned upon" (*glaza vsego naroda obrashchaiutsia*) high-ranking gentlemen, so they should behave in an exemplary fashion. The nephew marvels that Chistoserdov would dare to point out such a gentleman's sins "to his face" (literally "to say it into his eyes," *v glaza skazat'*). When Chistoserdov relates a story of how he has made some enemies after coming to the defense of a woman being harassed by a pack of "young scamps," the nephew responds that it is better to flee one's foes than to confront them (literally "to pry into their eyes," *v glaza lezt'*). Finally, their talk turns to the *shchepetil'nik* himself. Chistoserdov explains the shop owner's background: he is not a merchant but a former officer forced to retire for speaking the truth right to his superiors' faces (literally "into their eyes"—*v glaza govoril pravdu*).

Notably, the Russian idioms involving eyes involve a breach of boundaries, a violation of the eyes not present in English analogues of these expressions. This aggressive tonality itself draws attention to the eye. All of this emphasis on eyes prepares the way for the optical object lessons still to come. We recall worker Miron's visual/auditory confusion when he takes the spyglass for a musical instrument; it is echoed in the last transaction scene in the image of the eyeglasses that control one's hearing. This, too, is Lukin's own contribution. The sensory confusion in both cases speaks of an anxiety about using optical instruments properly, that is, about "seeing" correctly. Lukin's adaptation of Dodsley's play "to Russian mores" (*na russkie nravy*) places a far greater emphasis on the optical. This emphasis suggests a preoccupation with issues of seeing and being seen—and the artificial means of doing so—in the eighteenth-century Russian context.

It is important to consider *The Trinket Dealer* and the "optics" fad in the context of the Enlightenment, slowly making itself known in Russia through a series of advances in philosophical and scientific thought. Behind the invention and application of the optical lens lies a history of controversy and a dialectic of science and faith. Eyeglasses were already in use in some parts of the world before 1300, yet even in the early mid-fifteenth century there were many who balked at looking through Galileo's telescope, refusing to believe that it worked in the way it did. Daniel Boorstin accounts for some of the resistance with which the learned astronomer, not to mention the anonymous lens-crafter, met in the course of the development of optical lenses. He identifies two related obstacles to this development. The first had to do with the limited potential of the existing and enduring theories of how vision worked: "During the Middle Ages, Christian Europe was still dominated by the notion of the 'active eye' whose visual experience depended on the soul within, which meant that the eye itself was not merely an optical instrument, nor was light a phenomenon in physics."[128] The second obstacle was equally compelling: religious teachings pronounced light the creation and domain of God, not something for man to trifle with. As Boorstin writes, "Tampering with light, or treating light as a merely physical phenomenon was like inquiring into the chemistry of the Eucharist." Conventional wisdom united with religious orthodoxy to cast doubt upon the use of optical lenses:

> Why had eyes been given to men if not to know the true shape, size, and color of objects in the external world? Then were not mirrors, prisms, and lenses

> devices for making visual lies? And man-made instruments for multiplying, deflecting, enlarging or reducing, and doubling or inverting visual images were means for distorting the truth.[129]

During the Renaissance, devils wearing eyeglasses became a popular subject for painters. Because the manufacture of early spectacles for the most part lacked quality control, such spectacles conveyed blurred, distorted images of reality, and thus literally deceived the wearer; hence, they served as shorthand in artistic compositions to represent the notion of deceitfulness:

> Eyeglasses became the favorite equipment of demons who used them to sharpen their wits to ensnare men to sin and perdition. . . . What could be more appropriate than adopting the new technology, eyeglasses, to the evil purposes of the master deceivers? In essence, a device invented by men to better their lives and read the word of God was turned against them by evil spirits, who could certainly procure the best lenses![130]

Thus, it is possible for a common object such as a pair of eyeglasses to signify far more than its intended function; even in the action of a Commander Gudovich swiping the specs off a young man's face, the object begins to move into the realm of the symbolic.

The most precise information that we currently have regarding the origin of spectacles—in the form of "two convex glass disks enclosed in metal or bone rims with handles centrally connected by a tight rivet so as to clamp the nostrils or be held before the eyes"—dates the invention of this vision aid to around 1286 by an artisan living in or around Pisa.[131] Painters, however, did not shy away from anachronism in depicting bespectacled personages who had lived centuries before eyeglasses were invented, including Virgil, and Saints Peter, Paul, and Joseph; one painting even shows baby Jesus with a pair of glasses in his hand. In Vincent Ilardi's account, such figures merited eyeglasses because these vision aids were associated not only with advanced age but also with "*gravitas*, wisdom, intellectuality, and scholarship. They became the normal equipment, along with magnifying lenses and concave mirrors, of scholars' studies during the Renaissance. This prestige factor persisted over the centuries to our own time."[132]

The presence of spectacles was meant to confer upon the wearer an aura of dignity and wisdom; but the optical playfulness of glass ensured the instability of this carefully crafted image. Thus, at any moment the lenses might catch a reflected gleam of light, which would obscure the human gaze behind the spectacles and instill in the beholder a feeling of dread akin to that detailed by Goethe in the passage cited above. Closer to our time, Mstislav Dobuzhinsky's portrait of a contemporary art critic and poet, his eyes

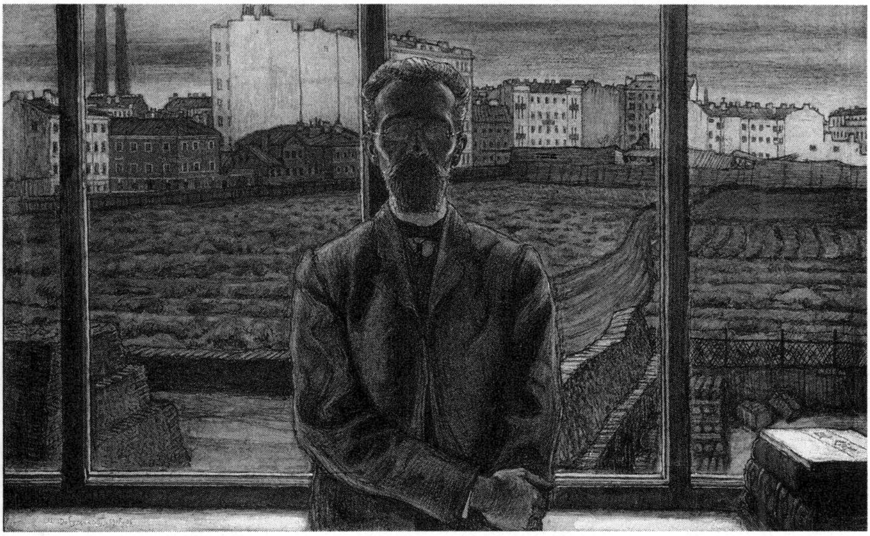

Figure 12. *Man with Spectacles*, Mstislav Dobuzhinsky, 1905–6. Tretyakov Gallery, Moscow. Photo credit: Scala / Art Resource, New York.

obscured by lenses and his body framed by an industrial landscape, titled *Man with Spectacles* (1905–6), vividly evokes the anxiety inspired by the bespectacled gaze. (See figure 12.) The landscape in the background signifies the advent of technology whose prospect is both exhilarating and ominous. Technological progress offers the potential to conquer the limitations of existing in a state of nature, but for human beings, the consequences of cutting themselves off from nature can be devastating. The glasses worn by the man in the portrait represent technology in microcosm. Optical glass offers a way to conquer nature by providing a new and superior way of seeing, which itself is essential to mastery—the link between vision and power is one that many thinkers (Goethe among them) have noted. Yet the glasses create a barrier that prevents human contact and epitomizes the barriers that human beings create between themselves and the natural world, as well as between one another, as they invent, build, and strive for machine-like precision and efficiency. That is one reason why this image by Dobuzhinsky, of the bespectacled figure who seems to have much in common with his bleak background, is so unsettling.

I will now touch upon a few twentieth-century literary texts that continue to reflect on this glass-induced anxiety; I focus on the early decades of the Soviet period because they mark a return to a preoccupation with glass that typified eighteenth-century writing. In this period, authors are particularly mindful of glass and its optical qualities as well as what glass objects, including eyeglasses, signify. The texts under consideration show how this wearable technology exceeds its utilitarian designation and ends up marking the wearer in a way that speaks to the biases and anxieties of the beholder.

In Yury Olesha's modernist novel *Envy* (1927), the desired and unattainable luster (*blesk*) of those who hold power in the new Soviet world takes the form of an oppressive light, embodied in the recurring image of industrialist food producer Andrei Babichev's eyes obscured by spectacles—as the protagonist Kavelerov describes in horror: "There were no eyes. There were two plates of a pince-nez, sparkling like mercury."[133] The pince-nez likewise plays a characterizing role in *Islanders* (1918), Yevgeny Zamyatin's novel set in England. The nearsighted Mrs. Dewley wears "a rimless pince-nez made of excellent glass with the cold luster of crystal. The pince-nez made Mrs. Dewley an ideal specimen of the class of bespectacled women from the mere sight of whom you can catch cold, as from a draft."[134] This description is markedly gendered: the woman with the cold glance is herself regarded with a cold, scientific gaze and classified as an "ideal specimen" of a particular class of "bespectacled women" (Zamyatin's text provides this phrase in English and glosses it as "*ochkatykh zhenshchin*"). Glasses serve here primarily not as a corrector of vision but as signifying costume.

A positive counterpart to the bespectacled Mrs. Dewley takes the form of a heavenly body: the moon (*mesiats*, a noun that is gendered masculine), sporting a monocle, which looks down at the residents of the town with "kindhearted irony" (Zamiatin, *Ostrovitiane*, 128). The pince-nez never enjoyed the popularity among the fashionable set that the monocle did; possibly the asymmetry, the "wink" of the monocle was favorably contrasted with the fixed glare of the pince-nez. (The pince-nez is also quite literally an instrument of repression, its "pinching" purpose spelled out in its name.) In twentieth-century Russia, the monocle lost its functional designation and became a prop of the dandy and a favorite affectation among artists of the avant-garde. A popular trick among wearers of monocles was to toss the eyepiece in the air and have it land in one's eye socket, all without the use of hands. Monocles waned in popularity among Russians during World War I, as they began to be associated with German officers.[135] The pince-nez, for its part, became a marker of bourgeois philistinism. Each kind of eyepiece had its own set of associations, a place in the fashion system.

In one of his autobiographical Odessa tales, Isaac Babel's narrator, in contrasting himself with the bold and virile gangster king Benya Krik, laments that he has "spectacles on his nose and autumn in his heart"—a formulation that speaks to self-consciousness about what one's eyeglasses signify to others. A later work by Babel illuminates the associations that eyeglasses had with intellectuals, and more specifically with Jewish intellectuals, in the early Revolutionary period. The Civil War was a period of heightened anti-intellectualism; as writer Konstantin Paustovsky recalls, "everyone treated people in glasses suspiciously in those violent times. They thought them cunning enemies and hated them bitterly."[136] This connotation of spectacle-wearing fuels the conflict in Babel famous story, "My First Goose" (1926), set in the period of War Communism. In the opening scene, a pair of spectacles becomes the object of bitter dispute: they belong to the narrator Lyutov, whom the officer Savitsky is reluctantly allowing to join a Cossack division as a war correspondent. Rather than affecting the way the narrator sees the outside world, they are a function of the way the world sees *him*: Savitsky warns, "In these parts they'll kill a man for wearing glasses," and the porter carrying Lyutov's trunk echoes him, emphasizing the perceived link between eyeglasses and the possession of an elite status that is intolerable, and potentially fatal, in the given setting: "Our fellows don't take kindly to glasses—nothing you can do about it. Around here, your man of distinction is as good as dead."[137]

Here, then, is the writer's quandary: he wants to wear glasses in order to "see everything," the better to write it all down; yet the glasses act as a sign of his otherness, and create preconceptions in his subjects and, perhaps, his audience. The motif of glass-enhanced vision links the narrator to the peasant woman who also wears glasses, and whom the narrator victimizes as part of his initiation into the world of the Cossack warrior—"sparkling with blindness and glasses," she is Lyutov's abject double whom he must destroy.

Thus, some of the ambivalent associations around the bespectacled gaze persisted from one century to the next. However, because glass is a form of technology, technological innovations can add new dimensions to the way in which glass objects signify. In the early decades of the twentieth century, the advent of cinema, which transformed people's way of seeing, brought about dramatic changes in both art and technology: film is an art form that necessitates the fusion of these two spheres, and glass made this union possible.

Sergei Eisenstein makes self-reflexive use of optical glass in his film *Battleship Potemkin* (1925). The eyeglasses of the ship's doctor are a key artifact in the opening sequence, "The Men and the Maggots." The doctor makes a point of donning his glasses, then taking them off and holding them up to the swarming meat, as he announces his professional opinion that the fare is perfectly acceptable. Eisenstein gives us close-ups of the glasses in the doctor's hand, and the meat (and maggots) seen through the lenses. This juxtaposition implicates optical glass, and by extension, cinematic lenses, into the vexed process of truth-telling, as well as the fabrication of lies. The film suggests an analogy between the lenses of the glasses and the lenses of the camera. The eagle-eyed sailors cannot be deceived by the doctor's deceptive lenses. The rotten meat combined with the brazen official lie leads to the rebellion and everything that follows in its wake. This sequence could be read as a self-conscious move on Eisenstein's part—he is concerned with conveying historical truth with his camera, and caught up in polemics with fellow directors (such as the documentarian Vertov) about the proper way to achieve this.

The final violent image in Eisenstein's film also involves great pathos: a schoolmistress in spectacles is shot in the eye.[138] We do not see the moment of impact, but are led to imagine it through the montage of woman—shooter—woman and aftermath.[139] This moment is witnessed by a young man whose image is doubled in a reflective surface (he is our stand-in; the doubling suggests, indeed, that he is the audience's "double"). He is horrified but can do nothing, a passive spectator. This is another self-referential moment, now dealing with the question of how exactly a film is meant to move an audience.[140]

In Eisenstein's film, spectacles themselves become spectacular; as in Lukin's eighteenth-century play, these vision aids function in a critical and meta-textual way as rhetorical objects. In the last two chapters we have examined the ways in which glass-to-be-looked-through can testify about the complex relationship between seeing and power. Let us keep that relationship in mind as we take another trip back to the eighteenth century in the following chapter, whose opening case study, the Ice House of Empress Anna, serves as a transitional object of sorts: while its transparent windows were meant to be looked through, the structure—a glowing spectacle lit from within—was designed to be looked at. The Ice House was a construction very much of its time, and yet it anticipated later twentieth-century developments in its capacity as an ideological spectacle. This eighteenth-century architectural marvel served multiple functions, both utilitarian and symbolic, and became a prototype of the glass houses that were imagined, and then built, in subsequent centuries.

Chapter Three

The Display of Power: Spectacular Glass in Imperial Russia

No forest fell
When thou didst build. No quarry sent its
stores
To enrich thy walls. But thou didst hew the
floods
And make thy marble of the glassy wave.
—William Cowper, "The Task"

ANNA'S ICE PALACE: CONQUERING NATURE, OR THE PROTO-GLASS HOUSE

In February 2006 a resplendent palace of ice, six meters high and covering an area of 328 square feet, was built in the center of St. Petersburg. Inside the palace were furniture, mirrors, and dishes, all made of ice—a building material in which the region abounds. The palace was created in less than a month by the country's leading ice sculptors using ice from neighboring lakes. Despite the subzero weather (–4 degrees Fahrenheit) about 300 people turned out to see the unveiling, and the fireworks and fashion show that went along with it. On St. Valentine's Day newlyweds would gather inside the building, while on other days, the palace would "offer various entertainments, including an ice bath, an ice bar, an ice cannon, and historical performances."[1] Notably, the organizers of the festivities arranged to have the palace taken apart rather than have it melt away—which would have created a very different impression.

Having the newlyweds gather at the ice palace echoes the myth around the original—and perverse—purpose of the palace's prototype. The original Ice House was built in January 1740, as legend has it, on the order of Empress Anna as a nuptial chamber for the "fools' wedding" that she organized for her favorite jester Mikhail Golitsyn. This building, with its dazzling interplay of transparency, reflection, and captive light, offered spectators the visual effects of a glass house at a time when the industry was not yet advanced enough to make possible the construction of such a house; it is productive, then, to approach Anna's ice palace as a structure that prefigured the ideological spectacles made of glass that appeared in Russia in subsequent centuries.[2]

After exchanging vows, the bride and groom rode on elephant-back from church to a palace on the Neva that was made entirely of ice. The facade of the house was decorated with eight cannons that actually fired; a working bathhouse (the classic Russian *banya*) likewise made of ice was situated nearby; and one can only imagine the reaction of the newlyweds when they discovered that the tables, chairs, clock, curtains, shoes, and even the bed in the bridal suite were all made of the same crystalline and mercilessly frigid material.[3] As we shall see, Ivan Lazhechnikov applied his imagination to this very same scenario in his historical novel *The Ice House* (1835), using spectacular ice imagery to convey the terror of Anna's time in visceral terms.[4]

Anna's ice palace was the centerpiece of an "amusing holiday" (*poteshnyi prazdnik*) orchestrated by the empress to divert the populace from the brutal conditions, both political and climatic, in which they lived; but it had a symbolic purpose as well: to celebrate the tenth anniversary of her reign and Russia's recent victory in the war with Turkey. The firing cannons in front of the palace explicitly alluded to military triumph, and the conquest of the elements in the creation of the palace itself underscored the omnipotence of the monarch and the nation that she represented. The ice cannons stood for both the military power of the monarch by whose will all of this was brought into being, and the defiance of nature—harnessing ice not only as a building material but bringing fire and ice together in such an unnatural way. What is more, Anna's act of forcibly employing some subjects to build this ice house—during a winter that was particularly frigid, even by St. Petersburg standards[5]—and others to spend their wedding night there in itself constituted a transgression against nature.[6]

In Lazhechnikov's novel, the empress gets the inspiration for the Ice House when she sees a mysterious ice statue in the manege near her palace. When Biron, Anna's closest advisor and the chief architect of the reign of terror bearing his name (the *Bironovshchina*), sternly asks what it is, one of the courtiers replies: "The grooms have sculpted an ice statue for your amusement." Struck by this comment, Anna conjures up a plan to "build an ice palace with various statues [*s raznymi figurami*]."[7]

What she does not realize is that the lifelike ice statue conceals an actual human being inside—a man who refused to divulge the whereabouts of a denunciation intended to reveal Biron's abuses of power to the empress, and underwent torture at the hands of the very same courtier who fabricates the story of the statue. The details of the torture are striking in their emphasis on the spectacular that anticipates the creation of the Ice House, and they show a parallel between ice and its man-made counterpart, glass. Outside in the freezing cold, the captors pour pail after pail of water over their bound victim: "Another pail of water doused the martyr from his feet to his head . . . the streams of water, seeming to turn into broken glass [*prevratias' budto v bitoe steklo*], spilled with a crackling sound on the snow. Another two or three pails, and it was impossible to recognize a human being beneath the hideous icy statue" (Lazhechnikov, *Ledianoi dom*, 58).

Lazhechnikov's novel associates glass with the pomp and ostentation of the oppressors in a description of Biron riding in his gold carriage, which is "covered in windows, so that the passenger can be seen from head to toe [*vsia v steklakh, tak chto sidevshii v nei mog byt' viden s golovy do piat*], like a splendid insect that an entomologist preserves in a transparent box" (Lazhechnikov, *Ledianoi dom*, 148). The earlier description of the "martyr" undergoing water torture (freezing water douses him "from his feet to his head") gets inverted in the image of glass-encased Biron, who is visible "from his head to his heels." In the former case, the transparent water turns to opaque ice, concealing the crime and its victim from the eyes of the empress; in the latter case, the transparent glass displays Biron, whose outward flashiness, "blinding the crowd" of onlookers, conceals a hideous inner core. Lazhechnikov thus uses the imagery of glass and ice to create a dynamic between display and concealment—a dynamic that structures the description of the Ice House itself.

Lazhechnikov sets up his description of the building with a nod to the conquest of nature at the heart of Russian cultural mythology:

> As if by magic, there arose in a few days a wondrous building the likes of which no country save Russia had ever produced and that could only be produced by our inclement north [*surovyi sever*] with the help of the cruel winter of 1740. . . . The foundation was laid using water; the walls, roof, windowpanes, and ornaments were crafted from it as well; everything was held together with water; water took all the forms that a fanciful imagination was pleased to assign to it. And when the sun turned its rays upon this ice house, it seemed to be cut from a single piece of sapphire, adorned with opal statues. (Lazhechnikov, *Ledianoi dom*, 173)[8]

In this rich passage, Lazhechnikov turns a minus into a plus by arguing that only in Russia could such a miraculous building appear, thanks to the extreme climatic conditions in that part of the world and, by implication, the ingenuity of the people therein. Nature does its worst—the winter of 1740 is particularly "cruel"; and in response, the Russian people make nature do their bidding (if only they could do the same with their cruel monarchs!), conquering the watery element itself by making it serve, against all odds, as a construction material for a glorious palace. In his poem "The Task" (1785), cited in the epigraph to this chapter, William Cowper conveys his wonder at a country in which such a building would arise. The ice, like glass, possesses the gift of mimicry; in this case it has the appearance of precious stones—sapphire and opal—when the sun strikes it at just the right angle.

At the front gates of the house, onlookers were greeted with the ice cannons mentioned above—six in all, which were "constantly being fired," according to the account by Academician G. W. Krafft, with the help of four pounds of gunpowder placed inside each cannon—as well as two artillery mortars and two dolphin statues; at night, the dolphins, thanks to cleverly placed pumps, spewed fiery fountains of burning oil out of their mouths, "which made for a pleasant and amusing sight." The building had a porch and two doors, leading to an outer entrance hall with four windows, and two bedrooms with five windows each; all the windows, complete with frames and panes, were made of thin, clear ice. At night, a multitude of lit candles were placed in the windows; in Krafft's description, "the radiance shining through the windows and the walls made for an utterly stunning and surprising view."[9]

Nearly all the windows in the ice house displayed "funny pictures" painted on canvas; surrounding the house were four-sided pyramids on pedestals with round windows carved in each side. These windows gave onlookers a peek at yet another amusing and edifying sight: an octagonal paper lantern with "all sorts of comical figures" depicted on each side.

In order to provide a good view of each picture, the lanterns were rotated by people concealed inside each pyramid. Hidden human beings were likewise responsible for animating a "cleverly made" elephant that spouted water twenty-four feet in the air in the daytime, and a fountain of burning oil at night, "to the great astonishment of all the onlookers"; the creature could even bellow like a living elephant, when the person hiding inside blew on a special trumpet. The interplay of display and concealment was intrinsic to the Ice House, which combined the spectacular effects of fire and candlelight interacting with the icy surfaces with people hidden inside the icy constructions, serving as their secret mechanisms. In Lazhechnikov's novel, Anna becomes inspired to build the titular House when she sees an ice sculpture, not realizing that it conceals a real person; that image anticipates the later one of human beings concealed inside the various parts of the Ice House who are making the machinery work while, presumably, freezing.

Entering the bedchamber of the ice palace, visitors would encounter a cozy scene: a lavishly decorated bed complete with a curtain, pillows and quilt, slippers and nightcaps, a dressing table and a fireplace with burning logs inside. Yet all of these trappings were likewise made of ice; the logs, smeared with petroleum, indeed burned, but they provided only light, not heat.[10] These chunks of burning ice pretending to be wood epitomized the defiance of nature that the Ice House embodied as a whole. Lazhechnikov's account of the bride and groom's wedding night is suitably chilling. They are locked inside the bedroom, with guards placed outside the door to prevent them from escaping.

> Everywhere they sit, anything they touch, all is ice . . . The cold blows upon them from every side, it draws closer, and finally begins to stifle and petrify them . . . They pound on the door, moan, and beseech the guards to let them out . . . Despair takes over. From entreaties they turn to anathemas: they curse everything that is human; they break and destroy everything that they can.

Finally they collapse on the bed and are near death by the time that morning arrives and their guard enters and revives them with a brisk rub of snow (Lazhechnikov, *Ledianoi dom*, 260). Lazhechnikov makes the ice-bound bedroom in which the hapless couple endures their grotesque wedding night into a microcosm of Russia during Anna's reign. N. Il'inskaia reads the Ice House as such a symbol, and the ice statue motif as "the embodiment of the suffering Russian people, who seem to have become petrified from oppression." She notes that such Western European works as Thomas Moore's poem "The Dissolution of the Holy Alliance" (1823) and Victor Hugo's novel-pamphlet "Napoleon the Little" (1852) likewise treat the Ice House as a "symbol of reaction,"[11] whether in response to Lazhechnikov's novel or (in the case of works that predate the novel) to the building itself.

Let us recall the transparent windows of the Ice Palace providing glimpses of octagonal paper lanterns with comical figures depicted upon them; these are an eighteenth-century precedent to the early Soviet "Windows of Satire" (discussed in chapter 1) as well as to another form of visual culture combining popular entertainment and ideology that invited passersby to peer through a window at comical and edifying images. The peep show known as the *raek* found popularity in Russia just at the time when Lazhechnikov wrote his novel; in fact, 1835 (the publication date of *The Ice House*) was the first year in which the definition of *raek* as a box containing images that one could view through a magnifying glass appeared in Russian dictionaries.[12] Dal's dictionary describes the lens through which spectators looked as a thick piece of glass (*tolstoe* [*briushistoe*] *steklo*—note the anthropomorphic tonality of "*briushistoe*," from *briukho*, belly); the images were "lit by a candle-flame or oil-lamp, while the operator, *raeshnik*, regaled [spectators] with salacious rhyming doggerel which purported to describe the pictures on view."[13] A newspaper sketch from 1842 describes the *raek* as a

> little box on a folding table . . . in the box are two lenses; behind it stands a retired soldier and shows various optic scenes to little boys and peasant men, who all crowd round his *raek*; shading one eye from the sun with a hand, while screwing up the other, they gaze intently and seriously into the little lens.[14]

This voyeuristic form of entertainment was a Western import: as Catriona Kelly explains, similar interactive spectacles "are attested in many Western European countries from the late seventeenth century onwards"; examples included the English *raree show*, the French *optique*, and the Italian *cosmorama*. A feature distinguishing the *raek* from all of these was its religiously inflected name (the diminutive form of *rai*, heaven) whose origins can be traced to two sources: the Garden of Eden scene, known as "das Paradiesel" ("the little paradise"), that was a popular component of peep shows mounted by German performers (although the *raek* images themselves were predominantly secular); and the presence of the lens, which would evoke or possibly consist of a glass prism that was itself known as a *raek* since the early eighteenth century.[15] Dal's definition indicates that these faceted prisms made objects seen through them "appear rainbow-colored." It is intriguing to consider that, in the Russian imagination, these prisms provided glimpses of an iridescent heaven; moreover, the notion of a glass paradise evokes the glass city of the New Jerusalem in the Book of Revelation, and did so for a good century and a half before the Crystal Palace was described in similar terms at its grand opening in 1851.

FROM INSCRIBED GLASSWARE TO MONUMENTAL GLASS: ICONOGRAPHY AND RITUAL

We will now move from a popular form of theater enabled by glass to the theatricality of glass itself—which is even made explicit by the way in which some inscribed glass vessels depict a monarch framed by curtains, transforming the glass surface into a kind of stage, as well as by the form of the Crystal Pavilion, a dazzling feature of the Hermitage Theater to be discussed below. The Ice House was a spectacular object, with its play of transparency and light, and as such it invited the gaze; it was a material object with a message, and it was indeed read, in a variety of ways, when it was built and in subsequent years. Glassware engraved with words and images constituted spectacles in microcosm, and as such, they served a purpose akin to Anna's Ice House; they carried similar associations of ritualized celebration; and fortunately, some of these delicate constructions have survived to our day, offering illuminating examples of imperial iconography.

What can we learn from the study of such small-scale objects of domestic use? As Lotman reminds us, "*all* the things that surround us are implicated . . . in social practice; they function as condensed forms of relationships among people and in this capacity they may acquire a symbolic character."[16] The tangible symbolism of Russian glassware is evident in a goblet from the late 1730s—a period when the art of glass engraving became more sophisticated—that shows the Empress Anna not as the fearsome ogre of Dolgorukaia's account, nor the weak and manipulated figurehead of Lazhechnikov's novel, but as a paragon of divinely sanctioned rule. The vessel features three portrait medallions depicting Anna flanked by saints Nicholas and Andrew, with Biron nowhere in sight.[17]

The glass industry developed rapidly in the second half of the eighteenth century, and it was at this time that all the major Russian centers of glass production were established. Many of the glass factory owners were members of the aristocracy, who had been enticed not so much by the promise of commercial gain as by the prestige and fashionable status of the material. Among these factory owners were the appropriately titled "most radiant" (*svetleishii*) Prince Menshikov, as well as the princes Potemkin, Golitsyn, and Orlov.[18] Potemkin built two glass factories on the Neva, one for manufacturing pharmaceutical dishes and another for casting crystal objects; he subsequently built a mirror factory as well.[19] Russian and German masters working side by side at this factory vied with one another, creating outstanding works of glass as a result.[20] Among the objects made at Potemkin's factory were pyramids, light fixtures, and the faceted prisms known as *raiki*.[21] The glass market expanded in the second half of the century, and a wide variety of objects were fashioned out of glass. The imperial glass factory in St. Petersburg produced such items as carafes, drinking glasses, saltcellars, vases, snuffboxes, inkwells, containers for sand used for blotting letters, globes, ice-cream dishes, fish traps, water pipes, candleholders, milk jugs, vodka glasses, and bottles of various sizes.[22] The beginning of the nineteenth century saw the introduction of a glass-cutting technique known as "Russian gem" (*russkii kamen'*), whereby a network of wedge-shaped grooves produced facets that sparkled with a diamond's fire.

The technique of engraving on glass was introduced in the early eighteenth century in Russia, later to become the main form of glass decoration in that century.[23] Engraved glassware made for the court depicted military insignia and other symbols of state power, floral motifs,[24] the monogram and portrait of the sovereign—usually together in the same composition. Thus, drinking glasses were objects meant to be looked at and even read.[25] (See figure 13.) The engraved, illustrated surface of the wineglass added an aesthetic dimension to the already ritualized act of drinking. The transparency

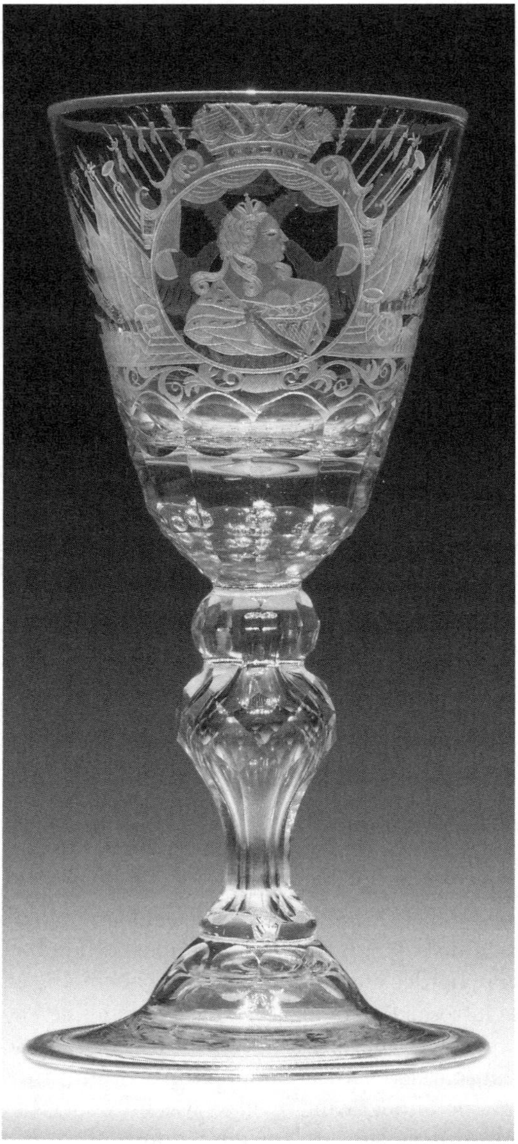

Figure 13. Goblet engraved with the portrait of Empress Elizabeth Petrovna, ca. 1725, Russia. Colorless glass; blown, cut, engraved. Height: 24.13 cm. The reverse side shows Saint George slaying a dragon against the background of the double-headed eagle. Collection of the Corning Museum of Glass, Corning, New York (2005.3.25).

of the glass created a superimposition of images, such that the shining face of the empress gazed at the beholder from behind a curtain of banners or flowers; the image had the illusion of depth. The act, whether real or imagined, of drinking from a glass engraved with the image of the ruler can be seen as a complex play of power relations: acknowledging the omnipresent power of the sovereign, while taking on some of that power through contact, as intimate as a kiss, with the sovereign's image.

These inscriptions on glass have a number of functions. At times, they preserved the idiom of a member of society for whom publishing was not an option. A glass bottle from the Izmailovskii works depicts a battle scene, most probably the capture of a Swedish ship by Russian forces in the battle at Hangö in 1714. The scene, painted with enamel, shows Russian soldiers marching across the tempestuous sea. This bottle is an early example of a historical event given a folk interpretation, and of the mode of its transmission.[26] Another example of an alternative folk aesthetic is a glass bottle whereupon the biblical tale of Joseph is told in panels reminiscent of a comic book, with images inspired by the popular prints known as *lubki* and extensive narrative text. One such bottle is in the collection of the State Historical Museum in Moscow. (See figure 14.) Some of the inscriptions are meant for an idealized imperial addressee; others aim for a popular audience. Some present narratives that serve as self-portraits of society—indeed, drinking vessels have a natural connection with sociability. (Thus, provincial decorative glass featured engraved dedications such as "I humbly request you to imbibe in the home of master Vasily Mikhailovich for many years to come.")[27] Others strive to glorify monarchs and the nascent Russian Empire through posed portraits and military theatricality.

Russian glass engraving reached a peak during the reign of Empress Elizabeth (1741–62). One engraved glass from this period constitutes a miniature "walk in the park": turning the glass by the stem allows one to visually stroll through an orderly, French-style garden, taking in such minute details as a bird-shaped fountain with splashing water. Glass artisans took advantage of the narrative potential of inscribed vessels to show an event unfolding in space and time. For example, a foot-tall goblet made at the Petersburg glassworks in the 1750s depicts a military parade (executed through a combination of engraving, gilding, and niello [*chernenie*]). We see horses and riders in the foreground, and buildings and trees in the background; the endless cyclical procession constitutes a parade-in-the-round.[28]

Throughout the eighteenth century, engraved, gilded, and filigreed glassware was manufactured to mark historical occasions, such as war victories, successful peace treaties, and military alliances. A two-foot-tall goblet dating to the late 1740s shows the monogram of Elizabeth, with military attributes radiating outward, evoking the image of the sun or the all-seeing

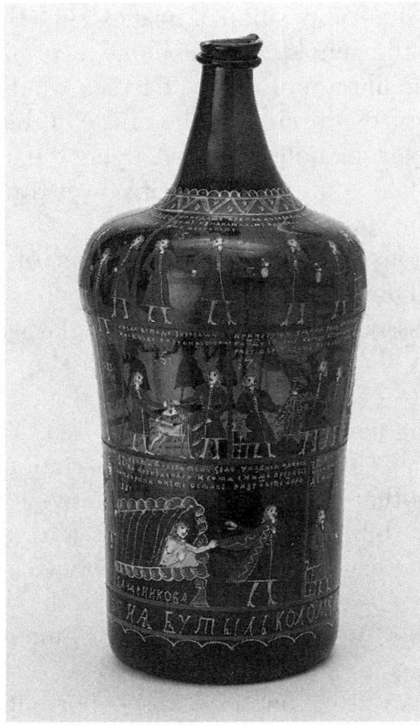

Figure 14. Bottle depicting scenes from the biblical tale of Joseph in fourteen enameled panels. State Historical Museum, Moscow.

eye design popular at this time. Another goblet shows a portrait of Elizabeth herself, this time with military attributes below her image; cupids hold a curtain-like mantle open around the empress, to striking theatrical effect.[29]

Glassware from the period of Catherine II (1762–96) frequently featured allegorical depictions and battle scenes. Engravers added figures to the basic ceremonial repertoire, which consisted of a portrait in profile (usually taken from coins), a monogram, and a double-headed eagle. One vessel depicts Catherine with two cupids holding a royal mantle about her, recalling the image of Elizabeth described above. Another features an allegorical representation of Catherine's triumph at sea over the Turkish navy. Tritons and Neptune appear in the composition; the double-headed eagle is framed by the ocean waves.[30] The triumphal function can also be seen in a goblet made in the 1760s at the imperial glassworks, showing a portrait of Catherine II in a cartouche and with military attributes. The all-seeing eye surrounded by rays of light hovers over her. The other side of the goblet depicts a female angel with wings; the transparency of the glass superimposes the image of the angel and that of the empress.[31]

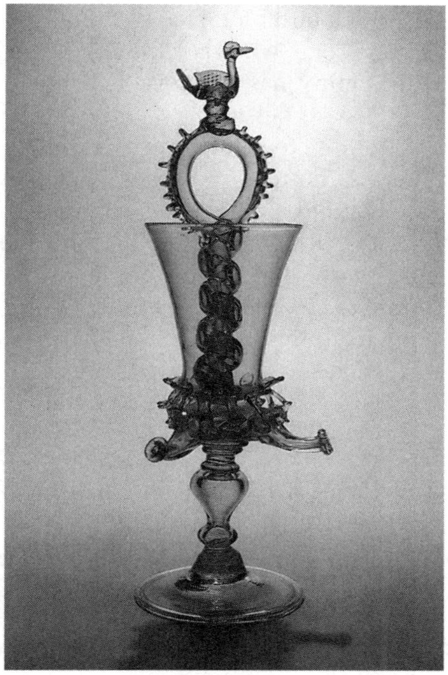

Figure 14a. *Shutikha,* early eighteenth century.

These stern ceremonial vessels had their less serious counterparts; indeed, glass is distinguished by its play of light, and thus it is in its nature to be playful. A striking illustration of this inherent playfulness is the phenomenon of the eighteenth-century "joke" vessel. Such vessels were produced at the imperial Izmailovskii factory (built near Moscow in 1668–69), where Russian glassmakers trained with foreign "Venetian masters," so named because they were skilled in Venetian glassmaking techniques. The Venetian influence translated into an emphasis on whimsy and plasticity as the most valued attribute of glass. Among the fanciful wares produced at this factory were drinking vessels and light fixtures adorned with blown glass animals, birds, and lacy molding. Many of the vessels were known as *shutikhi* (literally "[female] jesters"), or "joke vessels." (See figure 14a.) They contained an internal system of tubes that allowed a host to play a trick on an unsuspecting guest.[32] These vessels turned the ritual of social drinking into a still more codified performance. One had to know how to drink correctly from such a glass. The right way involved blowing into the tubes to create a miniature fountain—a spectacle for others. One wrong move would douse the guest with the liquid he was attempting to drink, creating no less an amusing spectacle.[33] Examples of such vessels include one from the turn of the eighteenth century, of clear glass with a bird on top, and several spouts to produce the fountain effect.[34] Another "joke" wineglass from the Izmailov factory, dating to the late seventeenth century, has a removable figure of an animal that resembles a ram with a peacock's tail attached to the pivot.[35]

Blown glass vessels often took the form of animals, traditionally the familiar folk motifs of horses, roosters, and doves. Examples include a dancing bear (such as the ones that often performed at country fairs) from the second half of the eighteenth century; and from the early nineteenth century, a rider on a three-headed horse. Judging by the rider's uniform, this figure is an idiosyncratic response to the Russian victory in the Napoleonic Wars. Art historian Nina Asharina reads this image as the folk artisan's way of creating a metaphor for an invincible Russian warrior.[36]

This glass horse and rider can serve as an example of how the playful can merge with the serious. The Russian jesting culture indeed has a serious side: at Peterhof, Peter the Great's splendid summer residence, "joke" fountains were part of a complex of water imagery that celebrates Russian imperial power. (See figure 15.) These fountains function just like the "joke" glasses (their miniature counterparts) that acted as fountains, dousing the unsuspecting drinker. Guests were invited to sit at a table and reach for fruit or sit on a bench; when they did, a concealed fountain switched on and drenched them.[37] The presence of numerous fountains at Peterhof underscores the association of water with Russia's new might, demonstrated through its victories at sea: thus, the glory of Peterhof finds a metonymical expression in fountains.[38]

Joking can take the form of serious play with profound implications. Hence the phenomena of Peter's "All-Mad, All-Jesting, All-Drunken Assembly" (a parody of Christian ritual, part of the emperor's campaign of secularization), mock weddings, and mock regiments; his propensity for jokes and games was manifested in carnivalesque displays that were used to consolidate the sovereign's power and institute change.[39] The confluence of serious play with the forces of nature harnessed in the service of the state takes us back to Anna's Ice House, whose creation, like that of Peterhof, underscores the importance of the watery element, and its conquest, in Russian cultural mythology.

In 1851, the London Crystal Palace was greeted as an iconic structure accommodating associations that were both pragmatic and transcendent, materialistic and spiritual; commentators worldwide rushed to interpret its significance, reading the language of iron and glass. Already at the beginning of the nineteenth century, Russia was making its own grand-scale glass constructions with rhetorical aims. We can catch a glimmering of the Crystal Palace in a now-forgotten crystal pavilion (*khrustal'naia palatka*), built some fifty years earlier to adorn the interior of the Hermitage Theater in St.

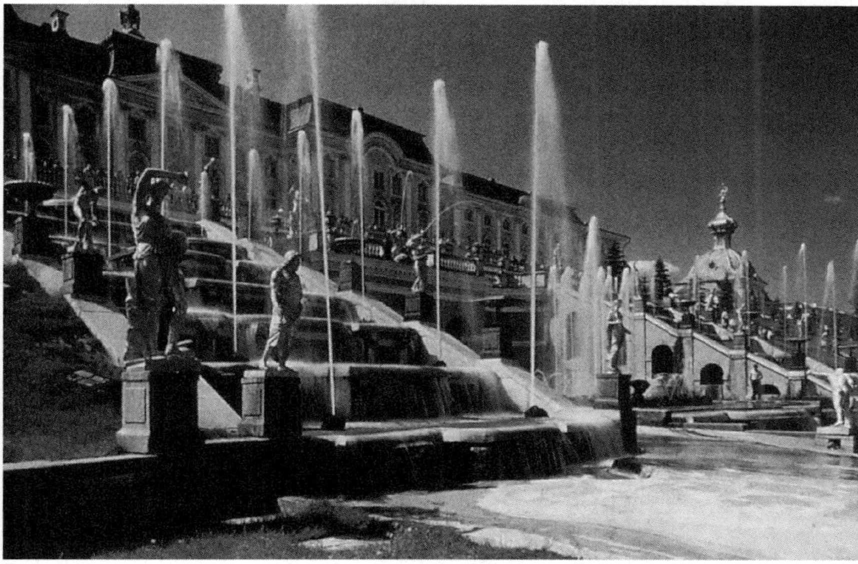

Figure 15. Peterhof Palace, St. Petersburg, Russia. View of fountains and facade. Photo credit: Art Resource, New York.

Petersburg. Plays and holiday ceremonies for the court were regularly staged at this venue. In 1808 a new theatrical tradition was introduced: New Year's Eve masquerades. A crystal pavilion was set up inside the theater for the occasion. The pavilion was lit up inside and out, and it sparkled with an iridescent fire. It was not only spectacular, but functional too: the interior housed a table set for twenty-five.[40] The Italian artist Pietro Gonzaga, the main scene-painter of the Hermitage Theater who created translucent screens for the stage that he illuminated with gas pipes to dazzling effect,[41] designed both the pavilion and the masquerades.

Gavrila Derzhavin attended one such masquerade in 1808 and penned a four-liner that would immortalize the fragile structure: "Is this not the house of the Sun? It is all aglow with lights! Nay! It is a cathedral lit up by hearts when the people are happy with their Tsar."[42] The title of this poem, "On the illumination of the Hermitage Theater, where a masquerade and supper took place," refers to a birthday celebration "in honor of the Grand Prince Constantine Pavlovich" (who had just turned ten).[43] The opening of the poem appears at first as a rhetorical question implying the answer: "yes, this is the house of the Sun," thus presenting the potential conflation of "house of the Sun" and "house of the Tsar" and the analogous equation of sovereign and celestial body. The third line clarifies the origin of the light: it comes not from the tsar, but from the enamored hearts of the populace—who have, through an act of the poet's imagination, taken the place of the small group of courtly elite actually granted access to the masquerade and its crystal heart. The burning heart, a trope of sentimentalist art, and the conflation of the monarch with the sun, coexist in the poem as two ways to read the dazzling crystal canopy. Either way, the result is glorification of the emperor and, through metonymic association, of the empire through visual means.

The crystal pavilion captures light, contains it, and orchestrates its movement. This object demonstrates how glass served to promote Russian imperial might through ceremony, spectacle, and the evocation of powerful elemental forces. Moreover, the presence of glass creates a kaleidoscope of meanings—one can imagine the wavering light refracted in the facets of the crystal: one interpretation arises, then another one takes its place. This play of light allows for multiple readings; thus, Derzhavin can create ambiguity even in the midst of lavish panegyrics.

The golden age of Russian glassmaking dates through the first half of the nineteenth century, if size and splendor can serve as measures of greatness.[44] From the crystal pavilion to the world's largest candelabrum,[45] ever more massive glass constructions were created; the enormous crystal vases, fountains, and columns of this period anticipate by a century the monumental style of High Stalinism. Glass was the ideal medium to add luster to the nation's self-image. Glass furniture appeared in palaces; a magnificent example is a cut glass table designed by Thomas de Thomon for Alexander I around 1808. (See figure 16.) The tabletop is an octagon of cobalt-blue glass above a spiral-cut amber glass column, which stands on a square amber glass base. The top is edged with gold and decorated with bronze acanthus leaves; the base rests on gilded lion's claws. Glass columns appeared in churches[46] and on the theater stage, both spaces for ritual and performance. The material moved from interiors to exteriors; its associations and social roles changed. As early as 1826, the Crystal Bed, which functioned as a strategic gift to a hostile political power and a spectacular illustration of Russian imperial might, was an artifact whose biography[47] marks this transition from interior to exterior.

In his *Russia and the Russians in 1842*, Johann Georg Kohl, a German traveling in Russia's capital, reported on the "luxury displayed in the plate-glass windows" among St. Petersburgians: "Finding the frames a great hindrance to the view, the people of Petersburg fill the whole aperture of the window with a single pane of plate-glass. . . . In many houses the windows from top to bottom are provided with these costly panes."[48] Kohl was struck by the use of glass in upper-class interiors and public gathering places. He contrasted the Russian appetite for mirror images with the customs that prevailed among his German readers:

> The colossal panes of plate-glass in the windows of houses . . . give them the appearance of transparent palaces built of crystal: in garden-houses, one whole side is frequently composed of the same costly material. In the interior of apartments, also, mirrors are lavished with unheard-of prodigality. In the coffee-houses of Petersburg you frequently see as many large mirrors as among us good copper-plates and pictures. In the private houses, too, the walls are covered with prodigious looking-glasses.[49]

In Kohl's account, Russian prefer the ambiguous and dynamic reflected image of themselves in real space, multiplied and fragmented, to the static and conventional images of the world offered by "good copper-plates and pictures."

The St. Petersburg glass factory, under imperial control during the first half of the century, produced the mirrors of which Kohl speaks and other spectacular objects for the wealthy, as well as ones, such as the crystal

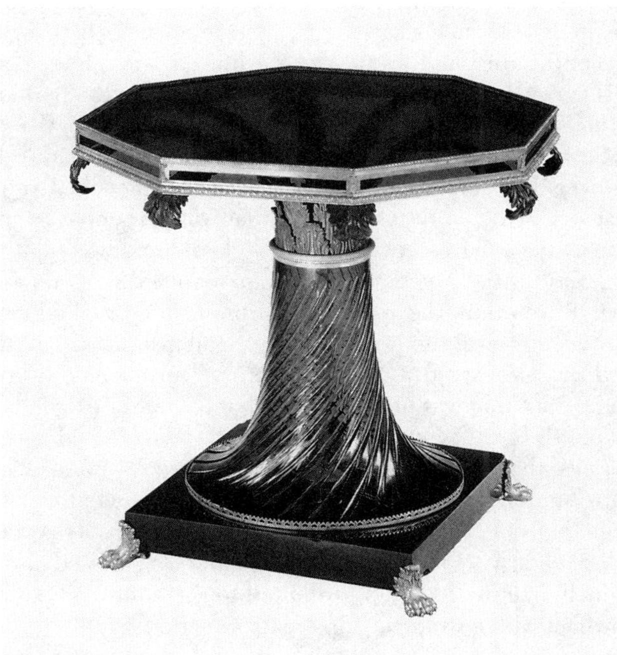

Figure 16. Cut glass table designed by Thomas de Thomon, St. Petersburg, Imperial Glass Factory, ca. 1808. Transparent amber, dark-blue glass, bronze, ormolu; blown, cast, cut, assembled. Height: 79 cm. Collection of the Corning Museum of Glass, Corning, New York, purchased with the assistance of the Museum Endowment Fund (74.3.129).

pavilion, that were oriented exclusively toward the needs of the court. In his book on the "forgotten past" of St. Petersburg, Pyliaev describes crystal columns made at the factory in the 1840s for the final act of the ballet *La fille du Danube* (taking place in the "underwater grotto" of a river god): "These columns, lit up from within by multicolored flames, created a striking effect, and all of Petersburg came out to see the columns, which they regarded as a great wonder."[50] The ballet, known in Russia as *Deva Dunaia*, starred Marie Taglioni, at the time the world's most celebrated dancer who performed for five seasons in St. Petersburg, from 1837 to 1842. Taglioni would take back with her tales of the magnificent stage decor. These columns thus had a local and an international audience.

Once again, glass had found a perfect fit in a theatrical setting. The crystal columns were an unprecedented creation in the world of applied art, glass on a monumental scale.[51] Art historians Batanova and Voronov propose that in Russia "the cold luster of faceted crystal most fully expressed the aesthetic conception of the Empire style in the decorative and applied arts."[52] One could develop this idea and suggest that the true effect—the Empire style as glorification of the Russian Empire—was achieved through the combination of "cold luster" with massive size. Resplendent glass was the perfect medium to convey through visual and visceral means the veneration of the state.

The St. Petersburg glass factory produced a number of other colossal objects over the years of its existence. At the turn of the twentieth century, the factory made a crystal fountain that was presented to the emir of Bukhara. In 1910, a palace covered with a glass dome was built for Grand Prince Nicholas on the Petrovskaia Embankment in St. Petersburg. After the October Revolution, the monumental impulse in applied art receded; it would not return until the period of High Stalinism. In 1949, the factory (now called the Leningrad Art Glass Factory) constructed a crystal-and-gilded-bronze vase that was nearly eleven feet tall and presented it to Stalin on his seventieth birthday. In the 1950s, the factory created another set of crystal columns, this time 16.5-foot-tall ones, carved with bas-reliefs, for the Avtovo metro station.[53] Perhaps the most famous monumental glass creation to issue from the St. Petersburg factory (Pyliaev mentions it, as does the English traveler Sears)[54] is also the most bizarre: the Crystal Bed (*khrustal'naia krovat'*), which, like the fountain presented to the emir of Bukhara, was an aesthetic artifact with a strategic, diplomatic function.

DIPLOMACY AND DANGER: THE CRYSTAL BED

In his overview of mid-nineteenth-century Russian glass, Kohl refers to *nargiles* (hookahs or water pipes) manufactured for export: "of these brittle commodities the Persians sometimes purchase lots amounting to 50,000 rubles or more, which they have then to convey by land, through the whole Russian empire, to their own country."[55] The production of glass hookahs originated in the 1830s with the Mal'tsev glass factory at Gus'-Khrustal'nyi, located about forty-three miles east of Moscow. This private enterprise went on to successfully compete with the imperial glassworks in the latter nineteenth century.[56] A scion of this glassmaking dynasty, Ivan Mal'tsev, served as the first secretary of the ill-fated February 1829 diplomatic mission to Persia headed by playwright Alexander Griboyedov, and was the sole survivor of the massacre in Tehran that took Griboyedov's life.

The massacre is the most infamous episode from the turbulent history of Russia's relationship with Persia in the nineteenth century.[57] According to several accounts, it was Mal'tsev's political double-crossing that saved him.[58] Upon his return to St. Petersburg, Mal'tsev wrote up a report that absolved the Persian government from responsibility, shifting the blame onto the angry mob and even Griboyedov himself. Mal'tsev did not just survive; he and his business actually thrived in the wake of the tragedy: "fearful of deteriorating diplomatic relations with Russia, the Shah lavished him with gifts" and granted Mal'tsev the right to sell crystal duty-free in Persia. When his usual factory output did not find a market in that country, Mal'tsev had several silver hookahs made and ordered the factory to produce glass copies. Subsequently he sold glass in Persia and Bukhara, while his stylized "Oriental" glassware sold well in Russia.[59]

As the story of the Crystal Bed will illustrate, glass played a key role in the diplomatic relations between Russia and Persia in the nineteenth century. The narrative of Lieutenant Noskov, whose job it was to deliver the grandiose gift to the shah in 1826, brings out the ostentation, illusoriness, and fragility of these relations, qualities that were embodied in the bed itself.

In the 1820s, Russia's military and political relationship with neighbors to the east was a volatile one.[60] Tsars frequently used diplomatic gifts to smooth over tensions and win the favor of foreign sovereigns.[61] Spectacular works of glass manufactured at the St. Petersburg factory were an important element in these delicate negotiations;[62] the most splendid among them were sent to Persia. The St. Petersburg factory at this time was the world leader in the creation of such one-of-a-kind, massive glass constructions.[63] In 1819 Russia presented a number of gifts to Fath Ali Shah, the ruler of Persia, chief among them a crystal swimming pool.[64] The pool was transported in parts, and the factory dispatched the glass artist Nikitin to assemble it on-site. The shah was very pleased with the swimming pool, and he requested a crystal bed to go with it. I. A. Ivanov, the artistic manager at the imperial glassworks from 1815 to 1848 who had designed the crystal pool, was now commissioned to draw up a plan for the bed.[65] Alexander I approved the project in April 1824. The cost of the construction was estimated at 50,000 rubles.

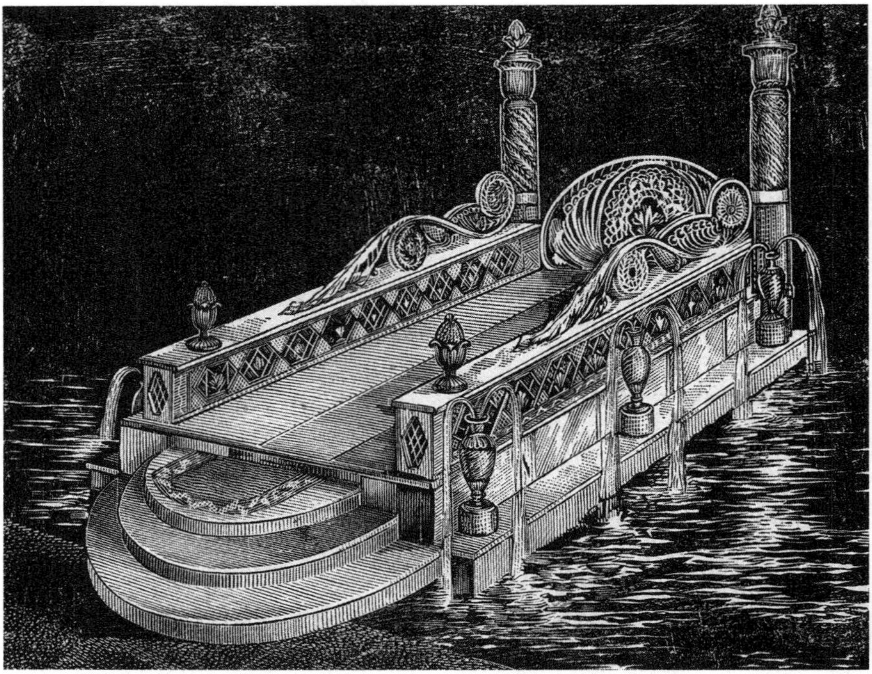

Figure 17. Crystal Bed, 1826. Aqua-colored glass and colorless faceted crystal.

The bed was designed as a spacious couch on a wide pedestal. (See figure 17.) A metal framework of silvered bronze served as the skeleton for the glass parts attached to it. The floor and semicircular steps leading to the bed were made of polished turquoise glass; the walls and armrests were of elaborately faceted transparent crystal. Carved crystal columns stood in each corner. Surrounding the bed were seven crystal fountains in the shape of vases. The bed was one of a series of gifts to Persia that also included a crystal fountain and the crystal swimming pool mentioned above. All three shared a water motif, which may be explained by the strong association between water and Russian imperial might, as exemplified by the famous fountains in Peterhof, the aquatic spectacle evoking the military conquests at sea that had helped make Russia into a world power. The fountains surrounding the bed and the turquoise color of the glass would underscore this association; we recall how crystal columns for the ballet *Deva Dunaia* created the ambiance of an underwater kingdom. When water and glass are combined, two transparencies play off one another, creating a sublime spectacle.[66]

It was a cold, wet bed with cutting edges; but where it failed as a bed, it succeeded as an astounding example of Russian artistry and technical achievement. The shimmering facets of crystal would convey the splendor (the Russian word *blesk* contains both the notions of literal and figurative luster) of the country that had produced it. Displayed in the shah's palace for visiting dignitaries to admire, it would transmit the glory and splendor of the Russian Empire far and wide.[67]

In January 1826, upon his ascension to the throne, Nicholas I sent Prince Alexander Sergeevich Menshikov, the Russian plenipotentiary, to Persia with a letter addressed to the shah in which he expressed his fervent hopes for the continuation of the peace established in 1813 by the Treaty of Gulistan (whose humiliating terms had forced Persia to cede territories to Russia).[68] Lieutenant Noskov of the General Staff followed a month later in Menshikov's wake with an assortment of crystal wares. Among them was the Crystal Bed, a gift that had already generated "all-around amazement" in its country of origin.[69] Like the swimming pool, it was sent abroad in disassembled form. Lieutenant Noskov brought with him a personal assistant and two artisans from the factory charged with watching over the fragile wares during the journey and reconstructing the bed once it had been delivered to the royal palace.

The journey, during which new hostilities broke out between Russia and Persia and the second Russo-Persian war began, turned out to be a perilous one for the envoys. They became ill with tropical fever;[70] Noskov had to fight off a dagger-wielding Persian official spurred on by mullahs who were "preaching hatred toward Russians";[71] the group crossed Mount Elbrus while dragging the disassembled bed in bullock carts that frequently broke down, so that a large part of the load had to be carried by hand;[72] in the large city of Qazvin, a "fanatically inclined mob" besieged the house where the Russians had taken refuge, throwing stones and, in what could only be a bad omen, shattering the windows. Then, in mid-August, the khan who had earlier attacked Noskov suddenly came to the rescue, transporting the incapacitated men on stretchers to Tehran; the debilitated envoys were now reduced to cargo themselves. While Noskov waited for the arrival of the shah, his companions succumbed to fever and bleeding one by one. At this point in the narrative Noskov at last refers to the Crystal Bed: "The crates containing all the things I had brought, including even those that did not constitute part of the crystal bed, and which I had been instructed to hand over to the English mission, were taken into the shah's palace, and in spite of my numerous subsequent requests were not returned to me."[73] In a moment of vexation Noskov for the first time in his account names the object for whose sake he, to say nothing of his doomed countrymen, had suffered so much. Its ostentatious beauty and sheer excess must have made a mocking accompaniment to the lieutenant's misfortune.

As Noskov was recovering from his own near-fatal illness, he was asked to choose a "seemly and suitable" place in the palace for the Crystal Bed, and then instruct two Persian masters in assembling and disassembling it. Noskov had to rely on sketches he had thought to copy in St. Petersburg to assemble the bed by himself, since, as Kachalov writes, "both of the nameless masters of the St. Petersburg factory already lay in the ground."[74] The Crystal Bed, which Kachalov describes as a "couch" (*lozhe*), in retrospect had foreshadowed a deathbed (*smertnoe lozhe*); after its makers carried it to its destination, they were carried off to their graves. The bed, on the other hand, was completely unharmed: "I fulfilled the shah's wish and set up this infinitely complicated thing, putting into proper order its parts, not a single one of which was damaged, neither during the journey nor during the assembly."[75]

The bed was given a place of honor in its own reception hall in the Golestan palace; the hall faced the chamber that housed the crystal pool and other diplomatic offerings that Russia had sent in 1817 and 1818. At last, on November 12, the shah made his entrance into the capital city and on the very same day came to see the Crystal Bed. The shah was delighted with the gift, and ordered that the room in which the bed stood be named in its honor "the temple of the crystal throne" (Amaret-takhte Bulur').[76] According to Noskov, the shah praised the gift as exceeding his highest expectations, then turned to the members of his court and said, "This truly magnificent thing is the best decoration of my palace; I am certain that even the Chinese padishah does not possess such a rarity. I should like to know, on what sort of bed does the Russian emperor himself repose?"[77]

It is curious that the outlandish gift was perceived by its recipient as both a bed (hence the jesting inquiry) and a throne (as evidenced by his renaming of the hall that housed it).[78] In fact, two centuries earlier the Persian shah had presented a throne to Tsar Michael.[79] The Crystal Bed, however, could not be used as either a bed or a throne; its function was purely symbolic. The Persian ruler may have felt compelled to deflate the pomposity of this Russian self-presentation with a joke, drawing attention to the uselessness of the gift as an actual bed, while basking in the knowledge that the Russians had been compelled to go to such extremes to deliver this "truly magnificent thing."

When Noskov met the shah, the ruler lavished him with praise, adding that this bed testified to the fact that glass carving in Russia had reached the peak of perfection.[80] He motioned to all the other creations of the St. Petersburg glass factory that he had received on previous occasions, then added: "I cannot gaze with indifference upon all this evidence of the goodwill expressed toward me by the Russian emperor, and with a feeling of profound regret imagine our present relationship, which has developed contrary to my own wishes."[81]

The giving of a gift obligates the receiver to reciprocate with an offering of even greater value.[82] Thus, the shah wished to bestow a number of rewards upon Noskov, including the Order of the Lion and the Sun (the same order that Mal'tsev would receive), two cashmere shawls, money in the sum of 1,000 tomans, and honorary Persian dress. Noskov replied, however, that he could not accept these gifts in light of the hostilities between Russia and Persia, adding that he would require permission from his emperor to do so. The shah did not take offense. On the contrary, he replied that he would petition the emperor with the appropriate request. In the meantime, he decided to add a little something to show that he was favorably disposed toward the envoy, and as a sign of his good intentions toward Russia as a whole: he would free the Russian prisoners of war being held in Tehran (250 remained alive of the 320 captured two months before) and present them to Noskov "as a gift."[83] Implicitly, the shah was offering to reimburse Noskov for the loss of his companions. The politics of gift-giving called for such a conflation of persons and things.

In spite of the deaths of all but one member of the expedition, the delivery of the Crystal Bed was seen as a diplomatic coup. Thus in 1828 a third monumental work of glass, intended as a gift for the Persian Prince Khosraw Mirza, was made to accompany it: a crystal fountain whose fanciful design and elaborate construction would top even that of its predecessor. Another delegation was set to deliver the crystal fountain to Persia when disaster struck. On January 30, 1829, an uprising led by the clergy took place to which the members of the Russian embassy, including Griboyedov, fell victim. The playwright, who held the post of minister plenipotentiary in Persia, defended the front entrance of the embassy "with saber in hand"[84] and was murdered by the enraged crowd. As diplomatic relations between Russia and Persia broke off, and sending in another delegation seemed out of the question, the crystal fountain was redirected to another addressee: King Charles II of France. Yet, as Kachalov suggests, "an ill fate of some kind hung over the fountain":

> Just as the solemn procession with diplomatic representatives, bricklayers, and cement had gotten halfway to their destination, the July Revolution broke out in France, and Charles II ended up as just a citizen with nothing much to do and absolutely no need for fountains.[85]

The delegation had to turn back, and the fountain was unceremoniously re-gifted to the tsar's brother-in-law. Even after this discouraging chain of events, the notion of a crystal fountain as a diplomatic gift par excellence persisted among the members of the imperial cabinet. In 1830 a second such fountain was manufactured, this time for the ruler of Turkey. During the cutting stage, the glassmakers were instructed, out of cultural sensitivity, to replace all human figures with dolphins.[86]

The creation of the Crystal Bed and the fountains that followed in its wake had its origins in the association between water, navigation, and imperial power as embodied in the Peterhof palace complex. This association also found itself reflected in a drinking custom that Kohl recorded while living in St. Petersburg. Around the beginning of April, when the ice breaks on the Neva sufficiently to allow the passage of a vessel from one side to the other, the commandant of the artillery at the Peter and Paul fortress along with his suite

> goes on board a splendidly decorated boat, to cross over to the emperor's palace on the opposite side. He takes up some of the clear [Neva] water in a large handsome crystal goblet, to present it in the name of Spring to the emperor. . . . He informs his master that the power of Winter is broken, that the waters are once more free . . . and hands him the goblet which the sovereign drains to the health of his capital.[87]

To complete the ritual, the emperor would fill the crystal goblet with coins. This goblet mysteriously increased in size over the years, forcing the emperor to consume ever larger quantities of the Neva; finally, he fixed a set sum of 200 ducats to be paid for the anticipated beverage. What is most striking is the symbolism of the act: the emperor takes in the water that is synonymous with imperial triumph as well as the triumph over nature (the end of the winter's reign), thereby taking on some of its elemental power.

At the center of this ritual was a "handsome crystal goblet" that served a symbolic as well as a functional purpose. It is one example of how nineteenth-century drinking glasses were involved in imperial self-fashioning. As had been the case in the previous century, Russian glassware was often used to record military triumphs; covered with images and words, it served as an easily readable text. Drinking glasses naturally suggest a ceremonial context; thus they make an ideal setting for iconic representations of imperial power. Glassware commemorating the 1812 victory featured satirical illustrations showing the retreat and flight of the French troops. These vessels were usually made of milk-white glass, the better to imitate the paper of satirical broadsheets (*lubki*) that served as the source of these images. One such vessel, intended for mass consumption, shows two Russian peasants mocking a Frenchman with Napoleon's face who is dancing before them. It bears the inscription: "You could not get us to play your tune; now, infidel, dance to ours."[88] Other more sober ceremonial glasses were made of crystal and featured inset medallions with images of war heroes, Alexander I, and such inscriptions as "Rejoice, Moscow, the Russian is in Paris. Taken

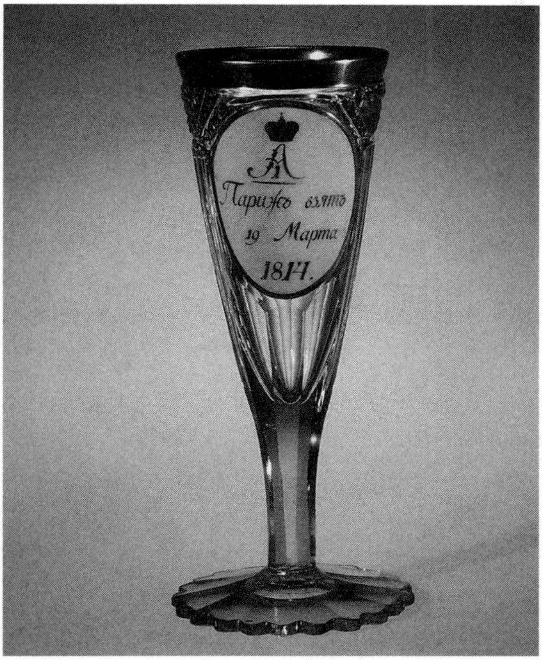

Figure 18. Flute glass, Nikol'skoe, Bakhmet'ev Crystal Glassworks, 1814. Colorless glass; blown, overlay, cut, gilded. Height: 17.3 cm. The inscription reads "Paris Is Taken, 19 March 1814." Collection of the Corning Museum of Glass, Corning, New York, gift of the Ruth Bryan Strauss Memorial Foundation (79.3.760).

March 19, 1814."[89] (See figure 18 for an example of glassware in the same genre.) The Bakhmet'ev factory (the largest of the privately owned ones) catered to a broad sector of the public with glasses that reproduced illustrations such as one showing a peasant chopping off his own hand before the eyes of the French, inscribed "The Russian Scaevola."[90]

At the end of the nineteenth century, the artist Elizaveta Bem designed glass drinking vessels for the Mal'tsevs' factory at Diatkovo combining imitation and inscription. The glassware featured a neo-nationalist style and folksy humor. A wine bowl (*bratina*) stylized to resemble thirteenth-century Russian wooden and metal tableware was inscribed: "Step aside, my dear, or I'll douse you! [*Postoronis', dusha, obol'iu!*]." A set consisting of a vodka flask, twelve conical glasses, and a round dish, all of green crystal with enamel decorations (dating to 1897), also imitates the style of ancient Russian dishes. The composition includes playful devils and imps as well as texts on the theme of drinking: "Greetings, little glasses, how are you, have you

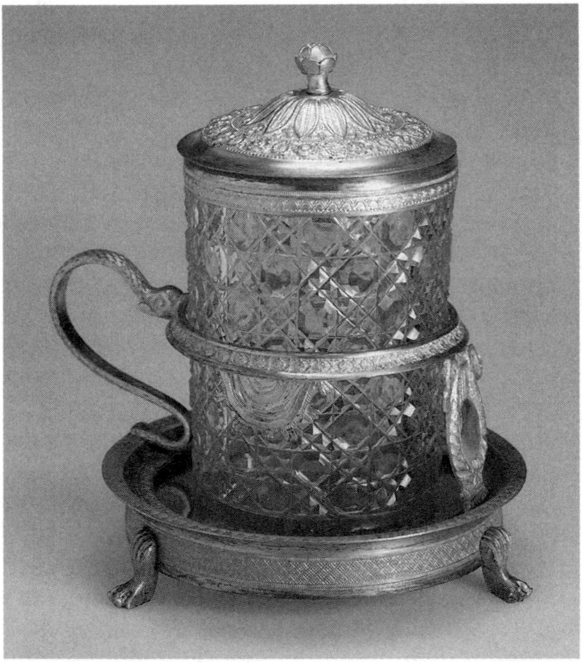

Figure 19. Drinking glass in glass-holder (*podstakannik*), carved in the "Russian gem" style, Imperial Glass Factory, 1820s–1830s. Colorless crystal, mirror, and bronze. Height: 19 cm (glass); diameter: 15 cm (glass-holder). The State Hermitage Museum, St. Petersburg. Photograph by Vladimir Terebenin, Leonard Kheifets, and Yuri Molodkovets. Copyright © The State Hermitage Museum.

been waiting for me?" and "Keep drinking and you'll see devils [*Pei, pei, uvidish chertei*]."[91] The "infidel" Frenchman, the demonized outsider, had given way to the beloved devils of national folklore.

In the late nineteenth century, when Bem's designs were all the rage, glass became an inevitable accoutrement of taverns. Nowadays Russians customarily drink tea out of faceted glass mugs, the better to show off the play of light in the beloved amber beverage, gladdening the eye. On trains, drinking glasses of tea cradled in filigreed metal holders—resembling jewels in metal settings—are a familiar and welcome sight. (See figure 19.) But how far back does this tradition reach? One historian of drinking customs writes that Russians customarily sipped tea from porcelain and faience cups until the end of the nineteenth century. It was then that tea became transformed into a drink of the masses, a "tavern" drink, and inexpensive drinking glasses (*stakany*) came into wide use.[92] Thus, lowlife, "cheap" associations displaced the earlier ones of luxury and social prestige.[93]

The late nineteenth-century proliferation of inexpensive glass is a manifestation of a democratizing trend whose consequences were diverse. We have seen Russian glassware evolve from ornate, symbolically freighted vessels created for the most privileged members of society to the mass-market glasses accessible to a much broader range of consumers. While the popularity of glass in taverns carried one set of associations, the architectural applications of the same material sparked the imaginations of utopian dreamers. In the following two chapters, we shall study the latter phenomenon in greater detail.

Chapter Four

Glass Architecture: Glimpses of Utopia

> [The] laws of nature need only be discovered, and then man will no longer be answerable for his actions, and his life will become exceedingly easy. . . . And it is then—this is still you speaking—that new economic relations will come, quite ready-made, and also calculated with mathematical precision . . . Then the Crystal Palace will get built. Then . . . Well, in short, the bird Kagan will come flying.

DOSTOEVSKY'S *Notes from Underground* contains a well-known attack on the Crystal Palace—both the real one in London and the fictional building it inspired Chernyshevsky to create in *What Is to Be Done?* Indeed, nowadays we are likely to view the latter Crystal Palace through the lens of Dostoevsky's ridicule. By attacking the palace, Dostoevsky attacked a set of concepts: the denial of free will, the advent of industrial capitalism, false unity, and the triumph of materialism over spirituality.[1] But how exactly does Dostoevsky depict the disputed building?

In the passage cited above, the Underground Man mocks the logical progression according to which the Crystal Palace will come into being when mankind achieves mathematical perfection. The Underground Man apes the rhetoric of his positivist opponents, then trails off into a perplexed silence. The ellipsis suggests that he regards their vision of utopia as a void, bereft of any real meaning or value. The bird Kagan, so incongruous in this context, had previously appeared in Dostoevsky's fictionalized prison memoir, *Notes from the Dead House* (1860–62). Dostoevsky first heard of this creature, a bird that brings happy tidings, while serving time in the Omsk labor camp. Now he sends the folkloric bird flapping its way into a scientific utopia.

The second reference to the Crystal Palace occurs near the end of part 1. Once again, the Underground Man addresses an audience of utilitarian-minded men of action:

> You believe in a crystal edifice, forever indestructible; that is, an edifice at which one can neither put out one's tongue on the sly nor make a fig in the

> pocket. Well, and perhaps I'm afraid of this edifice precisely because it is crystal and forever indestructible, and because it will be impossible to put out one's tongue at it even on the sly. Now look: if instead of a palace there is a chicken coop, and it starts to rain, I will perhaps get into the chicken coop to avoid getting wet, but all the same I will not take the chicken coop for a palace out of gratitude for its having kept me from the rain. . . . I will not take as the crown of my desires a tenement house, with apartments for the poor, with a thousand-year lease, and the signboard of the dentist Wagenheim just in case . . . Let my hand wither if I bring even one little brick for such a tenement house![2]

Here the Underground Man subjects the "indestructible" Crystal Palace to a rhetorical demolition. First, he makes it analogous to a chicken coop, thus cutting down the building's grandeur and associations with progress and civilization; in the meantime, the lofty bird Kagan has devolved into a flightless hen. Second, he replaces the crystal of the palace with the bricks of a tenement and the signboard of a German dentist. In the future, poverty will still exist; and so will toothaches—a suggestion of inevitable decay at the heart of the utopia.

The target of Dostoevsky's scorn is Vera Pavlovna's Fourth Dream, the culmination of *What Is to Be Done?* This passage introduces the Crystal Palace of Chernyshevsky's utopia, which is to be built some time after the revolution, and in which the "new people" of the future shall live. This edifice is informed by the communal dwellings known as "phalansteries" envisioned by Charles Fourier: the glass-covered galleries connecting the different parts of the dwelling—the private spaces connected to the public ones—offer protection from the elements, so people never have to suffer from extreme heat or cold as they travel to all the destinations that they need to reach. Strikingly, Fourier cites art museums, such as the Louvre, as a model for his phalansteries; the glass, then, offers comfort as well as an aesthetic kind of transport that is equally instrumental in creating a utopian society.[3] Another prototype for Chernyshevsky's Crystal Palace was the iron-and-glass building that housed the Great Exhibition in London in 1851 (see figure 20) and inspired utopian architecture for decades to come, including the circular Garden City, designed by Ebenezer Howard in 1898, at whose center would stand a crystal palace of the same shape, housing a garden and offering social services to one and all.[4] Vera Pavlovna, the heroine of Chernyshevsky's novel, exclaims:

> But this building—what is it, what sort of architecture is it? Nowadays there is nothing like it; no, there is already a hint of it—the palace that stands on Sydenham Hill: cast iron and glass, cast iron and glass, and that's all. No, that's not all: this is merely the sheath of the building, its outer walls; and

> there, inside, is the real house, a truly gigantic house: it is concealed within this cast-iron-and-glass building as if within a case; the outer building forms wide galleries around the inner building at each level. How light is the architecture of this inner house, how small are the piers between the windows—and the windows are enormous, wide, and as tall as the ceiling! Its stone walls seem a row of pilasters forming a frame for the windows that face the gallery.[5]

Chernyshevsky dwells upon the physical details; he takes care to emphasize the glassiness of the building, while Dostoevsky denies it. Why is glass so important for Chernyshevsky's utopian project? And what can account for Dostoevsky's avoidance of the same material? The answers may be found by looking at the material itself, at those of its functions, both practical and symbolic, that inspired utopian associations around glass, and at how these functions developed over the course of the nineteenth century. While scholars trace the genre of utopia back to Thomas More's foundational sixteenth-century text, the advent of industrialization and the attendant growth of cities in the late eighteenth and early nineteenth centuries lent particular

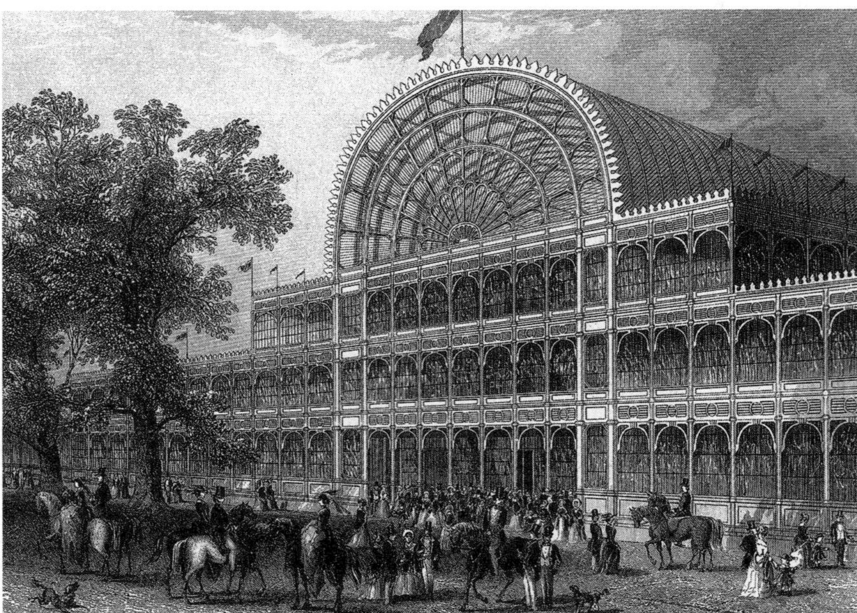

Figure 20. Exterior of the north transept of the Crystal Palace, built for the Great Exhibition in London, 1851. Oxford Science Archive, Great Britain. Photo credit: HIP / Art Resource, New York.

urgency to the utopian projects of writers, and subsequently architects, who sought to channel advances in technology and urban design into the liberation, rather than the enslavement, of humanity. Utopianism was a way to imagine cities free of the poverty, pollution, overcrowding, and disease that had become the consequences of rapid urbanization.[6] Crucial to utopian city planning was the question of what sorts of living spaces would not simply house but also nurture the teeming urban workforce. That is why both architecture and labor take center stage in this chapter and the next.

In what follows, I will first trace the literary linkage of glass and utopia in the Russian context back to a pair of early science-fiction works. Because, in its essence, a utopia depicts a just social order in which labor is a source of joy, I turn next to a consideration of how Russian glassmakers plied their trade; in this way, I seek to bring to life the creators of the artifacts I analyze as well as to illustrate the harsh working conditions that these glassmakers endured in order to sketch the context for the utopian alternatives conjured up by progressive thinkers. After taking a close look at works of glass and their authors, I will come back to Dostoevsky and *What Is to Be Done?*

In two literary works predating Chernyshevsky's novel by several decades, glass already appears as a futuristic building material. As early as 1824, in "Plausible Fantasies; or, A Journey to the 29th Century," arguably the first work of Russian science fiction, Faddei Bulgarin depicts a futuristic city with houses "built of thick masses of the purest glass." As the narrator's guide explains, "rather than employing imported products, we turn to our own industry. Our mountains abound in the materials needed to make glass,[7] and since it is simple to extract it from the earth with the help of fire, we have transformed mountains into glass by means of the powerful action of burning hydrogen gas, and with minimal labor we have the strongest possible building material." The latter may seem an odd claim; yet this story was written only twelve years after wooden Moscow had burned down. "Glass houses are sturdy, handsome, fireproof, resistant to mildew, and easily heated by small gas fires."[8]

Prince V. F. Odoevsky likely used Bulgarin's prosaic description as a point of departure for a much more fanciful vision of utopian glass in "The Year 4338: Letters from Petersburg" (1837–39). His future Russia is resplendent to the point of decadence. A comet is about to collide with the earth and possibly snuff out all life, yet the denizens of Odoevsky's utopia either assume that science will find a way to avert apocalypse or blithely welcome impending doom with an ironic smile: the fashionable women even wear electrical devices emitting sparks in their hair to create the coiffure "à la comète," described as "a beautiful electrical fountain in the shape of a comet's tail."[9] This shimmering aesthetic pervades Odoevsky's account (thus, the women wear dresses "made of flexible crystal in various colors")[10] and may be one reason for the prevalence of glass in his utopia. In St. Petersburg, an enormous city that has merged with Moscow to become "the capital of the Russian hemisphere and world enlightenment," the larger houses have glass roofs or are "covered with crystal tiles, while the name of the owner is shown in colored crystals" for the benefit of those about to alight from the sky.[11] At a high-society soiree, the narrator listens to haunting music produced by water falling onto crystal bells. Most compellingly, the future society is struggling to reconstruct the distant past out of the few texts that remain from ancient times. These surviving texts are "transcribed onto glass" in order to last forever. Odoevsky's story displays an anxiety about the fallibility of reconstructed historical narratives based on fragmentary and incomplete texts, and the destructibility of their medium. The narrator describes with regret an old library "filled with rotting bundles of writing paper" and contrasts his society to that of the ancients: "our writings will not perish. Here I saw books written a thousand years ago on our glass papyrus—as though they were written yesterday!"[12] Yet glass is itself so fragile a medium; perhaps it is relevant that the story is set on the eve of annihilation.

GLASS PRODUCTION: WORKS OF GLASS AND THEIR AUTHORS

Lomonosov's "Letter" is the best-known literary text on glass. Yet, as we have seen in the preceding chapters, Russia provides many examples of texts *literally* on glass (objects that are, in this sense, embodiments of Odoevsky's fantasy): thus, in museum collections we find glass vessels of all kinds with texts—from terse one-liners to entire narratives—carved into or painted onto the surface. Inscribed drinking vessels offer an explicit example of glass as text, but other works of glass can also function in this way. Indeed, the Crystal Bed was "read" by those who came into contact with it. Knowing the very real dangers that glassmakers faced in the factories deepens our understanding of the genealogy of the Crystal Bed, an object both beautiful and lethal. Turning from the consumption to the production side of glassmaking—factory conditions, moments of invention, factory facts and legends—takes us behind the scenes, putting us in touch with the "authors" of these works of glass.

Serf artisans played a leading role in designing the most original such works in nineteenth-century Russia. Konstantin Paustovsky's story, "The Master Glassmaker ("*Stekol'nyi master*," 1939), is about the continuation of the tradition into the twentieth century. In this fact-based story, a sketch set in Soviet times, a young glassmaking virtuoso named Vasya from the Gus'-Khrustal'nyi factory dreams of creating a crystal piano that actually produces music. The piano remains an unattainable dream, but the tiny blown-glass "toys"—"samovars, shoes, and flowers"—that Vasya brings to his grandmother's hut in the village have a remarkable acoustic quality all their own: whenever a visitor to the hut steps on a rickety floorboard, they "ring delicately for a long time, as if they were talking amongst themselves about something from their own world—something glassy and incomprehensible [*o chem-to svoem—stekliannom i neponiatnom*]."[13]

As these "talking" glass objects show, there seems to be something animate, even human, about glass. To an artist's penetrating eye, the visible liquid inside a glass vessel can be reminiscent of blood, making one mindful of the human body as breakable vessel. An extended simile in Gogol's *Taras Bulba* (1835) demonstrates this point. In the midst of a raging battle, a young Cossack suffers a fatal stab wound: "young blood gushed out in a torrent, like expensive wine that careless servants were carrying from the cellar in a glass vessel [*v stekliannom sosude*] and, having slipped at the very entrance, broke the expensive flask; the wine has spilled on the ground, and the master clutches his head as he comes running."[14]

In Paustovsky's account, Vasya's grandmother treats his blown-glass creations as if they were alive. She warns the local children, "You have to hold them very gently, as if they were baby sparrows." The author adds, "Aside from the glass toys, a ruddy dog named Jack *lived* in old woman Ganya's hut." Later, when visitors enter the hut, the glass toys "sing plaintively" to announce that the old woman has died.[15] Glassblowing, the very process by which the material is created, suggests the origin of these corporeal associations. In her work on transparency in nineteenth-century England, Isobel Armstrong juxtaposes the invisibility of the glassblower with the unseen bubbles left in the glass as traces of the worker's breath, his presence.[16] No other material is produced in this way—a rush of breath gives it shape; it receives the breath of life—as that of God into Adam. This process makes one aware of the relationship between breath and speech. Akin to its English analogue, the Russian word for inspiration, *vdokhnovenie*, literally means "breathing-in." The body and the spirit—the lungs and the breath—unite to pour the animation from one fragile vessel into another.

In the 1840s, traveler Johann Georg Kohl heard a Russian legend about a clever glassblower possessed of fairy-tale strength. Nicholas I had ordered the manufacture of huge round lamps to illuminate the Alexander column in grand style.[17] Glass, with its sought-after ability to contain and transmit light, found itself at the center of an imperial scenario of power. The factory workers, Kohl writes ominously, "blew all the breath out of their bodies" without success. Even after a reward was offered, no one could create a glass sphere of sufficient size. Finally a man stepped forward and claimed that he could do it: "Filling his mouth with water, he took up some of the melted matter on the blowing-tube, clapped his lips to it, and in a few moments a globe appeared, rising and swelling larger and larger, and presently surpassing the prescribed dimensions." At that point, his audience cried out for him to stop. Then they asked the proto-Stakhanovite how he had managed this incredible feat. The glassblower first demanded his bounty, then explained that he "had retained a few drops of water in his mouth, and blown it gradually into the glowing globe, where, transformed into vapour, it had done him this good service."[18]

The name of this legendary glassblower has been lost to us; but other names of talented serf artisans have survived. The self-taught glass master Alexander Vershinin from the Bakhmet'ev factory made a number of virtuoso glass objects for which Alexander I himself awarded him a gold watch. He created unique double-walled vessels containing straw, paper, moss, scraps of cloth, ladybugs and beetles, and tiny pieces of glass arranged into miniature landscapes.[19] The Bakhmet'ev factory museum still has one of his creations, a drinking glass showing a scene-in-the-round of gentlemen in satin caftans and ladies in silk crinolines out for a stroll. Aside from the incredibly delicate, detailed design, what strikes the viewer is the question of how such flammable materials could have withstood the blazing temperatures required by glassmaking. Vershinin figured out a way to make the glass appear single-layered, when in fact it has double walls, with the straw, cloth, and other materials placed inside, and the adjacent edges of the inner and outer walls soldered together in such as way as to make the joint undetectable.[20] The clarity of the glass, paradoxically, also helps to keep its secret. The Corning Museum of Glass has two more examples of Vershinin's double-walled vessels: a beaker of crystal painted with gold, from about 1800, depicting a high-society crowd watching a balloon ascension (see figure 21); and another such beaker from the same period, showing a rustic scene whose intricate design includes miniature log cabins and tiny swans. Both designs are composed of tiny bits of colored paper, cloth, and glass. In the Corning Museum's extensive collection of art glass from around the world, Vershinin's work stands out as utterly unique.

Vershinin may have found inspiration in a peculiar form of window decoration popular in Russia in his time. In wintry St. Petersburg, Kohl noticed homes with double-paned windows becoming spontaneous showcases—an example of art born out of necessity:

> In the intermediate space between the double windows, it is customary to place salt or sand. . . . The salt is heaped up in all sorts of fanciful forms, which stand untouched till spring; and the bed of sand is planted with handsome artificial flowers, which bloom for the same length of time in this cage. Every house has its own whims and devices, and whoever takes delight in

trifles, makes a tour of the streets some bright winter day, to observe the different ways in which the double windows are decorated.[21]

These windows may well have inspired Vershinin's virtuoso glassware. Vershinin worked in the provinces, but he made frequent business trips to the capital, where he would have had ample opportunity to view these window displays. An acquaintance of Bakhmet'ev's wrote to him after encountering Vershinin in St. Petersburg: "That master of yours is a splendid individual. His curiosity knows no limits; he examines everything, wants to copy everything, and has not idled away his time in the capital."[22]

In an analogous fashion, another glass artisan, Maxim Zubanov of the Gus' factory, was inspired by a winter-frosted window to create the "radiant flora" (*svetloe rastenie*) engraving technique. This style was typified by gently winding twigs with tiny leaves, creating a shimmering garland upon the clear

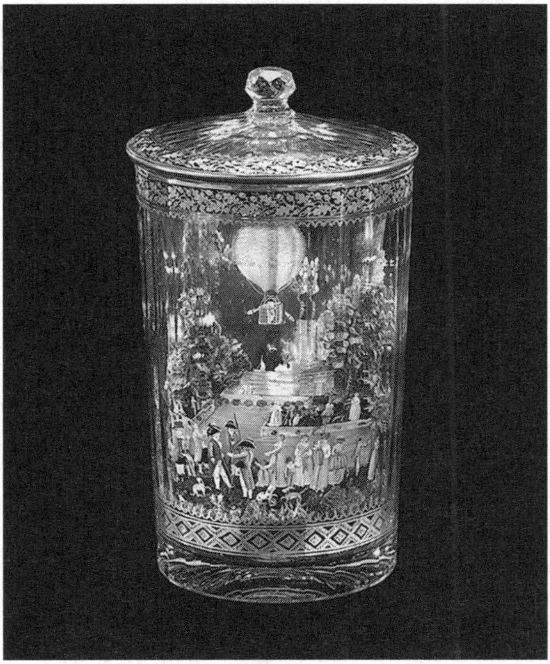

Figure 21. Double-walled beaker with a balloon ascension, designed by A. P. Vershinin, Nikol'skoe, Bakhmet'ev Crystal Glassworks, Russia, ca. 1800–1820. Colorless glass; blown, gilded, enameled, double-walled; paper, fiber. Height: 14.6 cm. Collection of the Corning Museum of Glass, Corning, New York (64.3.118).

glass surface. (One commentator remarks: "It stands to reason that this kind of ornament would be popular among glassmakers—yesterday's ploughmen.")[23] Serf master Zubanov came from humble beginnings; he was purchased from a landowner in Orel in exchange for some borzoi dogs. Legend has it that one winter morning the master was looking at a frost-covered windowpane in the workshop and thought to himself, "What a pretty design! It would be terrific to make another such design on glass." Zubanov got down to work in the polishing room, using a diamond wheel to cut grooves of various depths and widths on the surface of the glass. Stylized plants and flowers emerged from beneath the wheel, twisting in various directions, some narrow and sharp, like sedge grass, others, sprawling and soft, like the petals of a rose. This style of ornamentation made the vessel glow from within and appear light and airy—hence the name.[24]

According to another source, it was Maxim's son Pyotr who came up with the design as the two were engraving a Venetian ornament (a combination of straight and broken lines) on glass vessels. He, too, was inspired by a frosty windowpane "ornamented with silvery leaves. . . . The father doubted that such a pattern could be made with the wheel, but the son insisted that they give it a try. And so the patterns of the frost on the window were transferred to the surface of a crystal pitcher. Such a design had never before been seen anywhere. Instead of the stiff Venetian ornament, the crystal was adorned with the living lines of ethereal plants born of the frosty fairy tale of the Russian winter."[25] In this more overtly nationalistic account, the folk artisans reject the foreign design in favor of a "native" one whose origin lies in the inimitable Russian landscape.

In the last third of the nineteenth century a trend appeared of using windows to create a barrier between self and outside world rather than an opening into it, as had been the case with Classicist interiors; thus stained glass windows "screened off the residents from the outside world. . . . Special cloth, paper, and glass screens served the same purpose of not letting the surrounding environment intrude into the inner world of man."[26] The housebound dwellers whose windows Kohl describes created greenhouses of the imagination, thereby changing the window from something to look through to something to be looked at. Chernyshevsky's architectural vision also called for double layers of glass; and indeed, the windows of his communal house are there to be looked at—we recall that their picturesque beauty merits a "frame"; his work suggests that the creation of an ideal community calls for a transformed way of seeing.

After describing the remarkable productions of the St. Petersburg glass factory, Kohl gives a vivid sketch of the work environment therein: "The establishment for grinding glass is perhaps the largest of the kind in the world, for no fewer than 300 hands are here engaged in that horrible, screeching, scratching, grating, scraping, creaking, croaking, operation."[27] The refinement of the glass objects is counterpoised against the crude and barbaric noise that the unseen workers make, which sounds more like destruction than creation. Yet there is a grain of truth in the description; Russian glassmakers had to endure harsh working conditions that turned the workshop into a place resembling hell. The lighthearted tale of the clever glassblower does not hint at the brutal conditions under which glass was actually produced.[28] The workers suffered burns from the molten glass and had to cover their faces with rags to keep from breathing in the lime, dust, and sand that filled the air. At night, the work went on in pitch dark, punctuated only by an eerie glow whenever red-hot molten glass was removed from the furnaces. The following account of pre-revolutionary work conditions at the Vasiliev glass factory on the Volga River provides a vivid glimpse of the setting in which the workers plied their luminous trade:

> The work was carried out at furnaces that glowed red-hot; the temperature in the workshops reached 140 degrees. There was a solid wall of smoke, and the atmosphere was burning hot and yellowish-green. People did not have enough air, and when they stepped outside, they would collapse on the ground from charcoal poisoning and asphyxia. . . . At twenty-minute intervals, the workers would take "cold baths," that is, they would run to the Volga and jump in with all their clothes on. As long as their clothes were damp, the work was tolerable, but as soon as they began to dry, the workers' shirts would start to smoke in places.[29]

In Chernyshevsky's time, window glass was produced by blowing the molten material into a cylinder, then slicing the hot glass lengthwise and flattening it. (This was indeed the method used to create the glass panes for the Crystal Palace.)[30] At times, the production of window glass took a grotesque turn. Some panes of glass were as large as eight square feet; panes of that size could not be made by blowing alone, so artisans had to swing the blown cylinders, weighing as much as fifty pounds, over specially dug pits to stretch them out, and the workers had to be chained to pillars to prevent them from falling into the pits.[31]

Progressive thinkers dreamt of rectifying such injustices; they clung to visions of happy, gratifying labor, and glass houses were frequently at the center of such dreams. The Crystal Palace was a utopian dwelling conjured up by Chernyshevsky; but it was also a consumerist paradise that housed the first World's Fair. Looking at both manifestations can help us confront the meaning of glass—the fantasies and aspirations tethered to this material—at a particular historical moment. Walter Benjamin wrote of the "ambiguity attending the social relationships and products" of the nineteenth century, in particular the epoch of incipient modernity epitomized by brand-new structures of iron and glass—the arcades that served not only as prototypes for the modern shopping mall, but as inspirations for utopian dwellings within whose walls social justice would be realized. For Benjamin, "ambiguity is the pictorial image of dialectics, the law of dialectics seen at a standstill. This standstill is utopia and the dialectic image therefore a dream image. . . . Such an image are the arcades, which are both house and stars."[32] The arcade is a way to visually represent a unity of opposites, of "house and stars," which can be read as real and ideal, earthly and celestial, inside and outside, made by man and made by nature. Benjamin would not say "stars" were it not for the presence of glass, which allows the stars to be seen by those dwelling inside, and has the potential to shine as stars do.[33] Glass makes the dialectic possible and represents the dreamy, otherworldly side of the equation.

CHERNYSHEVSKY VERSUS DOSTOEVSKY: A WINDOW INTO *WHAT IS TO BE DONE?*

Tracing the parallel development of glass and literature can reveal the dialogue that occurs between these forms of cultural production. As the industry thrived,[34] large-scale glass constructions began to appear, and visionary thinkers could begin to imagine utopian glass palaces accessible to one and all. A shift occurred in the way that the spectacular function of glass was envisioned, from the glorification of the empire to the creation of communal living spaces—the democratization of the luster that glass confers.

Keeping in mind Benjamin's juxtaposition of dream, utopia, and arcade, let us now return to the crystal passage from "Vera Pavlovna's Fourth Dream." In her first dream, Vera imagined breaking out of a dungeon-like cellar; in her fourth dream, the notion of release becomes embodied in the glass expanses of the Crystal Palace. The endless windows open up the outside world to the gaze of those living within. Yet it is liberation with an asterisk, for the second, outer layer of glass both protects and contains the residents. In fact, the windows provide merely the illusion of release. The word that Chernyshevsky uses to name this outer glass shell is initially *obolochka* (which also means "cover" or "membrane" and is encountered in the phrase *zemnaia obolochka*, "the mortal body"). The second word that he uses to characterize it is *futliar* (from the German *Futteral*), meaning "case" or more specifically "etui" (an ornamental case for needles or other small items).[35] While *obolochka* has a number of organic meanings, *futliar* belongs strictly to the realm of artifacts. It carries connotations of a hard case used for safekeeping. Through this progression from the organic to the artifactual Chernyshevsky moves away from the corporeal associations of glass. By situating the communal house and its denizens inside the "cast iron and glass" walls that evoke the London Crystal Palace, Chernyshevsky turns them into commodities on display. Glass confers value on that which it encases; and the glass-encased communal house becomes a desirable spectacle.[36]

There is a tension in the novel between the mercantile and the socially progressive connotations of the glass house. The final chapter opens with the words "To the Passage!"[37] They are spoken by the "lady in black," now changed into a festive pink dress and riding in a carriage with a man who has just returned from prison—Chernyshevsky's alter ego. The implication of the chapter is that the long-awaited revolution has finally arrived. The Passage is the most famous of the glass-covered arcades in St. Petersburg; thus, the novel ends with a triumphant ride toward a building structurally evocative of the communal house that Chernyshevsky invented for Vera Pavlovna's dream.[38]

The tension within Chernyshevsky's text as to whether the Crystal Palace is appropriate as a utopian space is reflected in his heroine's language. As Vera Pavlovna attempts to describe the building, she changes her mind several times—anticipating the contradictory cadences of the Underground Man: "Nowadays there is nothing like it; no, there is already a hint of it . . . cast iron and glass, cast iron and glass—and that's all. No, that's not all." This ambiguity is engendered by the glass that she beholds and Chernyshevsky contemplates—it is seemingly monolithic, yet fragile; visible one moment, invisible the next.

Inside the Crystal Palace, "all the intervals between the windows are covered with enormous mirrors." Here the walls are hardly walls—what little wall there is recalls a "pilaster," in other words, the semblance of a column, a thin facade; the rest is all glass—mirrors pick up where windows leave off. This detail evokes the interior of a lavish eighteenth-century palace; indeed Benjamin notes that utopias, when translated into visual terms, are simultaneously forward- and backward-looking.[39] In such palaces mirrors alternate with windows; the illusionistic effect of glass makes the interior space appear larger, even infinite.[40] The mirrors not only expand the space but also make the objects within it proliferate, seeming to multiply the abundance.

The lush vegetation in Vera Pavlovna's dream house is a clear evocation of biblical paradise; this is, indeed, a backward-looking utopia. In an 1854 article,[41] Chernyshevsky notes that Paxton's specialization is in greenhouse and garden design, and the idea of the Crystal Palace "occurred to him in connection with his previous invention of an *enormous* glass hothouse for a *gigantic Victoria regia*, a water rose whose flower measures nearly a meter across, and its leaves—over two meters."[42] As in his novel, Chernyshevsky here equates the enormous with the marvelous, with progress and happiness. To extend Chernyshevsky's analogy, the inhabitants of the Palace in *What Is to Be Done?* are hothouse flowers too; and this serves as another source of tension: between the people working the land outside the palace (an image of dynamism) and the same people taking on the role of plants to be protected and cultivated inside the palace (an image of stasis). Glass, which plays with light, yet also traps and contains, embodies the conflict between the dynamic and the static that is crucial to understanding *What Is to Be Done?*

Chernyshevsky wrote his novel while imprisoned in the Peter and Paul Fortress; and the transparency of Vera Pavlovna's palace should be considered in this light. The palace's design can be seen as an expression of the author's elemental thirst for glass. Glass walls signify something quite specific to a human subject trapped in a windowless space, where the one tiny window is nicknamed "Judas" for its deceptive appearance and duplicitous function. In the Fortress, prisoners called the surveillance slot in the cell door *iuda predatel'* (Judas the traitor). The slot was covered by a thin strip of metal that could only be lifted from outside.[43] The windows facing the prison yard were painted to be opaque. The phalanstery of Vera's dream asks to be read as a happy inversion of Chernyshevsky's prison. Throngs of people live, eat, work, sleep here, side by side, yet they would not want to be anywhere else. The glass shell is what casts the spell, offering the ideal compromise of liberation and protection.

The novel contains several references to the window in Vera's room in her oppressive childhood home, which she initially threatens to shatter ("If you start to break down the door, I'll smash the window and call for help. But I won't give myself up to you alive"),[44] and later, in a standoff with her mercenary mother, vows to use it to commit suicide ("There's no way out! No, there is a way—here it is, a window. When it gets to be too much, I'll throw myself out of it").[45] This very same window reappears in the penultimate chapter; here, the woman in black reminisces with a group of friends about Vera's rebellion: "'Bravo, Vera Pavlovna! 'I'll throw myself out the window!' Bravo, gentlemen!' The lady in black clapped her hands. At this command, the young people began to applaud deafeningly and to shout 'bravo' and 'hurrah.'"[46] This applause suggests that it is a response to a performance; and indeed, Vera's histrionics around her bedroom window are theatrical to the extreme. Glass enables her theatrical behavior; this is another way in which the material is "spectacular." The window motif serves quite literally to frame the story of Vera Pavlovna's liberation; yet this window appears at times in danger of being broken, and at times as the site of suicide. By weaving this disturbing twist on the motif throughout the novel, Chernyshevsky reveals the ambiguity of windows, and of glass as such.

In his 1854 article, Chernyshevsky describes how Paxton's creation looks from a distance: "the bluish hue of the glass merges with the color of the sky, and the palace appears as a magical quasi-castle in the air [*poluvoz-*

dushnyi zamok]."[47] Glass is a material that tends toward invisibility, and here it makes the Crystal Palace appear to levitate. The English analogue of the expression *vozdushnyi zamok*, "castle in the air," connotes visionary thinking or daydreaming. The Russian version carries a connotation of groundless utopianism: Ozhegov's dictionary defines "to build castles in the air" as "to dream about that which cannot be." Chernyshevsky understands the appeal of the fairy tale. His description of Paxton's creation is telling: Chernyshevsky remains, like the palace he reveres, in a state of suspension.

Dostoevsky's reference to the folkloric bird Kagan in *Notes from Underground* foregrounds and mocks Chernyshevsky's vacillation between positivist "mathematical precision" and "castles in the air." Glass is at the root of this vacillation—it evokes both the test tube and the magic crystal. Let us return now to Dostoevsky's aversion to glass in the passages with which we began. In the first passage, the anticipation of a bright future trails off into an ellipsis. The Crystal Palace may be made of transparent glass, but nothing can be seen beyond it. This denial of the material recurs in the next passage, when the Underground Man transforms the crystal palace into an opaque brick tenement.

Other works by Dostoevsky reveal an apparent anxiety about glass. Dostoevsky does not mention the material unless it is broken, as in a vase (accidentally) or a champagne glass (for theatrical effect) in *The Brothers Karamazov*; or an icon cover (behind which a live mouse is placed, to heighten the blasphemy) in *Demons*;[48] or when it serves as a cruel barrier. Thus in "The Boy at Christ's Christmas Party" (1876), a sketch published in *The Diary of a Writer*, the word *steklo* (in the sense of "windowpane") becomes an obsessive litany, as if to underscore the boy's lack of access to such basic needs as nourishment, shelter, and warmth, while the invisibility of the barrier suggests that this arbitrary and unjust status quo does not strike the average eye as anything other than a normal state of affairs. As the starving orphan wanders the streets of Petersburg, he encounters a large expanse of glass. His awe at the sight of a well-appointed interior eerily echoes Vera Pavlovna's wonder as she beholds the Crystal Palace (its music, food, and even its plants all make an appearance):

> And what's this? Ooh, what a large glass window, and behind the glass there's a room, and in the room there's a tree stretching up to the ceiling . . . There's music too that can be heard through the glass. . . . Now he again sees a room through another glass window, there are trees there once again, and on the tables there are pies . . . But what's this again? A crowd of people is standing and marveling: in the window behind the glass there are three dolls . . . their lips are moving, they really seem to be talking—only he can't hear them because of the glass.[49]

The dolls enact a theatrical spectacle behind glass, and their illusion of animacy not only serves to condemn soulless consumerism; it also grimly alludes to the boy's fate. At the end of the story, a radiant vision of the boy in heaven is followed by the harrowing sight of the boy's frozen body lying in a courtyard. This is Dostoevsky's answer to Chernyshevsky's idea of heaven on earth.

For Dostoevsky, glass is never neutral, and often distressing. In *Crime and Punishment*, Dostoevsky estranges Raskol'nikov's murder of the old pawnbroker by depicting the victim's body as a glass vessel (recalling the extended simile in Gogol's *Taras Bulba*): "Blood gushed as if from an overturned glass, and the body toppled on its back."[50] Glass for Dostoevsky is emblematic of thresholds—between poverty and wealth, between life and death; thus he glimpses the frailty of the mortal body in a humble drinking glass. Dostoevsky's critique of the Crystal Palace is informed by a visceral response to glass as a material.

Once we take note of it, we begin to see that glass is an eloquent substance. Observing how it functions in a literary text can reveal unexpected things. According to Mikhail Bakhtin, Dostoevsky uses physical thresholds to point to moral ones: "the threshold and related chronotopes—those of the staircase, the front hall and corridor . . . are the main places of action in his works, places where crisis events occur, the falls, resurrections, renewals, epiphanies, decisions that determine the whole life of a man."[51] Glass is an invisible threshold, and when breached it can inflict bodily harm. A window is one such threshold in Dostoevsky; another is a glass door. In the final chapter of *Notes from Underground*, Liza leaves the narrator after he has insulted her, never to come back. This is the crisis event that shapes the rest of his life:

> "Liza!" I called in a louder voice.
>
> No answer. But at that moment I heard from below the tight glass outer door to the street creak open heavily and slam tightly shut again. The bang echoed up the stairway.
>
> She was gone. I went back to my room, pondering. I felt terribly grim.[52]

The glass door too is transparent, invisible, but a barrier nonetheless, representing the separation of the Underground Man from "living life." The echo of this glass door slamming rises up the stairs and continues to resonate years later; one could argue that it too has a part to play in the Underground Man's response to the Crystal Palace.

In the nineteenth century, the greenhouse—a crucial model for Paxton's Crystal Palace and the buildings that followed in its wake—came to be associated with the idea of the earthly paradise. After World War I, glass architecture participated in two diverging trends: the "radicalized utopia of Expressionism, according to which the subjective discovery of happiness succeeded only in the emphatic embrace of the whole of nature or of the individual" and, on the other hand, "a tendency toward a reinforced pragmatism" involving a "belief in the omnipotence of technology."[53] Through description and dialogue, Chernyshevsky's novel captures the ambivalence inherent to glass imagined as a utopian building material.

Artists from Chernyshevsky to the Constructivists have invested glass with utopian associations. Glass functions as a skin; glass vessels evoke the divided condition of being alive—the sense that our bodies are containers for soul, spirit, mind. We feel an affinity for this material as an idealized form of our own material. So we impose upon it utopian qualities that it can never hope to have. Glass embodies so many contradictions: strength, stability, a monumental potential—the promise of immortality; and at the same time, fragility always on the verge of annihilation. These contradictions speak to us of our own situation, poised as we are between safety and peril, desiring both protection and freedom.

Chapter Five

The Glass House as Dream and Nightmare

> To launch a building in glass would be a great shock to the European's innate sluggishness. . . . Glass architecture rules out the dull vegetative state of jellyfish-like comfort in which all values become blunted and worn, and it substitutes a state of bright alertness, a daring activity, and the creation of ever fresher, ever more beautiful values.
> —Adolf Behne, "Glass Architecture," 1918

IN 1882, THE All-Russian Artistic-Manufacturing Exposition was held on the outskirts of Moscow; the displays were housed in a complex of buildings, and "its central hall of metal and glass was an imitation of London's Crystal Palace."[1] On the one hand, Russians were watching and learning from developments in Western architecture—Chernyshevsky found inspiration in England and France for his Crystal Palace, and later, an exposition building was raised in Russia using Paxton's creation as a model; but, on the other hand, the influence went in both directions. If we look back a century, we discover that the idea for the prison known as the Panopticon was sparked by glass houses in the heart of Russia. In Armstrong's account, Jeremy Bentham designed the prison as a glass cylinder that was "almost all window": inmates housed at the periphery of the building would be under potentially perpetual surveillance by the jailer at the center. Bentham's brother, while working as an engineer on Prince Potemkin's estate, observed the semicircular conservatory at the Tauride Palace; Potemkin's greenhouse then gave rise to the idea of the Panopticon.[2]

The work of pioneering greenhouse designer John Claudius Loudon likewise demonstrates the far-ranging influence of Russian glass houses. Armstrong characterizes Loudon as "a visionary materialist [whose] philosophy held that people were energized by pleasure and desire" to whom glass walls spoke of emancipation (rather than incarceration). In 1812, Loudon traveled to Russia to study greenhouses there, including the conservatories on Count Razumovsky's estate. Most striking to the architect was "the

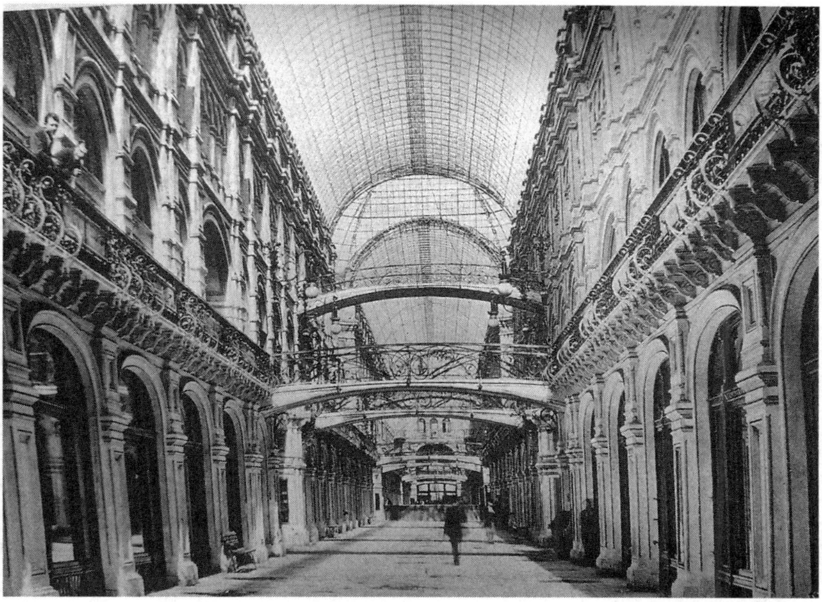

Figure 22. Upper Trading Rows, interior, ca. 1905.

glazed plenty of the Empress Catherine's strawberries amid snow at Tsaritsyn, which . . . spectacularly showed the way glass could transform the environment and be utilized for democratic equalization of resources instead of aristocratic consumption."[3] The sight of strawberries under glass spoke to Loudon of the potential that glass houses had for creating a world of plenty for all; and in associating glass with utopian social transformation, he was in good company.

If we could fast-forward through the history of glass in Russian architecture, we would move from its virtual absence, as evidenced by tiny windows covered with mica and animal skins, to the Petrine revolution in architecture, manifested in ever-larger windows as a sign of increasing receptivity to the outside world; the nineteenth-century vogue for enormous glass constructions adorning the interiors of privileged persons and institutions; and finally, the democratization of glass with the greenhouse-style emporia of the Upper Trading Rows (today known as GUM; see figure 22) at the turn of the twentieth century, followed by the dream of all-glass edifices in which man would work and live in the not-too-distant future.

The purpose of this chapter is to allow the reader to travel back in time to a historical moment that is difficult to imagine now: a period of seemingly infinite potential for making the world anew. In the early decades of the twentieth century, glass took center stage as the utopian construction material par excellence. In our day it may seem difficult to grasp how glass could have once been so precious and meaningful to so many. This chapter aims to answer that question, and related ones: Why did Russian architects, artists, and urban theorists of the twentieth century dream of building glass houses? What did glass mean to them? How did this meaning change over time? What can we learn from their fascination with this material?

After sketching the international context for glass architecture, focusing on the influential ideas of the German Expressionist poet Paul Scheerbart, I will articulate the meanings that glass held in early twentieth-century Russia by analyzing some key texts of the period. Constructivist architects, inspired by the notion that an ideal environment had to be built so that the ideal man could come into being within it, made a concerted effort to create the buildings that had appeared as utopian visions in the nineteenth century.[4] Artists had their own views on the subject. In this chapter, I will examine literary works, architectural statements, and two projects that existed only in the imagination: Khlebnikov's honeycomb-house of iron and glass, and Eisenstein's film *The Glass House*. Because every revolutionary idea has its detractors as well as its champions, I will juxtapose the sunny visions of an all-glass future as espoused by the Constructivists and the Futurist poet and visionary Velimir Khlebnikov with works by two artists with diverging political beliefs, yet united by their fear of glass houses: Evgenii Zamyatin and Sergei Eisenstein.

As the proponents of Constructivist architecture proclaimed in 1926, the very notion of architecture was undergoing a paradigm shift in which windows played a crucial part: the wall had evolved, growing gradually thinner over the centuries, until its function became transformed from a source of structural support to a mere "insulating shell" (*izoliatsionnaia obolochka*). The load-bearing points of the building could now be altogether hidden inside the building (as in a Mies van der Rohe project that had appeared in the Constructivist journal *Sovremennaia arkhitektura* [*Contemporary Architecture*], or in the Mostorg project published in the subsequent issue): "And thus there are no more technical obstacles to having a building be made entirely of glass, to its complete spatial exposure [*polnom prostranstvennom obnaruzhenii*]"—the last word means literally "bringing the inside into the outside."[5]

The attribute of glass that is of greatest relevance in the history of windows is, of course, transparency; yet of even greater interest to me are those elements, inherent in the same material, that interfere with it—most notably, the capacity to reflect. Transparency and reflectiveness were both important in shaping modern perception. Duchamp's painting on glass, *The Bride Stripped Bare by Her Bachelors, Even* (1915–23), played with the transparency of the medium, inviting the viewer to alternately look at and look through the work. Thus, glass has two kinds of inherent instability: it makes the human gaze waver between looking-at and looking-through, and it is fragile, always poised on the verge of shattering (indeed, Duchamp's *Bride* famously shattered during transportation, and the artist glued the pieces back together, thus preserving the moment of destruction). Or, to put it more positively, the way in which the transparency of glass invites the restless movement of the eye makes the material an ideal expression of the dynamism extolled by avant-garde artists.

However, the appeal of glass to the modernist imagination had to do not only with its futuristic associations, but also with a long-standing iconographic tradition that imbues glass with a magical aura. This tradition may be traced from the Old Testament to the Book of Revelation (a source for many of the mystical associations of glass) and medieval Christian and Arabic legends. German Expressionist architects embraced this tradition; for Peter Behrens, one of the first German architects to visit revolutionary Russia, crystal, epitomized by the bit of carbon transformed under intense conditions into a diamond, represented "the metamorphosis of everyday life into a heightened artistic experience."[6] Crystal was a material that many thinkers associated with glass even though the former is structurally distinct from glass on the molecular level. Russian artists were interested in crystal structure as an emblem of harmonious order; painter Nikolai Kulbin declared: "In the crystal lies the very greatest symmetry, the utmost regularity of position. The salt crystal, a cube, is but one example of the great harmony. In it all edges, surfaces and angles are equal; all its relations are exact."[7] Artists Mikhail Larionov and Natalia Goncharova used lines of color to represent reflected rays of light in order to create a shimmering crystalline effect in their "Rayonnist" works; one of Larionov's paintings from this period, titled *Glass* (1912), constitutes an attempt to capture the play of light on the surface of a crystal.

The 1920s were a period of an intense exchange between artists and architects across Europe; Russians journeyed to Berlin, Paris, and Prague and later shared their discoveries with colleagues back home. As in the case of glass architecture in preceding centuries, the influence flowed in multiple directions. Journals such as the multilingual *Veshch/Gegenstand/Objet*, published by Russians (Lissitzky and Ehrenburg) abroad, also had a powerful effect. Germans learned from Russians as well through travel and face-to-face dialogue, joint exhibitions, and such journals as *Sovremennaia arkhitektura* (which featured articles in Russian and in German translation). According to Anatole Kopp, progressive Soviet architects of the 1920s and early 1930s exerted a great influence on their western European brethren; moreover, "at the very moment that modern Soviet architecture was beginning to decline at home its influence in the West was on the rise."[8]

One might say that in the context of architectural innovation at the turn of the twentieth century, glass became an international language. In this period, and in subsequent decades, the notion of glass as a metaphor for language came to structure the work of various artists, and this chapter presents several key examples of that phenomenon. Earlier, I argued that Lomonosov's "Letter on the Usefulness of Glass" can be read as a celebration of his achievement in both crafts, his masterful manipulation of two sparkling and pliable materials. In the early decades of the twentieth century, glass again becomes an object of fascination for writers. Glass is man-made; it has a vast potential for expression and metamorphosis, as well as a capacity to magnify, reflect, embody, or distort visual reality; for these reasons, it offers itself up as a metaphor for literary language. While it is clear that working with glass inspired Lomonosov's literary production (in the sense of generating his "Letter," and possibly in more subtle ways as well), a number of twentieth-century artists make more explicit parallels between glass and language. Khlebnikov is particularly drawn to glass as a material whose potential for infinite metamorphosis echoes his own restlessly searching experiments with language, breaking or melting it down and creating new unprecedented structures. In Zamyatin's *We*, the language of the narrator struggles between clarity and opacity as the glass world around him shifts from transparency to distortion and reflection; the optical play of the very material of his surroundings pushes him toward the discovery of figurative language. Eisenstein's films compel the viewer to think about the links between glass, cinema, and truth-telling by drawing attention to such objects as glass windowpanes and optical lenses during key moments of narrative conflict.

Perhaps the most troubling attribute of glass is its fragility. In Khlebnikov's optimistic visions this attribute is elided, transformed into "lightness," that is, insubstantiality. In *We* it is used to underscore the true instability of the One State, while in Zamyatin's later work the fragility of glass takes on a much more poignant, human meaning. In Eisenstein it is used to target the "glass enemy" in the film *October*, to take one example: shots of Kerensky lingering lovingly over the lavish glassware with tsarist emblems are intercut with toy soldiers standing in formation; the shivering chandeliers shaken by artillery blasts anticipate the orgy of broken glass in the royal wine cellars at the end. Yet the utopian Sovkhoz in *The Old and the New*, designed by Constructivist architect A. K. Burov, is a modernist glass palace. Eisenstein had an ambivalent relationship to glass that can be seen as part of his ambivalence about filmmaking itself, an art that is dependent on glass as a material. Glass encountered some resistance in the architectural realm because of its breakability. In an essay from 1953, Soviet glass scientist Nikolai Kachalov refers to a scandal that caused glass to be temporarily discredited as a building material (in the wake of incidents in which glass plates used as surface decoration for buildings came detached and broke); decrying the apparent condemnation of glass, Kachalov calls for the material's "rehabilitation."[9]

Yet according to Robert Hughes, it was *precisely* the fragility of glass that helped it become the utopian building material par excellence in Europe. In the wake of the devastation of World War I, some architects came to believe that covering the globe with glass houses would bring about peace on earth because no one would dare raise a hand against such lovely, delicate constructions.[10] The beauty of glass would save the world.

An article on glass architecture in *Sovremennaia arkhitektura* (3, 1926) opens with a manifesto-like description of the houses of the future: "Instead of a sleeping, inert, stony and massive monument—a supple, dynamic, tense and reasoning organism."[11] *Sovremennaia arkhitektura* was the mouthpiece of the Constructivist architects, the leading proponents of glass in architecture; the attributes of glass listed here typify how the Constructivists regarded the value of this material. The authors pose the opposition between yesterday and today in architectural terms, and they present glass as a material that imbues a building with a peculiar animacy.

This article appeared in response to charges of "glass mania" leveled at architects whose projects, displayed at the First Congress on Civic and Engineering Construction, were judged to be materially and climatically unfeasible. The architects fought back, defending their work and accusing their critics of technological and psychological stagnation, typical of "specialists raised in petit-bourgeois coziness, within the cult of the secluded, individualistic way of life [*byt*], with its tightly curtained little windows, with its fear of air, light, and space." In contrast with this tableau of shuttered has-beens, the authors cited the exclamations of workers overheard debating the design of their new club: "More air, light, glass" and "We've lived in wood and stone [buildings], now we want to try living in glass [ones] [*Zhili v dereve i kamne, khotim pozhit' v stekle*]."[12] The architects linked glass with an open and communal spirit, and ascribed to it the potential for social transformation.

In the preceding year, an editorial entitled "New Moscow is Not a Museum of Antiquity" by Nikolai Popov, the chief of the Moscow real estate directorate, appeared in the newspaper *Izvestiia*; as such, it reached the mainstream Soviet reader. Popov, taking issue with architect Shchusev's appeal to preserve churches and other ancient buildings in the heart of Moscow, wrote:

> Miasnitskaia Street has no need of churches or hospitals. Miasnitskaia needs multistory houses of iron and plate glass [*zerkal'nykh stekol*]: as much glass and as little stone as possible. Miasnitskaia needs shop windows filled with machinery and flooded with light . . . Moscow is not a cemetery of the past

civilization but a cradle of the growing new proletarian culture founded on labor and knowledge. The revolution is guided by these great principles; these principles must be reflected as well in the outer manifestations of our life, in our tastes, art, style, and in our architecture. Our architecture is the style of labor, freedom, and knowledge, and not of luxury, oppression, and superstition.[13]

In spelling out the values of the new Soviet order, and articulating the privileged spaces of the new Soviet state (why no stone buildings? the material may be too evocative not only of antiquity but of the cemeteries Popov rejects as a model for Moscow;[14] why no hospitals? perhaps he associates these with weakness and infirmity, unthinkable in the utopia-in-progress), the author valorizes glass as the construction material of choice for the task of building socialism. Glass makes possible the vision of brightly lit shop windows stocked with "machinery" that for Popov embodies the principles of liberated labor, reason, and enlightenment in the concluding sentences of the article.

As early as 1920, El Lissitzky wrote a proto-Constructivist manifesto in which he declared that an unprecedented new architecture would "give a new face to this globe," a "dynamic architecture" providing a "new theater of life."[15] With the attention to the unique qualities of every building material that would become a hallmark of Constructivism, Lissitzky writes that "constructor-artists" will apply their painterly discoveries "to the whole of this still-to-be built world and will transform the roughness of concrete, the smoothness of metal, and the reflection of glass into the outer membrane of the new life."[16] Here Lissitzky isolates *reflection* as the essential attribute of glass in construction.[17] Later, however, Lissitzky shifted the emphasis to transparency as he took note of how avant-garde artists had come to invest modern building materials with symbolic significance: "Iron is strong, like the will of the proletariat. Glass is clear, like its conscience."[18] Leon Trotsky likewise imbued transparency with ideological meaning: he praised the toppling of the class system by "the Soviet dictatorship, transparent through and through [*naskvoz' prozrachnoi Sovetskoi diktaturoi*]."[19] Transparency for Trotsky was not only a political but also a personal ideal: "Man will set himself the goal of mastering his own emotions, to raise his instincts to the peak of consciousness, to make them transparent . . . thereby to raise himself to a new level—to create a higher social-biological type, if you will—a superman."[20]

Trotsky's rhetoric may owe something to the worship of transparency widespread among the artists of his time. According to John Bowlt, the origins of the modernist interest in transparency lay in "a search for a 'more transparent' reality" stemming from the popular fin-de-siècle belief in the false, illusory nature of the phenomenal world. Artists should therefore turn to see-through media that allow them to look beyond phenomena and catch a glimpse of the "real reality." Many artists concluded that "art should aspire towards the invisible."[21] Glass is a material that does just that. Its capacity to become invisible allows for both practical applications and magical associations.[22] Boris Arvatov, writing of a "materialized utopia" (*oveshchestvlennaia utopiia*) in the journal *LEF* in the 1920s, urged readers to view the idea of "towns in the air; towns of glass" not as fantastic visions but as "*optimized purposefulness*. In the air—in order to free the earth. Made of glass—to be filled with light."[23] Glass thus allows precious light to be captured, contained, and displayed. The conjunction of glass and light, also emphasized in Popov's article, was to become increasingly important in the 1920s with the advent of electrification in Soviet Russia and the sacral aura with which the common lightbulb became invested.

Even children's literature of the 1920s was caught up in the dream of glass as a utopian material: it is as if the very substance of glass, shimmering luxuriously like a diamond yet democratically accessible to all, evoked the bright communist future. In Innokenty Zhukov's "Voyage of the Red Star Pioneer Troop to Wonderland" (1924), a group of Young Pioneers stumble upon a glowing spot in a forest that turns out to be a glass aperture of sorts in the forest floor: "a brilliant opaque crystal surface" shines through the pine-needle debris, "radiating a milky white light extraordinarily pleasant to look at." The surface of the glass displays the mysterious digits "1957," and when the Pioneers' leader steps on the "window underground," he disappears, transported into that utopian year; the other boys follow him. Glass thus serves as the portal to the looking-glass world of the future, from a glass path leading out of the forest to glass houses in the city and the country: "houses of steel and opaque double-layered glass. Such houses didn't burn or collapse; they were hygienic, comfortable in all respects, and served people for an immeasurably long time."[24] This window into the future—a window identified not by an aperture but by an expanse of glass—may be seen as a variation on the theme of St. Petersburg as a window on, or into, Europe that Peter the Great created, with Europe standing for such values as progress, sophistication, and enlightenment.

In his memoir, *No Day without a Line*, Yury Olesha reminisces about the reconstruction of Moscow, and implicitly about the 1934 destruction of the Sukharev Tower.[25] Olesha focuses on a single window whose destruction embodies in microcosm the transition from Constructivist dreams to Stalinist demolition:

> I managed to see the Sukharev Tower. It was beautiful, fantastical, and pink. . . . I don't remember how the tower disappeared. Suddenly a broad, boring expanse was cleared. You couldn't even find a bit of glass [*steklyshka*]

> through which it might have been possible to catch sight of the past with Peter the Great and Leibniz as his guest.[26]

What is notable is not only that Olesha elides the historical facts of the tower's destruction—including the agents and the motivation—but that he imbues glass with magical powers, and makes it seem as if the window glass of the tower would continue to act as a portal into Peter's world (possibly playing on the famous association between Peter and his "window on Europe") long after that time had passed. In Olesha's account, the Soviet regime has erased not only history but also its material traces, and the glass with the potential to act as a time machine has been obliterated. Olesha gives us a glimpse of the destruction of historical buildings in the 1930s as well as the backlash against the material that had been emblematic of the future for so many.

HOORAY FOR GLASS HOUSES! VELIMIR KHLEBNIKOV, *PROJECTS FOR THE FUTURE*

In 1926, while staying in a dazzling glass hotel in Berlin, Eisenstein conjured up his vision of the film *Glass House* under the influence of what he called "recent attempts in glass architecture." What ideas and "attempts" in Russia and abroad might have inspired Eisenstein? I begin with the writings of a German artist whose influence resonated locally and abroad, then move to the sunny side of the utopian dream in Russia: the exuberant plans of Khlebnikov and the high hopes of the Constructivist architects.

In the first decades of the twentieth century, utopian architectural projects throughout Europe called for extensive use of glass, a material that took on a significance transcending its utilitarian value. Paul Scheerbart and his fellow thinkers wrote that replacing brick buildings with glass ones would bring about "a paradise on earth." Scheerbart, a German poet, science fiction writer, and eccentric visionary not unlike Khlebnikov, is now best known for his 1914 treatise, *Glass Architecture*. This text profoundly influenced such architects as Walter Gropius[27] and Bruno Taut, a member of the Glass Chain group who built the famous Glass Pavilion (Werkbund Exhibition, Cologne, 1914) in Scheerbart's honor and subsequently carried out important architectural work in Russia in the 1920s and 1930s. (See figure 23.) Several key passages from *Glass Architecture* illustrate the ideas that influenced a generation of architects and captured a fascination with glass that was in the air at the time.

Scheerbart proclaims that brick buildings should give way to glass architecture, which will adorn the face of the earth like "sparkling jewels;" then the world will become "as splendid as the gardens of the Arabian nights. We

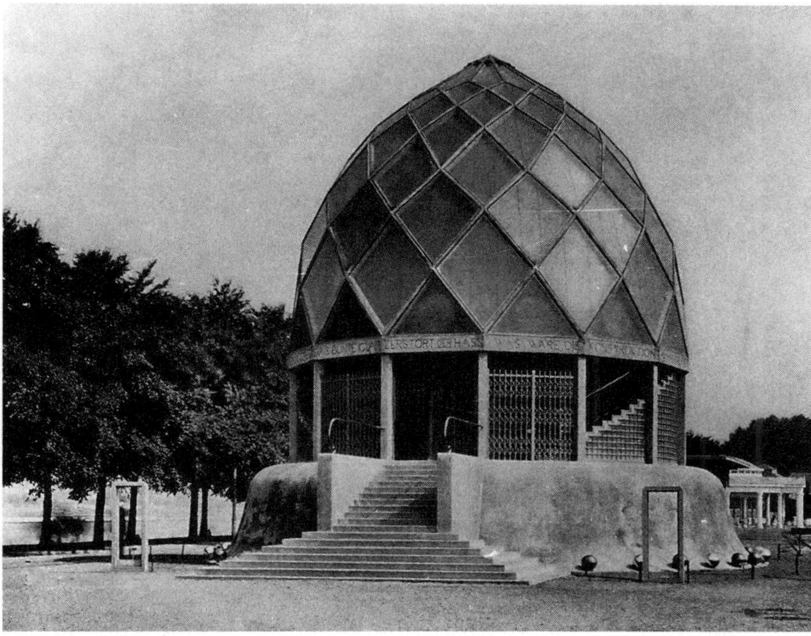

Figure 23. Glass Pavilion, Bruno Taut, Werkbundaustellung, Cologne, 1914. Cologne, Germany. Photo credit: Foto Marburg / Art Resource, New York.

should then have a paradise on earth, and no need to watch in longing expectation for the paradise in heaven."[28] He thus emphasizes the beauty and religious connotations of colored glass, evoking the centuries-old adoration of stained glass windows. Yet Scheerbart's is a revisionist religion: akin to many of his Bolshevik brethren, he rejects an ephemeral promise of a spiritual paradise in favor of an earthly Eden, and equates the creation of physical beauty with the attainment of paradise. The reference to "the *gardens* of the Arabian nights" resonates not only with the Old Testament paradise, but also with the greenhouses of the eighteenth and nineteenth centuries whose form inspired subsequent dreams of glass houses.

In later passages Scheerbart argues that life in and among colored glass houses will transform man into a more ethical being. The tentative first step Scheerbart takes toward that radical argument is in declaring that people would sooner throw stones at their fellow man than at glass mosaic; the implication is that that no one would dare shatter something so beautiful.[29] In the following passage, however, the tentative note is gone as Scheerbart proclaims the transformative qualities of glass; it is as if the glass house of the future will serve as a retort in which all base human qualities will be distilled out, leaving only luminous beauty and clarity, the qualities of the vessel itself. Scheerbart rues the fact that ancient works of glass have suffered abuse "from infamous hands." Yet he is optimistic that the very beauty which may have once courted destruction will, in time, do away with such delinquent tendencies: "Our hope is that glass architecture will also improve mankind in ethical respects. It seems to me that this is a principal merit of lustrous, colorful, mystical and noble glass walls. The man who sees the splendors of glass every day cannot have ignoble hands."[30]

The religious associations merely hinted at in the earlier passages come out into the open now that Scheerbart has raised the issue of moral reform. Scheerbart argues that the principle behind Gothic stained glass windows originated in the religious practices of Babylon and Syria, the first civilizations to use hanging lamps of colored glass in the temples, and subsequently in the Byzantine Empire, which introduced the use of glass ampullae (vessels for sacred ointments). Scheerbart concludes that the effect of light flowing through colored glass "on the human psyche can accordingly only be good. . . . Glass architecture makes homes into cathedrals, with the same effects."[31] All three artifacts—the lamp, the ampulla, and the Gothic cathedral—can thus be placed in the category of the sacred container.[32] Scheerbart ends on a cautionary note, mindful of the contrast between the aggression of stark artificial lighting and the subtle persuasion of natural light filtered through colored glass: "We must not strive to increase the intensity of light—today it is already too strong and no longer endurable. But a gentler light is worth striving for. Not more light!—'more colored light!' must be the watchword."[33]

Scheerbart's Russian contemporary, the visionary artist Velimir Khlebnikov, pushed the architectural infatuation with glass to the furthest limits of the imagination. Glass appears in numerous guises in his projects for the future, starting with the pre-revolutionary essay "We and Our Buildings" (*My i doma*, 1914–15),[34] which opens with a description of "cities made of glass, like inkwells. 'Sunward' is written upon them in the terrifying alphabet of iron consonants and vowels of glass!"[35] From the outset, Khlebnikov introduces an association between building materials—iron and glass—and language. In the later poem "The City of the Future" (1920), the first glass image is that of a building in the shape of a book with glass pages: "Here public dwelling-spaces, in a single layer, hang suspended like a page of glass."[36] Khlebnikov's urban vision is strikingly text-based, from the inkwell-city to book-shaped buildings. According to the logic of iron consonants and glass vowels, the vowels are analogous to windows. Fittingly, the breath that serves as the origin of every vowel parallels the breath of the artisan who breathes life into glass.

A recurring image in Khlebnikov's futuristic poems and essays is the honeycomb house, a structural framework of iron into which modular glass dwellings, transported by train and ship, may be placed at will.[37] The house of the future will be "a container of molded glass, a mobile dwelling-module" that can move from place to place with lightness and ease.[38] The iron skeleton-structures take various shapes, including sunflowers and poplar trees; here technology takes a page from nature.[39]

Khlebnikov's utopian architecture is based on the classic modernist combination, iron and glass.[40] The static iron structures are built by the state; the portable glass living modules are all that remains of private property. Glass in Khlebnikov's vision, which resonates with other such views among his contemporaries, is thus a key component of utopian social transformation. A striking feature of Khlebnikov's glass homes is their portability; imagined in response to World War I, they appear as a solution to the problems of geographic boundaries and national allegiance which seem to breed endless conflicts and strife. Khlebnikov's glass architecture offers alternatives to two oppressive systems—capitalism and imperialism.

Khlebnikov's buildings have tree-like and plant-like structures; for example, in "We and Our Buildings" the first view of the future city is conveyed in terms of "glass sunflowers in the iron shrubbery." At times the metaphor evolves from an organic into an anthropomorphic one: in the same essay, we read: "Every city had such a half-occupied iron framework waiting for glass occupants, like a skeleton without muscles."[41] Thus, in the buildings of the future, iron serves as the skeleton, and glass, the flesh. The anthropomorphic note sounds again in the poem "The City of the Future," which describes glass buildings on a mountainside crowned with a dome of colored glass, or possibly a clear dome that captures the hue of a sunrise: "and the scarlet-spherical summit is radiant with a wreath of glassy gray hair."[42]

The volume of glass that Khlebnikov piles up in his city of the future is overwhelmingly vast and varied, which underscores the capacity for metamorphosis that the material possesses. Thus, in describing the future house as "a container of molded glass or a mobile cabin . . . glass tent . . . glass hut . . . glass shell," Khlebnikov keeps changing the word to designate the house, as if enacting the restless perpetual movement that is intrinsic to his utopian vision.[43] This device serves as a reminder of the *lightness* of glass, hence the potential for mobility of dwellings and, in connection with this, the protean possibilities of glass as a material.

Khlebnikov's vision of glass dwellings as a means to attain infinite mobility reappears in "The Moscow of the Future" (1921), a poem that opens with the image of dwelling-spaces being transported to waiting empty frameworks and honeycombs: "With the skeletal frame of its tracery leaf, a palace of idleness raises its sail of canvas glass . . . This is a conference of dwellings of light and a congress of glass houses."[44] Here Khlebnikov defamiliarizes terms from the dull political register into something ethereal and transcendent. We will see a similar process at work in the design of Tatlin's Monument to the Third International, with its crystalline chambers for government congresses.

Khlebnikov's notion of mobile living spaces had an analogue in real-world Russia: it prefigured the "de-urbanist" movement among Soviet architects in the 1920s, who called for the blurring of boundaries between city and country, so that the life-giving benefits of the latter (fresh air, sunshine, space) could be accessible to everyone.[45] City dwellers would not depend on the countryside as a source of raw materials, nor would the village have to depend on the city as the industrial center. The de-urbanists believed that advances in transportation presaged a new, decentralized way of life just around the corner; goods and services as well as people could be transported to and fro effortlessly.[46] In his article "On the Problem of the City," leading de-urbanist Mikhail Okhitrovich argues that the "exceptional growth in the means of mechanical transport allows one to shun the centers . . . By eliminating urban overcrowding, we make short work of its by-products: queues, congestion, smells, noise, its visual and other traumatic effects."[47] Khlebnikov's essay "We and Our Buildings" features a profusion of fantastic glass-based architecture whose existence would be made possible by the very "revolution in transportation" of which Okhitrovich speaks; each structure constitutes a metal framework periodically filled with and emptied of nomadic tenants traveling in their glass mobile homes:

> The poplar-tree building consisted of a narrow tower sheathed from top to bottom by rings of glass cubicles. . . . underwater palaces built of thick glass blocks . . . The film-building [made] transparent by glass sun-spaces [*stekliannymi svetelkami*] . . . the goblet-building in the form of an open book . . . I thought about fairy-tale flying horses, about magic carpets; what *were* fairy tales really, I wondered: merely an old man's memory? Or were they visions of a future only children can foresee?[48]

In a nod to contemporary technologies already making dreams a reality, the film building (*dom-plenka*) evokes cinematic celluloid (designated by the same word, *plenka*); this building, then, becomes a variant of the book-shaped house.

Khlebnikov proposes "exchanging the street as a filthy container [*griaznyi iashchik*][49] for a street conceived as a single beautiful habitat." In "The City of the Future," dwellings are described as "a throng of transparently pure honeycombs" (*tolpa prozrachno-chistykh sot*).[50] The quality of transparency is linked with that of cleanliness or purity (the Russian *chistoe* conveys both). This "hygienic" association is a key to the way in which glass was perceived in early Soviet Russia. Mumford spells out the reasons for this association: "Transparent glass lets in the light: it brings out, with merciless sincerity, motes dancing in the sunbeams and dirt lurking in the corner: for its fullest use, again, the glass itself must be clean . . . So, both by what it is and by what it does, glass is favorable to hygiene."[51] The Russian lexicon itself makes glass into a signifier of purity and morality: thus, the expression "*kak steklyshko* [like a (bit of) glass]" means "sober," from the original "*trezv kak steklyshko*."

Khlebnikov's epic poem "Ladomir" (1920) presents a glassy cityscape with more obviously political overtones. The manifesto-like poem commands: "Sweep the filth of commerce from the face of the earth and level the castles and fortresses of trade; from the starry blocks you shall build a roof—the glass bell of capital cities [*stekliannyi kolokol stolits*]."[52] Once again, glass appears in opposition to "filth." In fact, glass is revealed to be made not out of the humble sand beneath our feet, but out of loftier material: the stars wrenched from the sky are transformed by Promethean human effort into an enormous domicile (the word *krovliia* can signify both "roof" and its metonymic relative, "house"). The firmament becomes a starry roof (a glass dome), "the glass bell of capital cities."

Khlebnikov's late poem "Russia and Me" ("*Ia i Rossiia*"—the word order reproduces that of *My i doma*; 1921) has the poet-persona, standing on the beach, peel off his shirt and compare his body to Russia itself:

> Russia has granted freedom to thousands and thousands.
> It was really a nice thing to do! People will never forget it.
> As for me, I took off my shirt
> And each mirrored skyscraper of the strands of my hair,
> Every pore
> In the city of my body
> Hung out their rugs and banners.
> . . .
> I have granted sunshine to the people of ME![53]

"Olgas and Igors . . . ecstatic at the sunshine" rush to the "windows of [the poet's] thousand-windowed hair" and look out through his transparent skin. The *lightness* of glass (as seen in the images of the infinitely mobile glass homes) is complemented here by the material's capacity to *let in light*; this is clearly what Khlebnikov treasures most about glass. The two attributes combine to make glass the most ephemeral of materials: inherently light, it can be blown to the thinness of a soap bubble; and when light shines through it, glass seems to disappear altogether. In an age that embraced materialism and dispensed with flimsy spiritual values, Khlebnikov valorizes the least "material" material of all.

In his zeal to assimilate nature and civilization,[54] Khlebnikov sees glass as the ideal material to aid in his quest. Glass can imitate organic forms, recreating them should the originals disappear from future landscapes; and its transparency grants human beings communion with nature, even while they are safely enclosed within four walls. This latter idea is one that the designers of greenhouses in preceding centuries knew very well.[55]

Khlebnikov's essay "A Cliff out of the Future" (1921–22) has much that is reminiscent of Scheerbart's and his disciple Bruno Taut's architectural fantasies, particularly the latter's *Alpine Architecture*, which describes mountainsides studded with sparking glass houses and the people who dwell there; the essay urges: "Let's undress our bodies, and our cities as well. Let's give them glass armor to protect them from arrows of freezing weather."[56] The seemingly paradoxical notion of "glass armor" (*stekliannye laty*) may derive from the old Russian word *zertsalo*, which means not only "mirror" and "Mirror of Law," but also "armor"—so named because it *deflected* blows akin to the way mirrors *reflect* images (the verb *otbrasyvat'*, literally "to throw back," accommodates both meanings).[57] Khlebnikov, as someone steeped in the heroic epic culture of old Russia, would certainly be familiar with this word. The notion of "glass armor," grounded in the Russian lexicon itself, is a denial of that material's fragility; thus it reinforces Khlebnikov's vision of the earth covered with glass architecture that serves to protect those inside, rather than needing protection itself.

The imperative of undressing at the end of the passage (which recalls the moment of disrobing in "Russia and Me," written in 1921) implies both the liberation that the October Revolution promised to bring as well as the openness essential for the revolutionary society to succeed. At the same time, the act of undressing suggests the enforced variant of openness, exposure/laying bare or the ideologically freighted "*razoblachenie*." This imperative of openness, making oneself visible, once again evokes transparency, the most cherished attribute of glass—the key material of Khlebnikov's sunny utopia.

Khlebnikov's ecstatic vision serves as a commentary upon other dreams of social transformation, in his time and beyond. Khlebnikov's optimistic embrace of glass as the ideal building material to house the new man and help him to flourish anticipates the views of the Constructivist architects of the 1920s, while it sharply diverges from that of Zamyatin, the author of the anti-utopia penned in the wake of the Bolshevik Revolution.[58]

DOWN WITH GLASS HOUSES! EVGENY ZAMYATIN, *WE*

In the novel *We* (1921–22), Zamyatin uses a glass world to show the utopian dream transformed into a nightmare. This novel can be read as a response not only to the contemporary fascination with glass architecture among the

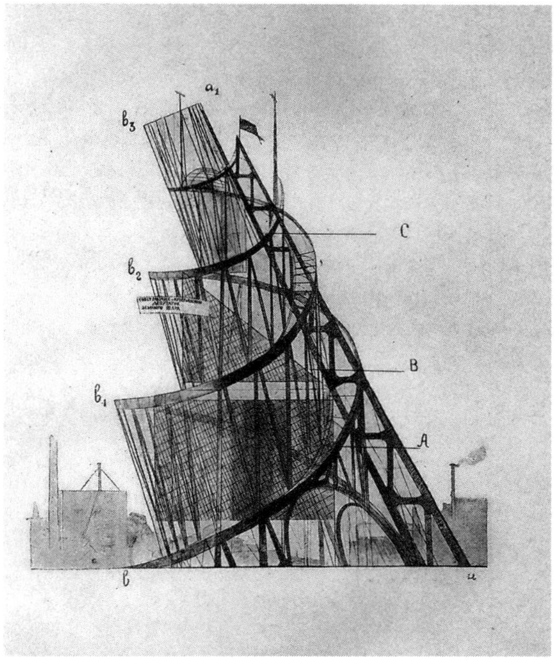

Figure 24. *The Monument to the Third International*, Vladimir Tatlin, in N. Punin, *Pamiatnik III Internatsionala*. St. Petersburg: Izdanie Otdela Izobrazitel'nykh Iskusstv, 1920.

Russian Constructivists, as well as their German counterparts in the Bauhaus and the Glass Chain, but also to nineteenth-century precedents: the phalansteries of Fourier, the Crystal Palace of Chernyshevsky, and the latter's critique in Dostoevsky's *Notes from Underground*.

Zamyatin wrote his novel before any major attempts in Russian Constructivist architecture, with one exception: the Monument to the Third International, which Tatlin was commissioned to design in 1919 by the Department of Artistic Work of the People's Commissariat for Enlightenment. The monument, planned to exceed the height of the Eiffel Tower, was to consist of two tilting steel spirals encasing a vertical series of revolving glass chambers in the form of a cube, a pyramid, and a cylinder (moving from the ground up, each chamber would be successively smaller). (See figure 24.) This construction, which later came to be known as Tatlin's Tower, was planned as a building to house the various institutions of a future world government. A statement of intent in a pamphlet, *The Monument to the Third International*, was published in 1920 to accompany and explain the appearance of Tatlin's Tower, which was presented to the public in the form of a wooden model. The author of the pamphlet was art critic Nikolai Punin, Tatlin's collaborator and spokesman. Without this pamphlet, viewers would not have known about the extensive use of glass intended for the built version—the model was made of wood, cardboard, wire, metal, and oilpaper.[59] The model of the tower was displayed in November 1920 in the Studio of Space, Materials, and Construction in the SVOMAS (Free Studios) building in Petrograd. In December of that year, the model was exhibited in Moscow, this time with a child concealed in the base whose job it was to turn a crank handle to make the chambers rotate.[60]

Several passages from Punin's text illuminate the meaning that glass held for architects in the 1920s and, more broadly, for the Russian modernist imagination in the wake of the Bolshevik Revolution. According to Punin, the basic idea underlying the construction of the tower was

> the organic synthesis of architectural, sculptural, and painterly principles [that would] yield a new type of monumental structure uniting pure creative form with utilitarian form. Therefore, the design of the monument consists of three large glass chambers [*pomeshcheniia*] erected by means of a complex system of vertical rods and spirals.[61]

While scholars usually discuss Tatlin's tower in terms of the symbolic spiral of its outer framework, Punin's description of the projected monument gives priority to the three glass chambers, the heart of the structure that illustrates the synthesis of "pure creative form" and "utilitarian form." The expressive intent of the glass material is elucidated in subsequent passages. First, however, Punin hastens to reassure readers who might question the practicality of this design: "The artist Tatlin intends the glass chambers to have double partitions with an airless space (thermos), thanks to which it will be easy to maintain a constant temperature inside the chambers" (Punin, "Pamiatnik III Internatsionala," 19). Punin then leaves realistic considerations behind as he moves on to the central part of the pamphlet: a section titled "The Artistic Significance of the Project." He attempts to imbue cold construction materials, glass and steel, with an organic life force originating from the clever design of the constructor-architect: "The entire form vibrates like a steel snake, constrained and organized by the impulse that all of its parts share—to rise above the earth. The form wants to overcome matter and the force of gravity; . . . straining its muscles, the form seeks an escape" (Punin, "Pamiatnik III Internatsionala," 20).

This passage is the first one in which Punin mentions steel, the other key component of the tower—up to now glass has been the only material discussed. The desire to "overcome matter" finds a solution in glass, a material that tends toward invisibility (we recall Bowlt's observation about modernists' belief that "the arts should strive to 'remove material'"). Punin upholds tension as the utmost value, and describes the architectural form in terms of organic life—echoing the motifs in the article about glass architecture in *Sovremennaia arkhitektura* cited above. The tension leads to release: "liberated life rises above the earth, above the raw earthly materials" (Punin, "Pamiatnik III Internatsionala," 21). The motif of desiring to leave the constraints of the earth's gravity, evoking other types of liberation, is a familiar one in this period; most often it is reflected in the fascination with flight. This passage introduces the idea of transcending "earthly material"; the anxiety about materials in a materialistic time is one that also appears in Khlebnikov's writings. The implication here is that glass *does not* belong among the "earthly materials."

Punin makes explicit the symbolic value of glass in the following passage, in which the glass chambers of the tower resemble the vials and test tubes of a vast futuristic laboratory:

> The monument is designed to concentrate the legislative (chamber A), executive (chamber B), and informative (chamber C) initiatives; moreover, these chambers, in keeping with the principle of expressing contemporary life, are erected into the upper strata of space. It is this, as well as the material (glass), that signifies the purity [*chistota*—literally "cleanliness"] of the initiatives, their ideality, freed from material dead weight. (Punin, "Pamiatnik III Internatsionala," 21)

Here the "purity" of the glass, a moral quality seemingly derived from its physical quality of transparency (as well as a long-standing symbolic tradition), is meant to reassure onlookers of the purity of the "initiatives" represented by the institutions housed in the tower.[62] Glass in itself carries a symbolic weight; glass in conjunction with steel has an additional value, producing a visual rhythm, the essential quality in a work of art and in life itself. The materials develop a type of syntax, behaving as units of language, and recalling Khlebnikov's "consonants of iron and vowels of glass": according to Punin, the artist's task is "to break down rhythm into the elements of material culture, the latter of which determine the growth and conditions of existence" (Punin, "Pamiatnik III Internatsionala," 21).

As John Milner writes, the tower "represented a vital extension of constructivism and social commitment."[63] The model took on great significance for visionary artists of the time, becoming an icon of dynamism, progress, and artistic and social revolution—in other words, a symbol of utopian aspiration embodied in architecture. Ilya Ehrenburg was mesmerized by the model, which appeared to him as a harbinger of an architectural revolution:

"a new architecture is coming into being [*nachinaetsia novaia arkhitektura*]." He praises the architectural use of glass for its "audacity" and, paradoxically, for its practicality (it is functional, rather than utilitarian—an important distinction for Ehrenburg), citing precedents from America to the Netherlands and playfully predicting that soon his readers will find themselves living in glass buildings:

> The material, alongside the iron that has already entered architectural life, is audacious glass [*derzkoe steklo*]. This is no stunt, but practical foresight. (In America over the last five years a number of workers' houses have been built out of glass. In Rotterdam, a joint-stock company of cheap housing estates, faced with a choice of building materials, settled on glass.) Today we have a model of a monument, but tomorrow the reader of this book will be giggling at the "futurist" Ehrenburg in the glass office of a glass house (thankfully not a transparent one [*khorosho chto ne prozrachnom*]).[64]

Yet there were dissenting voices as well, such as art critic Miklashevkii's remarks about how the building would only be fit to grow tropical fruit:

> The idea of placing state institutions into a glass vessel [*sosud*] cannot be recognized as successful. Anyone who has ever been in a film studio knows that a great drawback of glass buildings is their capacity to heat up when exposed to the sun . . . The Soviet of People's Commissars would flee from such a building on the first sunny day and, situating themselves on the grass nearby, would immediately issue a decree about putting Tatlin's tower up for auction and renting it out to horticulturists who can use it to grow pineapples.[65]

Miklashevskii refers here to the glass walls that were a requisite feature of early film studios, built in such a way (on the prototype of Georges Méliès's Star-Film studio) in order to use as much available light as possible. It is curious to consider that at the time, greenhouses, which were fantasy spaces where artifice met Eden, and film studios—factories of dreams—were, thanks to glass, architectural twins.

The utopian idea of glass houses did in fact find material inspiration in the greenhouses and conservatories of the eighteenth and nineteenth centuries; yet Miklashevskii is repelled by this association with the vegetable kingdom, greenhouses being perhaps overly redolent of the bourgeois decadence the Soviets were so eager to abandon. (The reference to pineapples further underscores the bourgeois association; thus, Mayakovsky's vicious 1917 couplet aimed at the "bourgeois" whose day of reckoning has come opens with the words "Eat pineapples, chew on grouse . . . [*Esh ananasy, riabchikov zhui* . . .].") Miklashevskii's choice of the words "glass vessel" (*stekliannyi sosud*) rather than Punin's original "glass chambers" (*stekliannye pome-*

shcheniia) shifts the emphasis from the neutral idea of housing (the word *pomeshchenie* itself contains the notion of containment; compare *pomestit'*, "to place") to the "laboratory" or "experimental" function of glass, thus evoking the specter of human subjects (government workers) trapped in gigantic glass retorts (as in Odoevsky's nineteenth-century "Motley Tales"), and ultimately rejects Tatlin's experiment as a misguided venture into alchemy. A more positive reading of the same "tower as glass vessel" analogy comes from Tatlin's biographer Milner: "Here was a social alembic: the evolution of human history was to be determined here, and corporate will condensed, purified and transformed into the energy of action."[66]

Architects such as Mel'nikov who advocated the use of glass in architecture were motivated in part precisely by the idea that inhabitants could be bathed in the rays of the sun.[67] Glass as building material thus entered into the discourse of sickness and health. The 1926 article "Glass in Contemporary Architecture" in the Constructivist journal *Sovremennaia arkhitektura* draws this connection explicitly. First, the authors argue that the costs of heating buildings with glass walls will be compensated by the lower lighting costs (artificial lighting will be replaced by sunlight) as well as "the condition of the organism as a whole, and in particular of the eyesight of the laborers working in well-lit buildings." Second, they declare that "the material forms of the new socialist way of life [*byt*]" will be based on "perfected technology and an abundance of light and air." Put simply, the human organism will benefit from glass architecture: "We assert the obsolescence of the old factories, industrial plants, offices, banks, shops, and residential buildings where workers go blind and destroy their bodies for the sake of stagnation and injudicious cost-cutting." Finally, a statistic running vertically alongside the article reads: "For every 10,000 residents, 84 persons died of tuberculosis given a window area of 1.8 square meters, while 13 persons died given a window area of 4.2 square meters."[68] Underlying the link between glass and health is the worship of sunlight shared by many creative thinkers, from poets Bely and Bryusov to architect Mel'nikov, in the early decades of the twentieth century.[69]

The ending of Mandelstam's *Egyptian Stamp* (1927), a work whose hero declares that life is nothing but "delirium, emptiness, and glass," shows how a window that lets in sunlight can have a stifling greenhouse effect:

> In Moscow he stopped at the Hotel Select—a very good hotel on Malaya Lubyanka—in a room where there used to be a store, with a chic glass shop window [*s shikarnoi stekliannoi vitronoi*] in place of a regular window [*vmesto okna*], heated by the sun to an improbable degree.[70]

This unsettling image makes for a startling contrast with the sunny shop window in Popov's article "Moscow Is Not a Museum of Antiquity." The location of the hotel on Malaya *Lubyanka* (the headquarters of the secret police was located on Lubyanka Street) suggests another kind of stifling oppression, not far removed from the enormous Bell Jar of Zamyatin's One State.[71]

What was the state of glassmaking technology, specifically window production, in Russia at the time that Zamyatin wrote *We*? My research indicates that glass in Russia was expensive and difficult to obtain in the early decades of the twentieth century, especially after the revolution.[72] The sort of large-scale production of transparent sheets of window glass that the buildings in the One State would require did not even become possible in Russia until 1926.[73] Even in that year, *Sovremennaia arkhitektura* bluntly reported that "today there is no glass on the Soviet market."[74] This might explain in part why most of the Constructivist all-glass fantasias either were not built at all, or were realized in an unrecognizable form as concrete boxes with tiny windows (e.g., "the dark, grim cube of the Lenin Institute" in Moscow that Zamyatin critiqued in his 1933 article "Moscow-Leningrad"). The factories did not become smoothly nationalized; during the Civil War years, their work temporarily halted. Glass production did not really pick up again until NEP; at this time, the focus of glass production switched from the bottle glass of tsarist times to window glass.[75] This shift in focus invites us to situate it within the context of a broader shift from the self-absorbed private consumer to the outward-looking collective.

Scheerbart notes the importance of glass architecture for the interpenetration of inside and outside:

> If we want our culture to rise to a higher level, we are obliged . . . to change our architecture. And this only becomes possible if we take away the closed character from the rooms in which we live. We can only do that by introducing *glass architecture, which lets in the light of the sun, the moon and the stars, not merely through a few windows, but through every possible wall*, which will be made entirely of glass—of colored glass. The new environment which we thus create must bring us a new culture.[76]

Anticipating Khlebnikov's utopian aspirations, Scheerbart hopes to reverse the alienation of modern man from the natural world by turning his gaze outward and fostering a cosmic consciousness. Closer to home, Mel'nikov envisioned glass as a democratic material that, by bringing together inside and outside, would make visible the labor that was heretofore obscured. His 1924 design for the *Leningradskaia Pravda* building was a motorized, revolving glass structure. Starr articulates the function of the glass:

> The newspaper workers themselves were to be put on view so that their movements within the glass-walled structure would merge with the mechani-

> cal exhibition provided by the building. Nor were Mel'nikov's workers to be mere spectators to the machine but its activators . . . In this way a sense of pluralistic vitality would be infused into the whole building and communicated to the public outside.[77]

It may seem difficult to argue with such visions of integration and equality brought about by the use of glass walls; transparency seems a key to a utopian society.[78] Yet this philosophy is demolished in Zamyatin's cautionary tale.

The fact that the denizens of Zamyatin's anti-utopia dwell in glass houses is usually read by scholars as a device to underscore the degree to which this future society is subject to surveillance.[79] The diarist narrator himself explains to his presumably naive reader that the glass walls of the houses in the One State are there to make it easier for the Guardians (secret police agents) to do their job. Indeed, a passage in the text that succinctly illustrates the role of glass in the One State's society of surveillance is the moment at which D-503, the narrator, tries to hide his self-incriminating manuscript from the approaching Guardians and despairs: "Nowhere to hide it—all is glass [*vse steklo*]."[80]

Yet Zamyatin does not stop with glass *houses*; his novel as a whole is glass-obsessed. Nearly every page is studded with shards of the material, which has become perfected, and ubiquitous, in Zamyatin's novel. D-503 speaks of glass as a material when describing his physical world, and uses it as a metaphor when turning inward. The only diary entry entirely free of references to glass is the very last one—after D has undergone the "Great Operation" to rid him of his imagination. Awareness of glass requires the mental flexibility to allow the eye to go back and forth between several visual/existential planes. Once he is perfectly integrated into the glass world, he stops being aware of it.

Glass has become the ideal building material in the One State. People live in glass houses whose transparent doors are embossed with gold numbers (Zamyatin, *My*, 341); but they also sit at glass tables and sleep in glass beds (328, 334); they wear uniforms of "glass silk" (342); they walk on glass pavements (310) and climb glass stairs (362); they travel through subterranean glass tunnels (371) in mirrored train cars (407). Their towers have glass parapets (382), and their auditoriums, glass benches (404). Their glass houses themselves dwell under a dome of "glass bricks" that filters the sun (318, 409)—a *matryoshka* effect of infinite containment, like the one that is evoked when D looks around at his fellow "numbers," suspended in their identical glass apartments and mirroring each other's every move (328, 378). The vast glass dome (the "Glass Crown" that covers the city in Scheerbart's fantasy, recast in a sinister light) is really a larger version of the Bell Jar that the State uses to inflict torture on dissidents. The dome forms a great glass wall that keeps out the green, primitive world. Similarly to this Glass Wall, the sheer volume of glass imagery in the novel threatens to become a wall against interpretation. Why does Zamyatin's anti-utopia make such extensive use of this material?

In an attempt to make sense of the pervasive presence of glass in *We*, S. A. Cowan argues convincingly that Zamyatin uses a structure of binary oppositions between "glass and crystallization" on the one hand and "fluids and dissolution" on the other to expose "the spiritual, philosophical, moral, political, and aesthetic calcification of the One State, while he promotes freedom and its related values, such as variety, imagination, passion, and dynamism."[81] The argument turns on the opposition between energy and entropy and places glass in the latter category. In Cowan's article, the attributes of "transparency" and "solidity" are taken as given and unchanging properties of glass; yet what actually happens in the novel is more complex. I do agree with Cowan that the central set of images in the novel all have to do with glass. I argue, however, that the *contradictory* qualities of glass were what appealed to writers such as Zamyatin and inspired them to use the material to create metaphors for the workings of consciousness and conflicting desires. In addition, Zamyatin found glass to be the ideal material by means of which he could express the paradoxes and perils of the new world coming into being around him; and the glass edifice he constructed in *We* ultimately helped him to glimpse the Stalinist future, as if through a telescope. In the analysis that follows, I will not seek to account for every reference to glass in the text, but rather will indicate several key motifs associated with the material in order to illuminate Zamyatin's authorial strategy.

In 1918, Adolf Behne proclaimed that glass architecture would compel mankind toward transformation, and eventually human beings would even come to share the physical aspects of the material that surrounds them: "Glass will transform [the European]. Glass is sheer and angular, yet in its hidden potential it is gentle and delicate. The new European will have these qualities too: clear determination and utmost gentleness."[82] In the One State, glass has become more than a popular construction material—it is an all-encompassing discourse, and an all-powerful paradigm. Those who are exposed to glass themselves take on its attributes.[83] Zamyatin takes note not only of the transparency of glass, but also its capacity for metamorphosis and its host of paradoxical qualities. Thus *We* lends itself to being read as both a topical novel and a prediction of the future; yet, more than that, this novel can be seen as a "materialist" approach to the problems of human perception, faith, and belief.

Glass plays a crucial role in the State's enforcement of mandatory happiness. Dissenters are tortured by asphyxiation in "the Famous Gas Bell," a human-scale bell jar, and the glass rocket ship *Integral* is designed to transport the One State's vision of perfection (by means of panegyric works "about the beauty and grandeur of the One State" [307]) to the furthest reaches of outer space.[84] In fact, the very first image of glass in the novel appears in the description of the *Integral* that D transcribes from the *One State Gazette*—the totalitarian State speaking through the narrator: the citizens are ordered to "integrate the infinite equation of the universe by means of the glass, electric, fire-breathing Integral." Both the *Integral* and the Bell are glass containers as well as means to propagate the mandatory happiness of the One State—the former is designated for the unknown inhabitants of other planets; the latter is for the "internal enemy."

In *Aelita, or the Decline of Mars*, a quasi-utopian science fiction novel written a year after *We* was completed, Alexei Tolstoi creates a link between the concrete material of glass (*steklo*) and the abstract notion of happiness (*schast'e*). As in Zamyatin, glass appears in Tolstoi's novel in both literal and figurative guises. One of the links in *Aelita* between glass and happiness is a recurring image of a bird singing a happy song in a "glassy" or "crystalline" voice. In the phrase *"khrustal'nym ot schast'ia"*—the culmination of the imagery at the end of the narrative—the ever-elusive happiness suddenly coalesces into substance.[85] Tolstoi's formulation links this emotion with clarity and stability—parallelling the vision of the One State.[86] The trope of "happiness" is an important one for early Soviet discourse; glass, as the key ingredient of the utopian future, is used to give tangible form to this abstract ideal. While Tolstoi appears to embrace this association wholeheartedly, Zamyatin (like Dostoevsky before him) shows socially engineered "happiness" in a much more ominous light.[87]

Glass is such a pervasive part of D's world that he looks to it when reaching for a metaphor to articulate his inner condition. The first such metaphor occurs in the second entry: D praises the blue sky, "unspoiled by a single cloud," calling it "sterile" and "impeccable." He then falls into an ecstatic reverie about what he believes is the clarity of mind that he has achieved as a citizen of the ultra-regimented One State: "On days like this the whole world is cast of the same impregnable, eternal glass as the Green Wall, as all our buildings." In the original Russian, the words *steril'noe* ("sterile"), *steklo* ("glass"), and *Stena* ("wall") appear in two adjacent sentences; Zamyatin thus uses sound orchestration to create an association between glass, walls, and sterility.

Vladimir Mayakovsky draws on the associations between glass and cold sterility in his vision of the future in *The Bedbug*. The hero of the play, Prisypkin, is frozen alive in 1929 (the year in which the play was written) and "resurrected" fifty years later in a world characterized by "sliding doors of frosted glass" and "glass-fronted buildings." The eponymous bedbug, which becomes Prisypkin's familiar, is caught by scientists and displayed in a glass case. And Prisypkin himself is held captive in a room with "smooth, opalescent, translucent walls"; he complains: "What kind of life is it when you can't even pin a picture of your best girl on the wall? The tacks break on this goddamn glass."[88] Here, as in Zamyatin, the glass wall functions as a denial of eros and human connection.

At the same time, in *We* glass emerges as a metaphor for "human material" in light of certain parallels between glass, the body, and architecture that D explicitly draws.[89] D extols glass as a sign of the superior technological achievement of his civilization and a symbol of the superiority of his fellow citizens. Yet the dangerous potential of glass remains—and D seems to be aware of this, as evident in his use of the word "shards" (*oskolki*) as early as his second entry. D's drafting tool becomes a blade-like weapon that I-330 wields during their programmatic conversation about energy and entropy: "she took from the desk my glass triangle and, as I talked, she kept pressing its sharp edge against her cheek—a white weal would appear on her cheek, then fill with pink color and disappear" (Zamyatin, *My*, 416). It is appropriate for the "heretic" I-330 to reveal the dangerous potential of the very material upon which the One State is founded.

The perfect transparency/purity of glass walls is put into question as D's diary unfolds. Disturbing optical phenomena such as reflections and glare manifest themselves; images of surveillance proliferate as D grows aware of the "Ideological State Apparatus" (ISA) and his position within it.[90] The optical effects of glass serve as a counterpoint to the transparency that the State values. Likewise, the fragility of the glass undercuts the "crystalline" stability that is so necessary to the ISA of the One State.[91] One of the most important optical qualities of glass overlooked by the One State is *reflection*. D starts noticing the reflective qualities of "the mirror-smooth pavement" during the episode in which he sees a woman who takes a tremendous risk in breaking from the ranks—a human "shard" whom he mistakes for I-330. He flings himself towards her but is relieved to see, at the last second, that "It is not she! Not I" (Zamyatin, *My*, 391) In the context of the "mirror-like" pavement, "I" can be read here as an aspect of D's own self.[92] The reflective capacity of the glass surfaces around D allows him to arrive at the realization that there are two selves inside him—a compliant self and a self that longs to rebel.

After an encounter with I-330, D has an epiphany, and declares: "I became glass. I saw—within myself. There were two of me." In the following entry D stands before a mirror and sees himself "clearly, for the first time"—sees himself as an unrecognizable "other" and the mirror, not as a flat reflective surface but a bottomless depth, so that he is looking simultaneously "here" and "there."[93] The mirror reflection that D contemplates plays a crucial role in his transformation from a conformist into a rebel. Zamyatin thus draws attention to the subversive potential of reflective surfaces, and this capacity to shift one's point of view in a dangerous direction is referenced in Scheerbart's manifesto, the sole troubling note in his celebration of glass: "the quicksilver-mirror . . . is dangerous—like poison.[94] Scheerbart turns the visual trickery of the mirror into a sign of its treachery, reinforcing the argument with reference to the toxicity of mercury (which mirrors did, at one point, contain).[95] His unease about mirrors is linked with their capacity to capture and convey the human likeness.

D's recurring references to the optical qualities of glass accompany his growing awareness of glass as the transparent medium through which he sees and that structures all human thought and behavior invisibly. D's language appears as a function of his environment to a striking degree. As Robert Russell notes, D strives for "a transparency of language that would correspond to the transparency of the buildings in the One State. Almost immediately, however, this ideal is compromised by the intrusion of metaphor, and as the diary proceeds, its style reflects the increasingly chaotic state of D-503's mind."[96] It might be more precise to say that it is D's language that becomes chaotic, as D grows more aware of the true nature of his reality and starts to recognize chaos where he once saw only order. The manifestation of the optical properties of glass leads to metaphor-making. Metaphors involve thinking in images: this becomes possible when D starts seeing reflections—representations of his world; in addition, metaphor implies one thing seen in terms of something different, therefore one thing turning into something else. This way of thinking also becomes possible once D starts realizing the changeability of the images in the glass surfaces around him according to subtle shifts of perspective.

Glass plays with vision and transforms it. It can allow one to change one's point of view in the form of windows, telescopes, and microscopes. Zamyatin provides a point-of-view shift that changes the way that his hero perceives the world around him when at the halfway point of the novel, D sees his city from above and compares the glass structures, previously seen as monumental and eternally stable ("crystalline, immutable, eternal—like our new glass"), to ice that is about to thaw and crack (Zamyatin, *My*, 385–86).[97] In the years prior to composing *We*, Zamyatin had worked on building icebreakers for Russia,[98] an experience that inspired his essay, "On My Wives, Icebreakers, and Russia." In the essay, Zamyatin calls the icebreaker an object as peculiarly Russian as a samovar, because only Russia needs icebreakers, surrounded as she is by ice-bound seas; were it not for icebreakers, Russia would be cut off from the rest of the world. Zamyatin calls the icebreaker an "amphibian" creature that dwells in water as well as on dry land—"because ice is, of course, dry land [*susha*]."[99] He opposes ice to liquid—in his view, it is resistant, a solid, immobile material. The descriptions of ice in the essay echo those of the glass structures in *We*: "blue, icy interiors, shards, floes . . . glittering, dispassionate, ruthless ice fields . . . in the dead, blind, indifferent ice."[100] These seemingly objective visual descriptions shade into emotional, subjective ones, attesting to Zamyatin's passionate stance regarding the physical properties of stasis and immobility, and to the degree to which he sees breaking through the ice as an unquestioned imperative.

Zamyatin's essay on icebreakers thus illuminates the metaphor of glass buildings as ice floes in *We*. Alan Myers points out that icebreakers in Newcastle were built in glazed sheds. It is in this environment that the inspiration for the themes and material surroundings of *We* came to Zamyatin.[101] The presence of the glass wall in his work environment may have spurred him to contemplate the scene in terms of oppression and un-freedom.

D's new perspective yields a view of the city as thawing ice, a new metaphor from the natural world that D has previously scorned. D's epiphany suggests that the structure of the State is not as stable and permanent as it seems.[102] Indeed, the ending of the novel proves this to be the case—the Wall has been breached, then repaired, yet rebellions continue to break out in the city. One could say that the One State is deceived by the monolithic appearance of glass, when by its very nature this material is in eternal flux. By analogy, the same is true of language. D begins his journal intending to praise the One State with predictable panegyrics, yet his writing becomes transformed and ultimately transforms him into something he never expected. Glass is not crystalline but amorphous in structure, poised on the boundary between solid and liquid: in fact, it is a solid with a chaotic molecular structure very similar to that of a liquid. It is widely believed that old windows are thicker at the bottom as a result of continual flow downward over the years, although recent research shows that glass flows much too slowly to account for this, and an explanation is rather to be found in old glassmaking techniques.[103] Yet the existence of the myth itself suggests the pervasiveness of belief in the idea that glass is perpetually in motion. In fact, the verbal root of *steklo*, *tek*-, signifies "flow." What material could better embody Zamyatin's permanent revolution?

In one of the final entries, D, studying his world from that same lofty perspective (now in his mind's eye), describes the pavement as a laboratory slide with "infusoria trapped in a drop as transparent as glass" (Zamyatin, *My*, 452). Glass, we are reminded, played a crucial role in the human conquest of nature. Yet this image also suggests D's realization that the world he is living in is still a social *experiment*, not the fully realized and static Eden that he once thought it was.

Glass as an element of material reality in the world of *We* is juxtaposed with glass as a metaphor sought by the narrator to articulate the intangible, yet equally visceral, aspects of his experience in the One State. Zamyatin chooses glass for its inherent ambiguity; its apparently monolithic stability conceals a fragility that threatens the very existence of the totalitarian state. The ending of *We* finds Zamyatin moving toward a way of perceiving glass as an emblem of the precariousness of existence.[104] From an oppressive, monolithic presence, glass becomes transformed into something fraught, tender, a material evocative of humanity rather than serving as its negation.

EISENSTEIN'S *GLASS HOUSE*: AMBIVALENCE ABOUT THE GLASS ENEMY

Khlebnikov and Zamyatin, we recall, were working during a time when fellow artists were captivated by the visual potential of transparent materials. In Russia, this fascination can be seen in Tatlin's counter-reliefs; Gabo's constructions; Goncharova's and Larionov's depictions of glass surfaces in paintings; Exter's set designs; and Rodchenko's photography of translucent surfaces. Bowlt places these projects within the broader context of "an international discovery of glass—of transparency and invisibility—as major artistic components."[105] At the same time, architects and city planners looked to large-scale glass constructions as a means to bring about the longed-for utopia.

> In its capacity to . . . connect the inside and the outside, glass serves a democratic purpose. Constructivist architects realized that glass could expose the function of a building, could emphasize the interconnectedness of human society and, therefore, undermine the notion of bourgeois privacy and individual space.[106]

These ideological implications were not lost on Sergei Eisenstein, who planned to ruthlessly expose the workings of bourgeois society in a film taking place in a glass skyscraper, using all-glass sets. A fusion of German and American modernist architecture served as the inspiration for Eisenstein's film project (1927–30), *The Glass House*. This dark and disturbing project resonates with Zamyatin's anti-utopia and throws into question the luminous dreams of Khlebnikov, in which the transparency and utter visibility enabled by glass walls appear as unquestioned ideals.

Looking at the work of Eisenstein brings to the foreground another crucial (and new) use for glass in the early twentieth century: filmmaking. Film, after all, was an art form and a technology that could not have come into being without the existence of glass. Even at the birth of photography, glass slides preceded celluloid in capturing fleeting images—akin to glass killing jars for butterflies. While architects dreamed of covering the globe with glass palaces, Eisenstein dreamed of making a film called *The Glass House* that itself would entail building a glass house. In this film, life in a transparent skyscraper takes the form not of utopia but of a grotesque tragicomedy. This latter characterization could well apply to Eisenstein's struggle, from the inception of the idea to the very end of his life, to make *The Glass House* a reality.[107] Ultimately I hope to show that fragments of his unrealized project can be glimpsed in his other films.

Eisenstein set out to make *The Glass House* a critique of bourgeois society, with the denizens of the skyscraper standing for a microcosm of Western capitalist society as a whole. He would use the transparent sets to create ideological montage within the same frame—something that he could not have done without glass. Here is an explicit instance of glass in the service of ideology. But his project can also be seen as a commentary on the society of surveillance coming into being in the Soviet Union.

The ambiguity around the political interpretation of the *Glass House* project resonates with a curious tension that exists in Eisenstein's filmmaking practice. On the one hand, he relied on glass in a variety of forms to promote his aesthetic and ideological agendas. Thus, he created expressionistic cinematic effects with the help of special lenses, lights, even mirrors: for example, Eduard Tisse, his cinematographer, used sunlight reflected off a large mirror as a spotlight of sorts, "marking out hard-edged blocks of space or endowing objects and faces with sculptural gleams."[108] What Eisenstein envisioned for *The Glass House* was to continue to use glass for meaningful visual effects, now on a larger scale—moving beyond lenses and mirrors to entire sets made of the material. On the other hand, glass in his films frequently carries negative associations: glass objects appear in association with negative character types; through montage Eisenstein constructs a "glass enemy." Yet there are moments when Eisenstein betrays a fascination with glass, perhaps because he realized that he would not be able to make films without this material.

Eisenstein particularly valued the 28mm lens because it allowed him to create ecstatic imagery, such as that found in Piranesi's architectural engravings and El Greco's depiction of bodies, as well as the "protoplasmic writhings of Disney's characters. [Eisenstein called it] 'the ecstatic lens par excellence.'"[109] But what exactly did he mean by "ecstasy"? For Eisenstein, the visual distortion enabled by optical lenses is a way to achieve the palpable illusion of his ideal—a body's endless metamorphosis, boundless potential for taking on new forms.[110] Eisenstein notes that in working on his film on collectivization, *The Old and the New*, he discovered that the 28mm lens, typically used by filmmakers to render objects in the foreground and background with equal depth of focus, had another capacity, "which previously had carefully been skirted, or at least carefully avoided during the late 1920s. It is the ability of this lens to produce perspective distortion."[111] Eisenstein cites examples of such distortion in his film and argues that the 28mm lens was what propelled the depicted objects

> "to go beyond themselves," beyond their natural bounds of volume and form. In this the theme of man resounded anew, with its own "plasticity," where aided by industry—under a new socialist regime—by means of his own creative effort, the age-old established norms and forms "of the idiocy of rural life" (Marx) were forced to go "beyond themselves," into new aspects, forms and qualities of socialist agriculture.[112]

Notably, Eisenstein links the aesthetic effects with ideological transformation. For the filmmaker, the optical effect of the 28mm lens contributes to a feeling of ecstasy, which he defines analytically as "being beside oneself," in the viewer. This out-of-body experience is a step toward a heightened political consciousness, and ultimately transformation of the self.

In April 1926, during a stay in Berlin, Eisenstein caught a first glimmering of *The Glass House*. Aside from a childhood trip to Paris, it was Eisenstein's first time abroad, and the director eagerly opened his eyes to everything around him. He and Tisse had been sent to Berlin by Soyuzkino to learn about advances in Western cinematography and to attend the German premiere of *The Battleship Potemkin*. They stayed at the Hotel Hessler, a glass high-rise building.[113] These living quarters put Eisenstein in a futuristic frame of mind, as did a visit to the set of Fritz Lang's dystopian film *Metropolis*. According to Oksana Bulgakowa, "The Glass House was intended as a polemical response not only to Lang's film, but also to Bruno Taut and Mies van der Rohe's glass architecture"; moreover, for Eisenstein the edifice served "as an architectonic image of America."[114]

In January 1927, he elucidated his vision into a film scenario: an ironic view of America (and American self-images perpetuated in Hollywood films) through the walls of a glass skyscraper. Subsequently this plan would evolve into something broader: an anti-utopia about the isolation of man in a technocratic capitalist society.[115] Eisenstein intended to take Hollywood by storm and film *The Glass House* in the United States; he even began negotiations with several glass factories in Pittsburgh to provide transparent floors, walls, and ceilings for the film sets (the factories reported that such sets could, in fact, be built).[116] The action of the film was to take place in an entirely transparent apartment building whose residents are unaware of their exposure and utter lack of privacy until a catastrophe awakens them to the truth. At that moment, however, eye-opening does not lead to a flourishing of conscience; instead, they become callous, voyeuristic witnesses of unspeakable crimes: the film shows images in which "walls, floor, and ceiling seem made of faces."

Eisenstein realized that the physical properties of glass would enable his ideological critique: transparent walls and floors would allow the filmmaker to capture perspectives in depth, overlapping images, and unexpected points of view, all of these visual devices helping to lay bare and problematize spatial and social relations—social stratification, poverty, and abuse existing side by side with luxury and wealth—that might have otherwise seemed normal. The transparency of the sets would make it possible for Eisenstein to achieve within a single frame the effects of juxtaposition and conflict that he had previously obtained through "ideological montage" of a series of shots. Eisenstein's original scenario for his early film *Strike* featured a montage sequence cross-cutting between two scenes: a worker drowning in a cauldron of molten metal and a woman bathing in champagne.[117] Now, glass sets would enable Eisenstein to achieve such shocking and tendentious juxtapositions within the same frame. For the premiere Eisenstein wanted to use a "monster screen" four times the size of the usual one, that would accommodate several actions occurring simultaneously, a juxtaposition that was essential to the driving conceit of the film: a transparent building as a model of a society.[118]

Eisenstein insisted that his project was not at all fantastic—such glass houses did exist, or soon would; he argued to his fellow filmmaker Ivor Montague that American workplaces were already characterized by total visibility of the workers, leading to a loss of privacy and an acceptance thereof. Montague comments: "Structurally, architecturally, his analogy did indeed exist. . . . But nobody could see it. Nobody could see that this was happening or could happen."[119] Eisenstein wanted to make invisible social relations visible, and the filmmaker shared with Khlebnikov and Zamyatin the gift of prescience.

Eisenstein's notes from 1928 elucidate the structure of the film: it is to be in five acts, from "Unconsciousness" to "Tragedies and Catastrophes," with an epilogue about the destruction of the house. These notes also show a shift in the direction of unmistakably ideological filmmaking, as Eisenstein searches for a way to realize his dream of an "intellectual cinema": thus, he remarks that what started out as a social comedy is becoming a "comedy of [Marxist] theses."[120]

This social critique via architecture can be compared with Mayakovsky's poem "Neboskreb v razreze" ("Skyscraper in Cutaway View")[121]—written in 1925, one year before the inception of the *Glass House* project. What Eisenstein planned to do through film and transparent sets, Mayakovsky does verbally, laying bare the seedy and sinister goings-on in the eponymous American skyscraper. In so doing, he plays with the inherent violence in "skyscraper," a concept retained in translation as "*neboskreb*," by coupling it with the slash of "*razrez*" (the root—*rez*—means "cut")—also underscored by the violent imagery in the poem. Conflict was a central component of Eisenstein's aesthetics, and he would recognize the inherent violence couched in the linguistic formulation of "skyscraper"/*neboskreb*.

According to a note Eisenstein made on September 17, 1927, *The Glass House* was "invented in Berlin. Hotel Hessler; Kantstrasse. Under the influence of attempts in glass architecture."[122] Four years later, Eisenstein came across an article in the *New York Times Magazine* (June 29, 1930) on Frank Lloyd Wright, who had just designed a tower (also fated to be unrealized) that struck Eisenstein as the embodiment of his own Glass House (Kleiman, "Stekliannyi dom," 106).

In the first set of notes, starting in January 1927, Eisenstein emphasizes the optical quality of glass, its capacity to mediate what one sees of the world (recalling Zamyatin's approach in *We*). Glass sets would allow him "to take the most commonplace actions and change the point of view. To take the most traditional types and psychological collisions and change the point of view" (Kleiman, "Stekliannyi dom," 96). One of the ways he planned to "change the point of view" was to film from unfamiliar angles, for example, from underneath, which would render familiar actions grotesque—thus exploding the status quo. Indeed, he writes in his notes of the following year that his film would do battle against automatism. In the preceding quotation, the phrase "to change the point of view" appears in English; Eisenstein thus jarringly switches languages mid-sentence to underscore the idea of changing the point of view. He uses a total of four languages in his notes, while the title of the work oscillates between the English "Glass House" and the German "Glashaus"—pointing to the two architectural traditions that had the strongest impact on his project. Thus the ideological montage within the same frame that Eisenstein envisioned for this film has its analogue in the linguistic code-switching that seems like second nature to the director.

Again recalling Zamyatin's practice, Eisenstein frequently associates glass with coldness: "The coldness of things. The coldness of glass par excellence [*Kholod veshchei. Kholod stekla* par excellence]" (Kleiman, "Stekliannyi dom," 96). (Later he makes the synesthetical suggestion of "lyrical scenes with frosted and corrugated glass" to counterbalance "the coldness of smooth glass walls" [Kleiman, "Stekliannyi dom," 98].) He also speaks of "a nightmare of smooth glass" in his later notes. What Eisenstein may have seen as nightmarish about an expanse of smooth glass is the reflective capacity whereby the human image is held captive, and the seemingly endless expanse of ice wherein life itself is trapped (this would echo Zamyatin's glass/ice analogy). Indeed, Eisenstein himself felt trapped throughout his career, and never yet as keenly as in the year in which he wrote this note.

Eisenstein imagined a prologue to the film that shows glass as infinite metamorphosis: "Prologue—symphony of glass (objectless). Glassblowing gives shape to all the forms. Glass strands and filaments are stretching out." At this point the melted glass, with its boundless potential, recalls the foam from whence Aphrodite emerged and to which Mandelstam urged her to return in his 1910 poem "Silentium." Then gradually the quality of "ecstatic plasmatic plasticity" so highly valued by Eisenstein gives way to concrete constructions: "surfaces, facets, objects, a glass automobile (saw it once in a magazine)—a house" (Kleiman, "Stekliannyi dom," 96).

In an essay from 1940, Eisenstein argues that the appeal of Walt Disney's animated characters stems from their changeable quality: they possess the capacity for what he calls "'plasmaticness," able to cast off one form and take on any other and thus behaving like "primordial protoplasm."[123] Subsequently he defines ecstasy as the overcoming of the boundaries of embodiment: "Ecstasy is the perception and experience of the initial 'state of infinite potential' [*pervichnoi 'vsevozmozhnosti'*]—the element of 'becoming'—the 'plasmaticness' of existence out of which anything can develop."[124] The very word "plasmaticness" illustrates Eisenstein's principle of ecstasy, as he has to overcome linguistic boundaries in order to coin it.

In a later version of the film's prologue, the history of glass is presented from its earliest times, with "decorations, glass beads, glass chandeliers, monocles" typifying what Eisenstein called "silly uses of glass" to contemporary times when glass took the form of "cashiers' booths, glass automobiles, glass coffins, glass catafalques, glass furniture, a glass wall, glass . . . glass . . . glass . . . a glass house." This description recalls Lomonosov's sense of wonder at the way in which glass gives rise to "proliferating forms" (to use Barthes's terminology) and Khlebnikov's celebration of the protean qualities of glass. At the same time, these objects are problematic, and freighted with oppressive potential, evoking commerce and commodities accessible to only a few (thus, cars were seldom seen on the streets of Moscow in the 1920s, and they belonged only to the privileged); dynamism gives way to stasis and its ultimate manifestation—burial.

In Eisenstein's film scenario, glass evolves from infinite potential into discrete, isolated forms. The motif of isolation (of things and ultimately persons) is a crucial element in Eisenstein's strategic use of glass. This material oscillates between visibility and invisibility and makes palpable the unseen walls that divide human beings in society. In a set of notes dating from December 1927 to January 1928, Eisenstein includes a shot of falling snow juxtaposed with the "tropical" furnishings of an interior. By using the word "tropical," Eisenstein lays bare the bizarreness of greenhouses that allow tropical plants to flourish in wintry climes, and underscores the use to which glass has been put in the modern world: it is that which allows us to create *divisions*, as in the case of the arbitrary, abusive divisions between the classes (Dostoevsky used glass for a similar purpose in "The Boy at Christ's Christmas Party," discussed in chapter 4).

Eisenstein also plans to make heavy objects, such as a piano, seem as if they are soaring or hovering ("*effekty 'reianiia'*") by shining a light onto the glass surface that supports them, and thus making it seem to disappear. (Eisenstein planned to alternate the scenes of "hovering" with ones in which the glass glimmers with light effects, creating a contrasting psychological ambiance—"the 'play' of all the glass objects [*'igra' vsego stekliannogo*]"—switching the invisibility on and off.) Why would he want to achieve this "hovering" effect? From a personal perspective, it may have something to do with the desire to transcend the self and one's limitations that always accompanies the urge to take flight. From a more consciously political point of view, the "hovering effect" may be linked with the attempt to take commodities that have such weight, gravity, importance in the life of the capitalist society, and to expose how insubstantial they really are. In a later set of notes from 1928, Eisenstein describes a room in the Glass House "with furniture in the petit-bourgeois style. A room with ultra-thingy things [*s ul'traveshchnymi veshchami*]" (Kleiman, "Stekliannyi dom," 108). It is the materiality and weightiness of these commodities that the "hovering effect" aims to dissolve.

The above strategy can be seen as part of Eisenstein's overall aim of exposing the capitalist bourgeois status quo as constructed and artificial, and to show the poverty of the capitalist, "individualist" way of life, the spiritual emptiness behind the lavishly appointed interiors—the nakedness of the emperor. (Eisenstein himself alludes to that fairy tale in his notes.) Indeed, nakedness is a central leitmotif in the planned film. Thus, the second set of notes describes a scene in which a character serving as a Christ figure preaches to a well-dressed audience that gradually becomes naked as he implores them to "bare (their) souls"—a typical moment of playful blasphemy. Visibility for Eisenstein seems to be linked with voyeurism and more specifically nakedness. Is this laying-bare more about eroticism or violence—the humiliation, vulnerability of the exposed body? Subsequent evolution of the project suggests that Eisenstein was more interested in the latter interpretation.[125]

While Eisenstein stated that he had never read Zamyatin's *We* (true or not, this would be a politically expedient claim), there are, as we have seen, a number of parallels between the two works. Eisenstein's project also resonates with Zamyatin's novel in its treatment of opacity. In the latter work, the lowered shades that are used to conceal sexual activity, a relic of bourgeois respectability, constitute the only non-transparent architectural element in the One State; in the former work, Eisenstein's first set of notes specify that the doors in the Glass House be opaque, as a dig at philistine conventionality that is, at heart, meaningless: "As for the doors, make them solid [*A dveri sdelat' material'nymi*]. A strong symbol of conventionality" (Kleiman, "Stekliannyi dom," 97). Note that he uses the adjective "solid" (*material'nyi*), literally "material" to signify "not made of glass." Indeed, the manifesto explicating the Monument to the Third International did not count glass among the "earthly materials"—the material, in that text and in Eisenstein's scenario, offers a way to transcend the earth, an ecstatic transport out of earthbound captivity.

What seems paradoxical about Eisenstein's plan to show things from unusual vantage points that would only be enabled by the all-glass sets (for example, a woman hides a clandestine lover beneath a pile of laundry, and we watch his undignified contortions from beneath as he attempts to stay hidden) is that by so doing he would make the viewer be guilty of the sort of voyeurism for which the film condemns its characters; consider the sketch that shows a love scene rendered vulgar by being viewed through a "water closet," thus framing the sex act by the lavatory. (See figure 25.) Eisenstein sketches another scene in which a crowd watches an act of violence and the glass wall becomes all eyes, then all hands—as the viewers cannot bear to look anymore—and then all hands with eyes peering through the fingers, as curiosity takes over. In a later set of notes (written in English in New York, just before his ill-fated visit to Hollywood), Eisenstein plans a scene from act 1: "the man who beats his wife and 4 rooms around—seeing, but not noticing it" (Kleiman, "Stekliannyi dom," 107). It is important for Eisenstein to establish early on that the transparency of the walls does *not* lead to a moral regeneration in those who dwell within, contrary to the hopes of the architects of his time.

The Glass House becomes a container for bottled-up violence; the very fragility of its walls hints at potential destruction. When violence breaks out, it is always accompanied by voyeurism, either explicitly, as when a crowd watches "a society lady burn up" (Eisenstein adds a telling detail: "the glass doesn't crack"—the harrowing scene has no effect on the impassive upholders of the status quo), or implicitly, when, in the early scenes, the apartment dwellers are oblivious to one another, and the film viewer is placed into the position of the voyeur. In another projected scene, a broken faucet causes a man's cubicle to fill up with water; afraid of opening the door and flooding the adjacent rooms, the man "drowns in front of everyone" (Kleiman, "Stekliannyi dom," 99). The victim is done in by the indifference of others, as well as by his own misplaced sense of propriety. In this episode, water takes the place of fire, but the violence is ever-present.

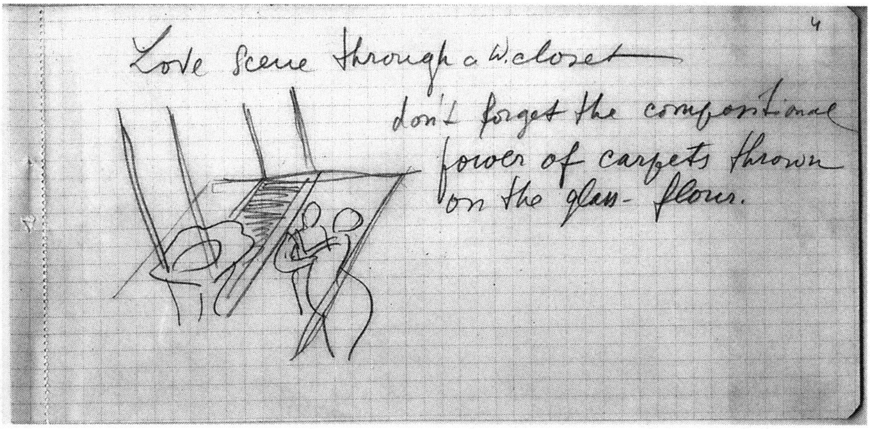

Figure 25. Love scene from Sergei Eisenstein's *The Glass House*, 1927–30. 1923-2-162, l. 64, Russian State Archive of Literature and Art (RGALI).

Eisenstein strives to use the glass sets to achieve other visual effects aside from that of ideological montage within a single frame. A few are purely expressionistic, such as the cubical rooms filled with smoke alternating with empty ones. More often, Eisenstein aims to shock the viewer out of his complacency, as in a scene in which a resident hammers a nail into the glass wall out of "philistine convention" (Kleiman, "Stekliannyi dom," 99) to take place just when the viewer may have gotten used to the glass surroundings and begun to take them for granted. At that moment, the sharp shock assails the viewer; indeed, in his polemic with Vertov, Eisenstein declared that film should function not as a "cine-eye" but as a "cine-fist." In a variation on the hammer-and-nail image, the second set of notes includes a "machine gun tracing a design of bullet holes across the glass" (Kleiman, "Stekliannyi dom," 101). Here, the motifs of violence and voyeurism are brought together in a new way: the medium of viewing itself is shattered, thus doing violence to the viewer.

In the set of notes written in America, the last substantial piece of writing devoted to *The Glass House*, Eisenstein develops the pathos of the early scene in which a man beats his wife. As before, "no one notices"; but then, suddenly, one man tries to intervene: "Mr. X rushes to help her and hits his head against the glass. Down below, a woman is ironing (she raises her head). Up above, [someone] washes the floor and looks" (Kleiman, "Stekliannyi dom," 108). Here Eisenstein uses the transparency of the glass sets to juxtapose several kinds of motion: striking (the man hitting his wife, her rescuer hitting his head) and stroking (the woman ironing—the Russian word, *gladit*, also means "caressing"—and another washing the floor). The simultaneous exposure of the contrasting actions allows Eisenstein to show how easily a tender touch can turn violent, how quickly good intentions can go bad. The sexual violence in a variant of the scenario—the same Mr. X "sends the Robot to rape the poor girl who does not reciprocate his feelings"—casts the moments of nudity and "laying bare" in the film in a sinister light.

At the end of the film Eisenstein imagines the Glass House smashed to pieces at the peak of conflict and uncontrollable passions: his note from May 1930 reads, in English: "Part 5. Impossibility to continue like that, smashing of the house"; the House is eventually replaced by an "ideal communal settlement," an idea he himself sheepishly admits is *"un peu orthodoxe"* (Kleiman, "Stekliannyi dom," 97)." It seems that Eisenstein was more interested in the breaking of the Glass House than in what might be built in its stead; indeed, the smashability of glass was one of the attributes compelling him to explore this contradictory material.

The story of the glass house was to begin as a "new paradise" (a parallel to the "glass paradise" in *We*) ("first, life in nakedness [*zhizn' v obnazhenii*], then the nightmare of the eyes and visibility, and the panicked desire to be covered") and end with a new apocalypse. In a note dated May 22, 1946, in his last written reference to the project, Eisenstein called *The Glass House* his "mystery play"; this can be understood to refer to the architectural, multilayered setup that presents social life in cutaway view, to the combination of satirical and sermonizing elements, as well as to the subject matter: the miraculous creation and apocalyptic destruction of the Glass House.[126]

During his 1930 visit to Hollywood, Eisenstein opened up to fellow director Josef von Sternberg about the dangers Soviet artists faced back home. Von Sternberg recalls:

> When I asked him how his country rewarded good films he told me jokingly, though he might well have been serious, that when a director made a good film in Russia he was rewarded by having a window added to his room and if a film was bad he was shot for treason. I enquired as to the numbers of windows in his room, and he answered, one.[127]

Eisenstein's irony is telling: the image of the window here suggests an illusory freedom (visible, but not otherwise accessible) granted to filmmakers whose vision happened to match that of their state benefactor—indeed, a window, by virtue of its frame, constructs vision in a very particular way.

The Glass House may have been overtly "an ironic view of America through glass walls," but it was more than that. It was Eisenstein's most obsessive contemplation of his own craft, which taught people the right ways to "see" but also trained them to become voyeurs ("Major line can be built on the gradual growth of 'seeing' by the inhabitants," he wrote in 1927). And

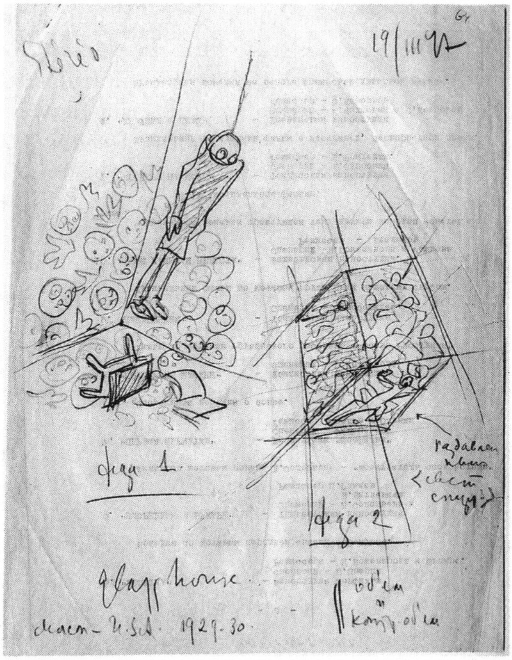

Figure 26. Suicide scene from Sergei Eisenstein's *The Glass House*, 1927–30. 1923-2-162, l. 4, Russian State Archive of Literature and Art (RGALI).

although Eisenstein insists that the surveillance he depicts is "characteristic of the American way of life," it is hard not to find echoes of life closer to home in passages such as the following: "Suddenly they realize that [the transparency of] these walls can be 'used.' . . . A series of crimes takes place. Blackmail attempts . . . Spying on neighbor's documents, affairs, break-up of families . . . Suicide in a single room with light on. He sees no one, but all eyes are on him."[128] (See figure 26.) Indeed, increasing censorship and official surveillance were already plaguing the Soviet film industry by 1927.[129] In the fall of the preceding year, mass arrests had swept up many of Eisenstein's fellow film workers, including Alexander Khanzhonkov and Yakov Bliokh, two of his former associates.[130]

Upon his return to the Soviet Union, Eisenstein encountered a hostile ideological climate in the arts, which were coming increasingly under the sway of state functionaries clinging to the party line. Eisenstein found it impossible to continue work on *The Glass House*, let alone to hope that it would ever be made in his lifetime. For years he struggled to win back the credibility he had lost as a Soviet filmmaker, ultimately triumphing with

Alexander Nevsky, a historical pageant read at the time as a glorification of the Stalinist regime (the same was true of the reception of the later *Ivan the Terrible I*, though not its successor). Before this miraculous comeback, however, Eisenstein experienced the depths of despair. In May 1937, pilloried for his work on the never-completed film *Bezhin Meadow*, Eisenstein took a rest cure for the sake of his frayed nerves and ailing heart; immediately afterward he was to begin work on a new, politically acceptable screenplay. It was then that he wrote to his wife, Pera Atasheva: "I feel like I'm in a glass coffin, could that be why I dreamed of the Glass House?"[131]

Eisenstein could only survive by turning his talent to the craft of panegyric. *The Glass House* was many things—a caustic critique of society (but which one?), a psychological drama, an unprecedented visual experiment—but it was no panegyric, and thus, Eisenstein would never see it built. Yet fragments of his longed-for project can be glimpsed in several of the films that Eisenstein brought to completion, all done prior to his trip to the West, when the director could still hope that Hollywood would someday make *The Glass House* a reality.

In Eisenstein's first feature-length film, *Strike* (1925), depicting a strike from 1905 as a paradigmatic example from the history of the workers' movement, glass imagery frequently has self-referential associations with the equipment and craft of filmmaking. Indeed, Eisenstein noted that in *Strike* his attention was focused on "mastering the 'specifics' of cinema and on re-educating [his] thinking away from the theatrical to the cinematic."[132] Here Eisenstein uses glass for optical effects, most prominently reflection. This technique can be read as an implicit commentary on the debate about documentary versus fictional cinema, the question of whether filmmakers should merely record and reflect reality, like a mirror, or whether they should use creative editing techniques to craft tendentious messages out of the collision of unrelated images.

In *Strike*, a series of mirrors command the camera's attention, but each of them deviates from its conventional function as a reflecting surface in which an individual contemplates his own image; this is fitting in light of the film's depiction of what happens when workers go on strike, and their machines stop. The mirror is, after all, a form of technology, and its function, too, gets subverted by Eisenstein's film. When the strikers' luck begins to change, a desperately poor worker is shown taking his family's only mirror to the flea market to be sold: he tosses it down on the floor on top of a pile of clothes, and the mirror lies face-up, chaotically reflecting the space around it. Reflecting surfaces dominate the screen at the beginning of the following sequence, gesturing at the reversal of fortune that is a major structuring motif throughout the film. A factory spy checks his reflection in an oval street mirror; we next see a large glass sphere in which the bustling street life is reflected and the spy Fox is "caught," allowing the two strike leaders to spot him. These workers use mirrors in a strategic way—not to study their own faces, but to watch for danger and protect the collective.[133]

In the transparent sets of *The Glass House*, Eisenstein hoped to represent unjust social relations spatially, and more broadly, to create ironic juxtapositions within the same frame. We can already see him striving for such an effect in the final sequence of *Strike*, "The Liquidation." The workers' building under siege is shown in a cutaway view: we see several stories at once, the mounted police attacking the scurrying inhabitants, violence on top of violence. This sequence, which allows us to glimpse "through" the house to the nightmarish goings-on within it, can be seen as a precedent to *The Glass House*, for it creates precisely the sort of effect, and social critique, that Eisenstein wanted to achieve with that project. The sequence allows us to look into the building as if with X-ray vision, to see the oppressive social relations that are usually obscured.

Even in his earliest film, Eisenstein was intrigued by the possibility of multilayeredness in cinematic depiction. He explains his use of "trick photography" in a sequence in *Strike*:

> The scene showed how a "mobile meeting" of the future strike committee was held, under the guise of an innocent evening's ramble through the countryside . . . In those days I was altogether fascinated by double exposure, and in particular by the double exposure of objects differing widely in scale. Perhaps this was a lingering sympathy for Cubism's use of multi-level space.[134]

In this sequence, the double-layered image makes literal the duplicity of the conspiring workers. Eisenstein declares that this layering is essential to the process by means of which "every phenomenon reveals itself" as being made up of "two inseparably united levels . . . (1) a depiction of the phenomenon itself through which (2) a generalization about its content also emerges as though by double exposure."[135] A year after the completion of *Strike*, Eisenstein began his search for a way to achieve the ultimate multilayered depiction of phenomena within the transparent sets of *The Glass House*.

Eisenstein's first set of notes pertaining to *The Glass House* date from January-February 1927, a time when he was consumed with the filming of *October*.[136] This convergence of projects can help to shed light on the riot of glass imagery that appears in the latter film, consistently in an ideologically motivated fashion. In a sequence in which Lenin goes underground, we do not actually see the great leader (just his shadowy outline), but we do see a close-up of his little teakettle hanging over a campfire. Lenin's humble kettle, metonymically linked with the Bolshevik leader, is implicitly contrasted with the lavish emblem-embellished glassware from which the

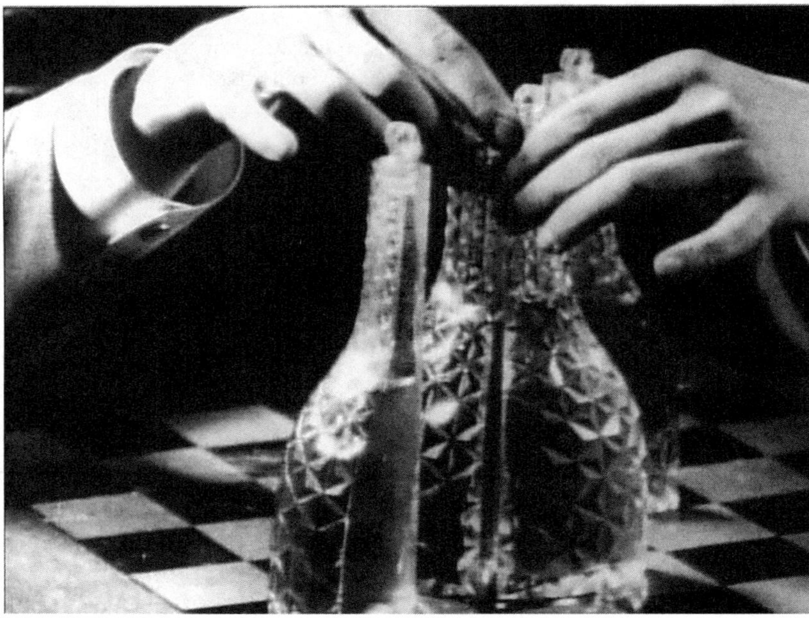

Figure 27. Kerensky's hands assembling the crystal decanter, from Sergei Eisenstein's *October*, 1928.

enemies of the revolution drink.[137] This Lenin sequence is followed by the one depicting Kerensky in the chambers of Empress Alexandra. Then, a shot of a crystal chandelier (which will later shudder at the salvoes of the revolution) acts as the seed crystal for the next sequence. Following a shot of Kerensky juxtaposed with Napoleon, images of tall crystal wineglasses bearing tsarist insignia alternate with those of armed toy soldiers. Both wineglasses and soldiers stand in formation at a diagonal to the screen. After a series of such juxtapositions, we see hands moving together the four chambers of a crystal wine decanter that stands on a chessboard, followed by extreme close-ups of the detailed cut crystal pattern on the surface of the decanter.[138] (See figure 27.) The hands take an imperial crown out of a secret compartment in the chessboard. Now we can see that it is Kerensky fitting the crown to the top of the assembled decanter. He places the crown on top and gives it a twist. Then there is a jump cut to a factory whistle, a close-up of the crown, and another shot of the whistle. An intertitle reads: "The Revolution is in danger!" Kerensky lets go of the decanter and folds his hands.

What do we make of this emphasis on glass vessels in this central sequence of the film? As Bordwell notes, "The toys, cutlery, plates, glassware, and other luxury goods are evidently in the palace, but they are filmed in such intense close-ups or framed against such neutral backgrounds that they seem to hover in a purely symbolic space."[139] Through this emphasis, it is clear that Eisenstein intends to imbue the glass objects with significance and to force viewers to consider what that significance might be. The objects take on particular meaning in juxtaposition with other images.[140]

Eisenstein's close friend Victor Shklovsky objected to the way in which the director made pieces of imperial crystal into key players in *October*. In a 1929 lecture, he argued that the accumulation of "dishes" ended up obscuring what really mattered: "Beyond the objects one could not see the 'insignificant' event of the October Revolution." Three years later, in an article, Shklovsky addressed Eisenstein directly with a withering characterization of his film as "Your rebellion of the dishes in *October*—that amazing battle against things in the Palace."[141] The great critic would have dismissed the sequence of toy soldiers juxtaposed with glassware as a particularly egregious example of Eisenstein's distraction from the human actors in the revolution in favor of inanimate bric-a-brac. Yet I would argue that this sequence, far from misguided, is integral to the film and shows Eisenstein in full control of his artistic strategy. Eisenstein carries over his insight about the "coldness of things" and "the coldness of glass par excellence" from the *Glass House* notes into the scenario of *October*.

Eisenstein's trademark "montage-image" is the result of the collision of two images. As Yury Tsivian explains: "in Eisenstein's art theory the smallest indivisible unit always consists of two things, not one. What constitutes the structure of the work is for him not A or B, but the difference, the tension growing between them in their twin cell . . . The montage-image harbors mutually conflicting features."[142] Thus what is important is the way the glassware is juxtaposed against other elements, that is, the toy soldiers, the Napoleon statue, and Kerensky. The sequence conveys that the leader of the Provisional Government is flashy, fragile, and empty. If we ignore the surface luster, we can see right through him. The linkage of the toy soldiers and the drinking glasses suggests that his power is illusory.

Notably, imperial emblems appear at the very beginning of the film, when the statue of Alexander III is about to be pulled down, with shots of the orb and other imperial attributes with which the statue is covered. *October* is, in fact, about a battle between different iconographies.[143] The film is replete with mythological, allegorical figures, statues of emperors and gods, and military crosses. The trick sequence in which the Alexander statue reconstructs itself, symbolizing the onset of political reaction, can be seen as prefigured in the image of the four imperial decanters coming together in Kerensky's hands.

The destruction of glass is what signals the impending wave of violence that will topple the old regime. The sequence begins with shots hitting the facade of the palace. Streetlights are smashed. The women of the "death battalion" throw down their guns one by one. During a barrage of gunfire at the palace, we see a shuddering crystal chandelier in close-up: the revolutionary violence has penetrated inside the imperial stronghold. Later Eisenstein would admit that this effect was the most successful of all his attempts to viscerally communicate the echoing sound of the blasts outside. Indeed, the crystal chandelier shivers as a human being would, glass conveying the sensitivity of skin or psyche. Peasant women try to raid the wine cellar, but Aurora sailors wrest the bottles away and demonstratively smash them. The destruction of the imperial wine bottles serves as the climax of the shattering glass in this sequence (a visual answer to the earlier sequence linking wineglasses, toy soldiers, and Kerensky)—a way to convey through the senses the enormity of what has really been shattered.[144]

Eisenstein's work on *The Old and the New* (1929), as was the case with *October*, again coincided with a feverish bout of note-taking on and thinking through *The Glass House*. It was at this time that the director composed the first comprehensive outline of *The Glass House*. As in earlier films, in *The Old and the New*, the privileged classes are associated with glass objects upon which the camera dwells: a shiny windowpane and a kvass barrel from which the barrel-shaped kulak takes a leisurely drink. Both examples embody the accusatory way in which Eisenstein planned to use glass in *The Glass House*.

Yet this material is not consistently presented as negative in the film. Vast amounts of glass are to be found at the Sovkhoz where the cattle are housed. Kleiman characterizes the Sovkhoz as a utopian fantasy: Eisenstein's script imagines it as an organic union of a high-tech dairy farm, mechanical station, and breeding lab. The set of the Sovkhoz was designed by Constructivist architect A. K. Burov, who "gave it the appearance of a palace of glass and concrete."[145] Eisenstein instructed Burov to build the set "in the style of Le Corbusier's buildings."[146] This set was the closest that Eisenstein came to building his *Glass House*—but what a difference ideologically. Rather than expose social abuses, here the glass walls juxtapose indoor and outdoor scenes of harmonious labor, embodying ideals of communication, honesty, and purity; akin to mirrors, they act to multiply the bounty.

The mirror images in Eisenstein's films resonate hauntingly with the director's account of a cryptic episode from the time he served in the Red Army in the spring of 1919, recorded in his memoirs from the 1940s:

> I sleep on the surface of a mirror in Dvinsk. In the flat hastily allotted to me—after the Red Army has taken Dvinsk—there are no beds left. . . . But a mirrored wardrobe stands proudly in the empty room. The wardrobe lies

> on its back. A straw mattress lies down on top of the mirrored surface of its doors that reflect the world. On the mattress I lie. My God, how much I'd like to make a metaphorical interpretation or an image out of this! But nothing comes. So I shall leave myself lying on the straw mattress, placed between me and the mirrors of the wardrobe doors.[147]

No "image" comes to Eisenstein as he contemplates the memory, and indeed, by covering the mirror "that reflected the world" with straw and then with his own body, the future filmmaker effectively prevents any image from emerging; the straw mattress, the Red Army's contribution to the decor of the expropriated room, serves to block his access to the mirror world. At the same time, sleeping on a mirror is akin to sleeping atop an abyss—not only because of the fragility of glass, but because the space beyond the mirror, *zazerkal'e*, looms as a chasm in literary works and folklore stretching back in time for centuries. The concluding lines of this passage suggest that the terrifying sensation of lying stretched out over an abyss is still with the middle-aged Eisenstein as he writes these lines, a coded reference to his fate as a visionary artist under the Stalinist regime.

Chapter Six

Light in Captivity: The Glass Object as Ideological Spectacle

> Depending on the weather and time of day, the star on the Vodovoznaya tower has the most varied hues. In the morning, when the sun shines, its gold mounting shimmers, and its red glass panes grow brighter. At midday, the color of the glass panes becomes more concentrated. At twilight, they take on yet another hue.
> —*Pravda*, October 4, 1937

IN 1925, NIKOLAI Popov, the chief of the Moscow real estate directorate, published an editorial in the newspaper *Izvestiia* in which he called for "as much glass . . . as possible" in the cityscape of the new socialist metropolis.[1] But, as we have seen, not all architects and officials championed glass at this time—it was, in fact, a polarizing material. The controversy over glass architecture in Moscow continued into the 1930s. A key example of this controversy was the Tsentrosoiuz (Central Union of Consumer Cooperatives) building, extolled as the expression of a "new communist culture" when it was first commissioned from architect Le Corbusier in the 1920s.[2] (See figure 28.) For Le Corbusier, a building flooded with natural light was essential to express the spirit of the new socialist world under construction, and his design gave pride of place to horizontal windows. In *Sovremennaia arkhitektura* in 1926, he reported: "Experiments have shown that buildings with such windows get eight times as much light as buildings with vertical windows." The building took on an iconic status by virtue of its location, on a street meant to become "the major boulevard running toward the Kremlin." As Blair Ruble explains, the Tsentrosoiuz and two neighboring buildings designed in the late 1920s "were intended to provide a triumphant new entrance to socialist Moscow."[3] Yet during construction, the architect and the style that he represented fell out of favor with Soviet officialdom, and the extensive use of glass in his building came under critical fire at home and abroad.

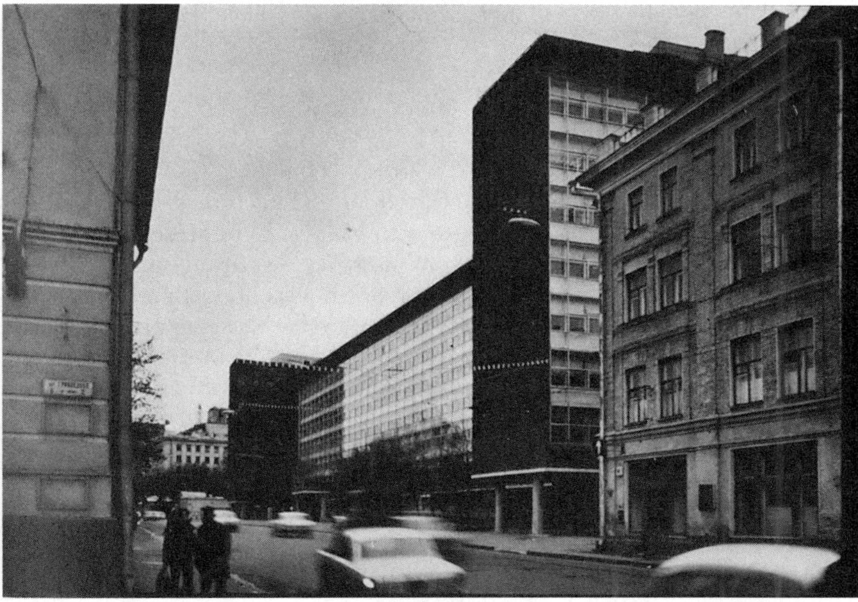

Figure 28. Tsentrosoiuz building by Le Corbusier, 1933. View from Miasnitskaia Street, photographed in 1973 by Jean-Louis Cohen.

In 1931, architect Hannes Meyer called the Tsentrosoiuz "an orgy of glass and concrete" that would never be completed. Two years later, a German observer spoke of a neighboring building whose extensive use of glass made it not so much a "machine for living in"[4] as a perpetual motion machine, with the workers inside scurrying about in desperation, seeking refuge from heat and cold, and pondered whether the completed Tsentrosoiuz would have a similar effect: "The reinforced concrete skeleton . . . was left unfinished for two years . . . while the people prayed for sanity." Now construction has resumed, and "the horror of glass walls . . . may yet become reality."[5] This critique was echoed in 1934 by architect Sergei Kozhin, for whom the "enormous glass walls" of the building made it seem "cold, monotonous, and disagreeable" and gave rise to fantasies about dreary *Metropolis*-like working conditions inside:

> It seems that inside these walls people must work in a tense, automatic, gloomy, joyless way. This is Americanism, which is alien to us and unacceptable in Soviet conditions. Furthermore, the continuous glazing of the walls is incompatible with the climatic conditions of Moscow. In the winter it will be

> cold inside these walls, and in the summer people will not know how to save themselves from the scorching rays of the sun.[6]

This attack came less than a decade after the Constructivists had emphasized the *benefits* that glass buildings would bring to workers in particular.

A later condemnation of the Tsentrosoiuz building, from 1947, reads, mixing its metaphors: "We saw the music of architecture dissected like a corpse when Corbusier built a house with glass walls in Moscow on Kirov Street."[7] Transparency, the attribute of glass that was at one time invested with such positive associations, now took on an aura of death and dismemberment. In fact, while the quality of transparency was condemned, a different feature of glass—its capacity to contain light—was exploited by official image-makers; and the origins of this practice can be traced back to the beginnings of the Soviet state.

Maksim Gorky, in his journal from the early 1920s, recounts a story about a priest named Zolotnitsky who was imprisoned for thirty years "for some sort of heretical thoughts." The priest's one consolation was a fire in the stove in his cell. After he was released "in the first years of the century," he began to worship fire and lived to watch the dancing flames. When he encountered an electric lightbulb for the first time, he was horrified at the sight of "the white, bloodless fire imprisoned in glass":

> The old man peered at it, began to wave his hands and mutter piteously: "And him too—oh!—and him too . . . What did you [imprison] him for?" . . . Tears poured from his dull eyes, he shivered all over and, sighing sorrowfully, appealed to those around him: "Oh, slaves of God . . . You are holding a little sunbeam captive . . . Oh, you people! Fear His fiery wrath." And with his trembling, thin little hand he cautiously touched his listeners, sobbing: "Oh, let him go."[8]

In the early decades of the twentieth century, written sources in Russia celebrated electric light as a technological discovery that would liberate mankind—literally, from the relentless alternation of day and night, and figuratively, from ignorance and other vestiges of the oppressive past. Against such a background, Zolotnitsky's response to the lightbulb is unorthodox, to say the least. Gorky presents the mad priest as a representative of the old world who cannot understand and is frightened by this icon of the New Epoch. But if there is a grain of truth in madness, as the Russian literary tradition attests, can we then think of Zolotnitsky as a holy fool with an insight into the perils of progress? His contemplation of fire puts him in touch with the divine; the notion of fire "held captive" in glass seems unnatural and evil to him.[9] The priest's reaction to the bulb reveals a spiritual, emotive potential in an otherwise common technology. This potential was recognized by the young Soviet regime.

In the 1920s and 1930s, the Soviet state used the visual power of light in glass to construct a variant of what Jean Starobinski has called the "solar myth" of the revolution, and thereby to present an exalted vision of Russia's transformation. Glass lets in, captures, and manipulates light, and the spectacle that it creates can be used to serve those in power. With the growth of the glass industry in Russia, this spectacular potential was harnessed with ever greater success, culminating in the twentieth century with such massive constructions as the Kremlin stars. Even the lowly lightbulb took on a sacred aura and was implicated in the Lenin cult; the *lampochka Il'icha* (Lenin's Little Lamp) lies on the same continuum as the Kremlin stars as an attempt by the Soviet state to lay claim to the domain of light.[10]

The Soviet version of the revolutionary "solar myth" transformed the electric lightbulb, a humble everyday object, into an ideological icon, as we can see by considering its treatment in Soviet popular culture as well as in several literary works of the late 1920s. The Kremlin stars serve as a monumental manifestation of the Soviet lightbulb and a case study illustrating the state's ideological use of captive light. One of my conceptual points of departure is Richard Wortman's term "*scenarios of power,*" which refers to performative mythmaking meant to consolidate autocratic power by appealing to "the symbolic sphere of ceremonies and imagery" in imperial Russia.[11] The phenomena under consideration here also have a theatrical dimension; scholars have noted the ideological significance of ritual and performance in the early Soviet period.[12] Borrowed religious symbolism lent these displays and performances much of their power. Richard Stites has documented how the Bolsheviks plundered the symbolic treasure trove of both Russian Orthodoxy and pagan rites in creating Bolshevik rituals in the period immediately following the October Revolution.[13] Ready-made sacred light imagery was applied in written works to Vladimir Lenin and "his" lightbulbs to invest both with a religious aura and to make Soviet technology seem miraculous.[14] In the 1930s, the official discourse around the Kremlin stars strove to transfer religious meaning to the Soviet state's own creations. The Kremlin stars were raised in the very period when cathedrals were being demolished on official orders, including major churches in the Kremlin itself.[15] The man-made stars would take their place; they would become the new beneficiaries of the people's devotion.

As the preceding chapter has shown, at the turn of the twentieth century many believed that the very essence of what it means to be human could be changed through the transformation of our material environment—and glass was *the* material to effect that transformation. The dream of glass architecture became a worldwide phenomenon. Artists, architects, and other visionaries believed that the transparency of glass was good for body and soul. Glass houses would expose the populace to the beneficent rays of the sun.[16] At the same time, the transparency of those buildings was associated with moral purity, openness, and democracy, attributes that the inhabitants would take on as well. Thus the literal would somehow magically become the figurative.

While the vast crystal palaces of which the Constructivists dreamed did not, for the most part, materialize in the Soviet Union, another use of glass on a monumental scale did come to the fore and played a significant role in shaping the country's self-image. The new Soviet state used objects such as the Kremlin stars to create and consolidate its mystique. These stars were lit by the most powerful lightbulbs in existence; but their low-wattage, household counterparts themselves loomed large in the Soviet imagination in the 1920s.

LENIN'S LITTLE LAMPS

In 1925 Osip Mandelstam wrote a children's science book titled *Primus*, with illustrations by Dobuzhinsky that included an image of a blond boy in a sailor suit cradling the top of a glowing lightbulb with his hand. (See figure 29.) The bulb is the size of the child's head; the rays of light radiating from the bulb echo the child's long lashes; while the text invites readers: "Go ahead and touch; your palm barely feels warm . . . The little glass lamp does not give heat, but glows [*lampochka stekliannaia ne greet, a gorit*.]" The navy emblem on the boy's shoulder glows with the same yellow as the electric light. The visual and textual elements combine to create a striking portrait of intimate contact with a power that seems both animate and otherworldly; glass allows for the existence of, and communion with, a mysterious, paradoxically "cold flame."

Human beings have an instinctive response to light; though incandescent bulbs seem unremarkable nowadays, their initial appearance caused quite a stir in Russia, in both the city and the countryside.[17] This elemental response was amplified by descriptions in literature and the mass media that gave these objects an aura of adoration and sanctity. Light imagery with sacred associations was used to promote the Soviet state from its very beginnings.[18] As early as 1919, Ilya Ionov's poem "The Future Yet to Come" featured the displacement of religious iconography by the Bolshevik symbol of the red star.[19] In the visual realm, Dmitry Moor's poster "Christmas" (1921) juxtaposes a procession of counterrevolutionary characters following the three Magi toward Bethlehem against another procession of workers, peasants, and Red Guards walking in the opposite direction, following a beaming

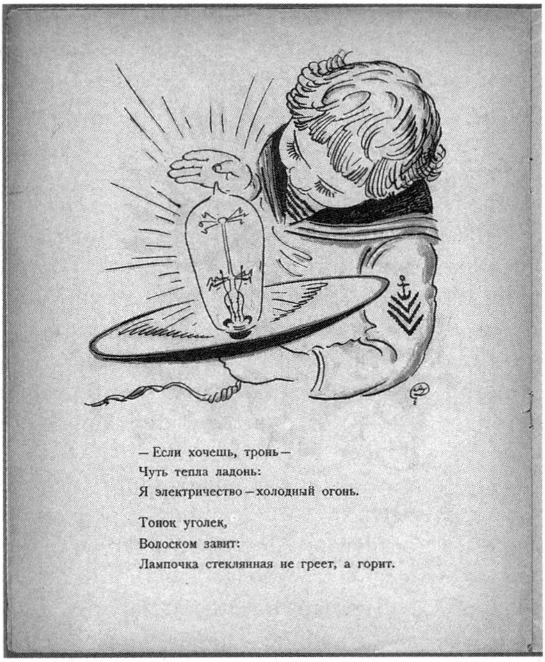

Figure 29. A page from *Primus*, with illustrations by Mstislav Dobuzhinsky and text by Osip Mandelstam, 1925. Houghton Library, Harvard University, fTyp 958.25.555. Russian texts of the works of Osip Mandelstam. Copyright © O. E. Mandelstam and heirs.

red star. Underneath the illustration is a poem by Demyan Bednyi with the lines, "The star over the Kremlin has eclipsed the Star of Bethlehem."[20]

The official appropriation of sacred light imagery became crucial in the case of the most important symbol of all: Lenin, who came to represent the Party in the 1920s;[21] as Vladimir Mayakovsky put it: "When we say Lenin, we mean the Party; when we say the Party, we mean Lenin." The Lenin cult took on particularly religious overtones in the wake of the attempt on his life in 1918.[22] The radiant star motif recurs in the representation of Lenin in his capacity as leader. On the occasion of Lenin's death, the Union of Railroad Workers of the USSR wrote to the Central Committee of the Communist Party: "Lenin's name is a star. The Communist Party follows the light of this star. We shall walk with it through the storm until our victory is complete."[23] Associating Lenin with the sun (often as *solnyshko*, "dear little sun") in poetry and official slogans reinforced his mythical aura.[24]

The notion of Lenin as a light source combined traditional religious iconography with the topical project to "electrify the countryside." Electric light had profound symbolic meaning in the context of the October Revolution. Russia had possessed electric power since the 1870s, but its use was almost completely limited to large urban centers.[25] Bringing light from the city to the ignorant (*temnye,* literally "dark, dim") peasantry came to be seen as a way to resolve the "contradiction between city and country." Lenin led the effort to electrify the entirety of the vast Soviet Union. He threw his support behind the State Commission for the Electrification of Russia (GOELRO), which strove to link up city and country, to kick-start wholesale industrialization, and to produce a literate rural populace, all with the help of electricity.[26]

Yet these practical goals, which envisioned electricity as a means toward modernization, coexisted with a set of aspirations based in symbolism. As Stites formulates it, electricity represented, among other things, the dawn of light and knowledge in a benighted land: "In the Russian Revolution—as in ancient religions—light was a metaphor for everything good, just as darkness was for poverty, evil, and prejudice."[27] This association of light with "everything good" recalls Starobinski's formulation of the "solar myth," which he applies to the imaginary at the heart of the French Revolution, but which also resonates in the Russian context: "Metaphors of light triumphing over darkness [are] charged from time immemorial with religious values . . . Once the old order had been symbolically reduced to the semblance of a dark cloud or cosmic scourge, the struggle against it could, by the same process, represent its object as the advent of light."[28]

A description of Lenin's visit on November 14, 1920, to the village of Kashino—the site of one of the first rural power stations—claims that the expression "lampochka Il'icha" originated here:

> When Vladimir Il'ich finished talking, high above him, on a gray pole trimmed with fir branches and scarlet ribbons, an electric lantern flared up [*vspykhnul*] with a bright light. At the same time light flared up in the peasant huts as well. People stood as if under a spell and stared at this "unnatural" light that had flared up over the village of Kashino. One of the peasants exclaimed: "Lenin's little lamp has lit up [*zazhglas' lampochka Il'icha*]!"[29]

Although the phrase was most likely invented by an official writer, it was recast as a spontaneous expression of joy and gratitude from the simple folk; the triple use of the verb *vspykhnut'* (to flare up) sets the tone for the peasant's outburst. Notably, in this account of the phrase's origin, the expression is said to arise from the folk, an unprompted display of emotion. Like the term *solnyshko*, *lampochka* is a caressing diminutive that conveys the simple folk's love for Lenin.

In a March 9, 1920, issue of *Bednota*, a peasant from Kashino testified that electrification was initiated in his village under peer pressure: the peasants in the already electrified neighboring village had been taunting them, calling them "rural ignoramuses" (*temnota derevenskaia*, literally "dim rural folk"). Tellingly, the peasant lists only one advantage of electrification: the artificial lighting allowed the neighboring villagers to work through the night. Just as greenhouses had done their part in lengthening the working day, lightbulbs now showed another way in which glass enabled the mastery of nature for the sake of increased productivity.[30] To make electrification more appealing to the public, official writers resorted to magical motifs. In a jolly folk song written by Mikhail Isakovsky in 1925 that depicts lampposts "striding hastily" through the village, the lightbulbs are heavenly bodies brought down to earth, leaving the heavens green with envy:

> We've never seen such a thing, not even in our dreams,
> That the sun would light up atop a pine tree,
> That joy would befriend a *muzhik*,
> That everyone would have a star beneath the ceiling.
> In our village there is merriment and beauty,
> And the heavens envy us.[31]

Apart from its winning melody, what is most appealing about this song is the celebratory mood and the egalitarian promise of "a star under every ceiling." Poet Nikolai Starshinov testifies to the success the song enjoyed in his village when neighbors brought the record, and a gramophone, from Moscow. Half the village came to listen, and in a few days, the song had seamlessly become part of the local repertoire.[32]

In this song, glass, in the form of the lantern and the lightbulb, holds light in captivity and grants culture the status of nature: glass globes masquerade as sun and stars. An advertising poster from 1923 by Mayakovsky and Rodchenko presents lightbulbs as domesticated heavenly bodies: the central image of a lightbulb, tilted at a jaunty angle, is accompanied by the text: "Let's have the sun at night! Where to find it? Buy it at GUM! It's cheap and blinding."[33] As late as 1939, in a Stalinist "pseudo-bylina" by A. M. Pashkova titled "You Are Our Bright Sunshine," lightbulbs again appear as heavenly bodies: "Little stars from the heavens / Have descended on our peasant villages."[34] There is a subtle difference between this image of lightbulbs as stars or suns and earlier examples: rather than boasting of the state's ability to create stars of its own, the later poem states that actual stars have come down "on our peasant villages"—an even more grandiose claim.

"Lenin's little lamps" appeared in visual propaganda as well, although not without controversy as to how these lightbulbs were to be "read." A

1934 poster by Konstantin Zotov depicts a family of beaming collectivized peasants with a gramophone in the foreground and a lightbulb in the background—a fitting illustration to Isakovsky's song cited above. Yet the electric lamp is, curiously, not illuminated. A contemporary reviewer listed this as one of the faults of the poster.[35] The bulb is situated next to the profiles of Lenin and Stalin, on a diagonal reminiscent of Orion's Belt. Hence the leaders, it is suggested, are the source of enlightenment made literal in the reflected glow on the faces of the mother and child.[36] At the same time, placing the leaders so suggestively close to the dim bulb made for a provocative juxtaposition and was likely what made the reviewer uneasy.[37] No such ambiguity existed in the "industrial carnival," a popular kind of mass spectacle from the late 1920s featuring puppet figures of positive and negative characters of the Soviet regime. In one such carnival, the phrase "lampochka Il'icha" was reified: "above the Leader's head a real electric light was shining, like the nimbus of a saint."[38]

By the mid-1920s, the discourse of *lampochki* was in the air, and the phrase "lampochka Il'icha" had moved beyond the context of the village and developed into a universal Soviet slogan.[39] The unassuming lightbulb thus became a key element of the Lenin cult. The metaphor of Lenin as light source underwent a transformation: now Lenin was both a god and a humble electrician. The lightbulb, as a necessary component of *byt*, is the perfect propaganda object: it is so small, so utilitarian, that it begins to seem "natural" in no time at all, just as ideology comes to seem like a part of the natural order of things; but all the while, the mythical association remains.

In the first decades of Soviet power, electric lightbulbs were depicted as part of the official portrait of the fledgling state's astounding success in the areas of technology, creature comforts, and all-around enlightenment. What happens to these images, with their aura of beaming enthusiasm, when they are refracted through an ambivalent writer's imagination?

In 1924, Mikhail Zoshchenko published a feuilleton titled "Electrification" under the pseudonym Semyon Kurochkin; a year later, the piece appeared in a revised version under his own name as the story "Poverty." In the feuilleton, the residents of a communal apartment are appalled when the bright light of the newly installed electric lamp reveals the squalor in which they live: the light illuminates torn shoes, shredded wallpaper, scampering bedbugs and fleas, and various pieces of trash. The narrator tidies up his corner as best he can, but the landlady, who cannot stand to look at "how poorly [she] lives," ends up cutting the wires in despair. The piece ends with the following meditation: "Brothers, light is a good thing, but it's tough to live with it! Now we have to turn our whole lives around. To have cleanliness and order. To get rid of rot and vileness once and for all. Everything that's good in the dark is bad in the light! Am I right, fellows?"[40]

These ambivalent words were cut in subsequent editions of the story. Other changes are notable as well. The sentence "They began to install electric light" is followed in later versions by "soon after the revolution." The landlady is more clearly delineated as the narrator's antagonist and a negative example for the reader.[41] Most striking is the change in the narrator's attitude toward the lightbulb that causes such turmoil in his life. In the original feuilleton, he admits that he grew depressed after seeing the true state of his living conditions, and upon coming home, "I wouldn't turn on the light and would just hit the sack." In the revised version, on the other hand, he writes that upon his return, "I'd turn on the light, feast my eyes on the light bulb [*poliubuius' na lampochku*]" and only then go to bed. Notably, the narrator gazes lovingly at the lightbulb even *before* he decides to fix up his corner of the apartment. Gaston Bachelard has contrasted the primal flame with the gaslight that came to replace it, noting that the latter does not lend itself to contemplation.[42] The same could be said of the still more modern light source, the incandescent bulb. Zoshchenko gives us the odd image of someone contemplating a blinding electric light as they would an open flame.

In 1930 Zoshchenko wrote a story whose narrator takes issue precisely with the intensity of Soviet lightbulbs: 400-watt bulbs in the hallway and toilet generate "such a senselessly bright light [*takaia bessmyslennaia iarkost'*] . . . that you just start to feel bad." A chatty electric meter reader reveals to the narrator that this is a result of the command economy: factories are turning out lightbulbs with grotesquely high wattages in order to meet the assigned power quota in time. In this context, the idea of gazing in adoration at "Lenin's little lamp" becomes even stranger.[43]

Zoshchenko's stories featuring the unceremonious home invasion of the too-powerful lightbulb address the effects of electrification in urban settings, while Andrei Platonov's stories take place in the village, where electrification efforts were particularly important. The official version of the wonders that a *lampochka* could achieve is embodied in this testimonial by a peasant: "Lenin's little lamp has made me look at many things with a different set of eyes. . . . For one thing, I got a hankering for books because of Lenin's little lamp. And it's much tidier inside my hut thanks to that same little lamp . . . I began to want to live and work better, in a more cultured way. I began to want to read and to learn things."[44]

Platonov wrote several stories about the electrification of the countryside. One of these was originally called "About the Extinguished Lenin Lamp" (1926); later it was given the more upbeat title "How Lenin's Lamp Was Lit."[45] The instability of the title hints at the ambivalent attitude toward the symbolically freighted lightbulb at the center of the story. The narrator is a Red Army–trained electrician who brings electric power to his village. His venture is initially met with some doubt—one peasant fears that "we'll all burn up from your electricity" while another expresses suspicion toward "inventors who want to plaster the earth with lipitricity [*zemliu lipistrichestvom mazat' khotiat*]"—but eventually the villagers are won over.[46] The narrator and his work crew fashion a five-pointed star studded with bulbs, place ten lanterns along the street, and stretch a garland of lamps across it. When, at two in the morning, the village is illuminated with electric light for the first time, the incandescent moment is compromised by the people's ambivalent response. Peasants wake up "in confusion"; children burst into tears, and their mothers carry them outside only to find that they cannot escape the blazing electric light: "A fever broke out in the village. The people ran to the station, rejoicing and worrying, threatening and wondering. An anxious feeling seized everyone, and sleep vanished in the village" (Platonov, "O potukhshei lampochke Il'icha," 331). We recall that the peasants of Kashino village said that electric light allowed them to work through the night, forsaking sleep.

The grand opening of the station "coincides" with the anniversary of the October Revolution, and the local Bolshevik cell organizes a holiday to mark the occasion. Crowds of people gather to view the miracle of electric light as they used to marvel at "icon processions" in the old days (Platonov, "O potukhshei lampochke Il'icha," 331). At the grand meeting, a local official declares: "Lenin's lamp is about to flare up, and it will give light to the Soviet village for centuries, like the eternal memory of our great leader." On cue, the narrator pulls the switch: "Light fell into the dark room like a cloudburst . . . Everyone screwed up their eyes and hunched over—it was as if hot water was pouring down" (Platonov, "O potukhshei lampochke Il'icha," 332). For the second time, the story invokes the anxiety of being burned by electric light.

Several years before Platonov's story, Ivan Simakov's poster *Electrification and Counterrevolution* (1921) mocked this sort of confusion as a signifier of political backwardness. (See figure 30.) The poster depicts the hand of a robust proletarian grasping a bright electric bulb that beams like a sun in the sky. Meanwhile, the enemies of the revolution, including a priest and a White Army general, ineffectually try to extinguish the light with a fire hose, by blowing, and with a bucket of moonshine. Apparently unaware of the lightbulb's protective glass shield, they misunderstand the nature of electric light and treat it as an open flame.[47] What is comical in the poster becomes poignant in Platonov.

At the meeting in Platonov's story, another official addresses the crowd:

> Comrades! . . . We have discovered the lamp of the so-called Il'ich, that is, our beloved comrade Lenin. As we all know, he taught that kerosene lamps

> cause fires, create stuffiness in our huts and harm our health, whereas we need physical fitness. . . . And I say to you: remember the precept of our eternal Il'ich, and carry his wise face in your unhappy hearts. (Platonov, "O potukhshei lampochke Il'icha," 332–33)

Here the speaker bursts into tears and sits down. Once again, the display of light leads to a display of emotion.

These ambivalent moments anticipate the story's bleak conclusion. For "one happy year," the power station is up and running; then, the kulaks who own the windmills that have been rendered obsolete by the new power source sabotage the station, burning it down one night. The lightbulbs remain in the peasant huts, but now they are empty, dark glass globes covered with flies (*zasizheny mukhami do potuskneniia stekla*)—evoking not adoration but disgust (Platonov, "O potukhshei lampochke Il'icha," 334).

The image of a lightbulb that has gone dark figures prominently in Yury Olesha's novel *Envy*, published two years after Platonov's story. A glimpse at the beginning of the novel reveals that Olesha is very attentive to the effect of light captured in glass.[48] The first thing that catches the eye of antihero Nikolai Kavalerov is "an oval piece of translucent glass" set into

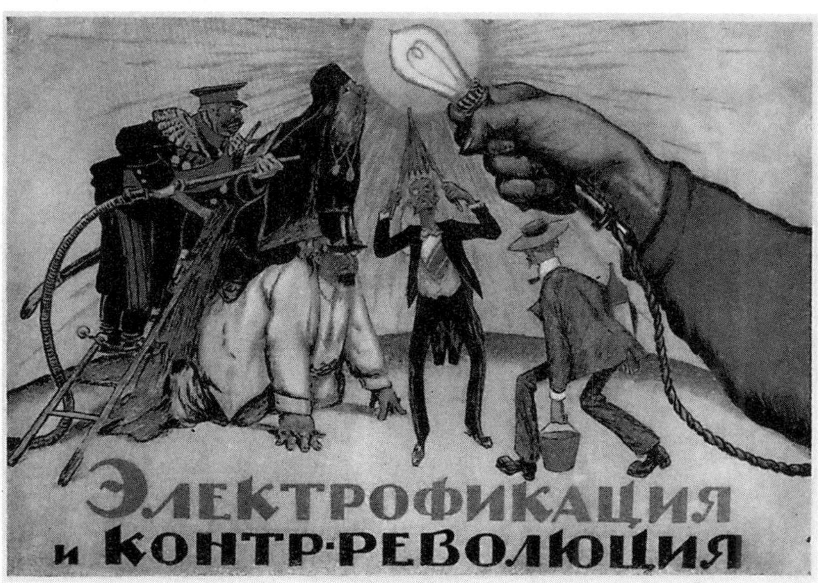

Figure 30. *Electrification and Counterrevolution*, Ivan Simakov, 1921.

the door of the toilet where Andrei Babichev, his benefactor, sings his vigorous songs. "He turns the switch, and the oval, lit from within, becomes a splendid opal-colored egg. With my mind's eye I see that egg, hanging in the darkness of the hallway."[49] Kavalerov's description of the glass oval as spectral and ethereal provides a counterpoint to Andrei's too-solid flesh, mere inches away from the door. We already see how Kavalerov tries to dematerialize the material world, in which only men of action such as Andrei feel at home.[50] Kavalerov is drawn to glass because it can become invisible, losing its oppressive materiality in a flash. This glass oval, lit up from within, behaves as a light source. As such it anticipates a central image of the novel: a lightbulb on the verge of burning out.[51]

When Ivan Babichev, a representative of the old world and a politically suspect rabble-rouser, is arrested at his brother Andrei's command, he is questioned about his attempts to gather disciples and his "conspiracy of feelings." When the police inspector asks him what he hopes to achieve through this conspiracy, Ivan hunts around for a metaphor, possibly seizing upon the bare bulb in the interrogation chamber.

> It sometimes happens, you know, that a light bulb suddenly goes out. Burnt out, you say. And if you take this burnt-out bulb and give it a shake, it will flare up [*vspykhnet'*] and burn for a while longer. There's a disaster going on inside the bulb. The tungsten filaments are breaking off, but when the pieces touch, the bulb comes back to life. A short, unnatural, obviously doomed life—a fever, an overly bright incandescence, a brilliance. . . . I want to shake up the heart of a burnt-out epoch, the heart-bulb, so that the fragments of filament will come into contact again . . . and call forth that momentary bright splendor.[52]

Ivan asks us to read this lightbulb image as a eulogy to the dying epoch to which he proudly belongs. Yet Olesha takes care throughout the text to show that Ivan is not to be trusted. Ivan's interpretation is not the only one possible; in light of what a *lampochka* would signify to readers of the time, Ivan's analogy can be read as an irreverent swipe at the imagery of the Lenin cult.[53] First, the lightbulb is made to represent not the new era but the old decrepit world. Second, the very idea of a *lampochka Il'icha* meant to glow with an eternal flame, "suddenly" going out, betraying its imperfect construction, cracks the veneer of this bright Soviet icon.[54] As Olesha worked on his novel during the 1920s, he imbibed the iconography of the new regime in the making.[55] Trying to engage with the new order, Olesha incorporates the new imagery in his writing,[56] and his playful approach to the official symbolism verges on the subversive.[57]

Throughout his novel, Olesha contrasts images of light in captivity and mobile, dancing light, using the latter to point to moments of optical play in the text, and by extension, to potentially liberating ways of seeing. The street mirror that appears halfway through the novel is an example of reflective glass with the potential for liberating optical play.[58] Kavalerov loves such mirrors because they allow him to study the vibrant world around him; and because the world is in motion, the mirror generates the illusion of time moving backward.

> Suddenly, for an instant, it becomes clear to you—unprecedented changes have taken place with the world, with the rules of the world. Destroyed are optics, geometry, the nature of that which was your walk, your movement, your desire to go precisely where you were going.[59]

By such means as lenses, test tubes, and slides, glass helped scientists discover the rules of the natural world, yet here the same material subverts the very rules that Andrei and others like him hold dear. Even the linear nature of time is altered: a tram and a straw hat that had already disappeared from view now swim back into Kavalerov's field of vision. These details are poignant because Kavalerov is a man who has missed his chance; he is one of the "has-beens," or as the literal Russian has it, "former people" (*byvshie liudi*).[60] When Kavalerov's mentor Ivan approaches the mirror, he brushes off a caterpillar clinging to his shoulder. At the moment of infinite potential with which part 1 ends, the caterpillar suggests metamorphosis, whether it be the changes that the material world undergoes when seen through Kavalerov's eyes, or Kavalerov's desire to become other than he is. This chapter, the last one in part 1, concludes with Kavalerov's meeting with Ivan, mediated by the street mirror, which has the power to reverse time; it ends on a note of pure possibility—this incandescent moment can be considered the "alternate ending" to the novel itself.[61]

Thomas Edison, metonymically associated with the lightbulb,[62] is invoked a number of times in the novel. Andrei's protégé Volodya confesses that he envies the machine and vows to become "the Edison of the new century"; Ivan mocks Volodya with the same epithet; and Kavalerov even repeats this formula when he imagines begging for Andrei's forgiveness ("I am also young, I too will be an Edison of the new century"). In the context of the burgeoning Lenin cult of the 1920s, the metonymic association between lightbulbs and Edison coexisted alongside with the one between the lightbulb and Lenin. Three years after completing *Envy*, Olesha expressed in his journal his wonder at the gifts that Thomas Edison had bestowed upon the world: "the electric light bulb, the telephone, the tramway." Then he pondered: "What then has changed and what hasn't changed? What is illusory and what is real? *Why hasn't the electric bulb brought any order into the human soul?* How much time—centuries!—do we need for technology to change the human psyche, if it is even capable of changing it at all, as the Marxists say it is!"[63] Olesha takes issue here with those who uphold technological progress as that which will "re-forge" human nature and with those who believe scientific laws govern behavior and historical change. The wording in Olesha's journal entry underscores the idea that his use of the lightbulb image in *Envy* is polemical.[64]

In his play *Conspiracy of Feelings* (1929), Olesha tried to undo the ambiguity of the characterization in *Envy* and create clear-cut good and evil characters for the era of the Five-Year Plan. He imbues Andrei with Kavalerov's aesthetic sensibility, while making Ivan admit to being a "counterrevolutionary." Ivan's speech about the lightbulb now takes place in a "petit bourgeois" interior featuring a gaudy lamp with a lightbulb that actually burns out.[65] The change of venue is part of Olesha's attempt to show that even though the scene depicts the last gasp of "Lenin's lamp," the target of his attack is the *old* world.

As if the ideological agenda of *Conspiracy of Feelings* were not clear enough, Olesha proclaimed in the statement "The Author on His Play" (1929): "My aim was to show that the people of the old world do not have a monopoly on pathos, . . . that the builders of our new world and our new way of life are the most humane of all, and that what seems to the doomed man to be the stone face of an idol is in fact the beaming face of the new man, incomprehensible to the doomed one, terrifying and blinding him."[66] Olesha's use of the categories "old world/new world" as if they are givens and the assumption that the representatives of the former are "doomed" are chilling. But most chilling of all is the notion of "the beaming face of the new man" that terrifies and blinds the doomed man incapable of understanding this light source. The "light that burns the enemy/outsider" is a motif that would appear nearly a decade later in a poem praising another Soviet light source: the Kremlin stars.

THE KREMLIN STARS, VERSIONS ONE AND TWO

The five red stars on the Kremlin towers are high-maintenance beauties; powered by an intricate system of lamps, ventilators, air pumps, and other mechanisms concealed inside each tower, the stars are perpetually in need of repair. In the words of Mikhail Topolin, an engineer who spent thirty years looking after them, "the stars are like living beings; they need constant care and the warmth of human hands."[67] One calm sunny day, Topolin recalls, two workers climbed up to inspect the star on the Troitskaya tower. The men had to finish all repairs by nightfall, when the star was to shine once more

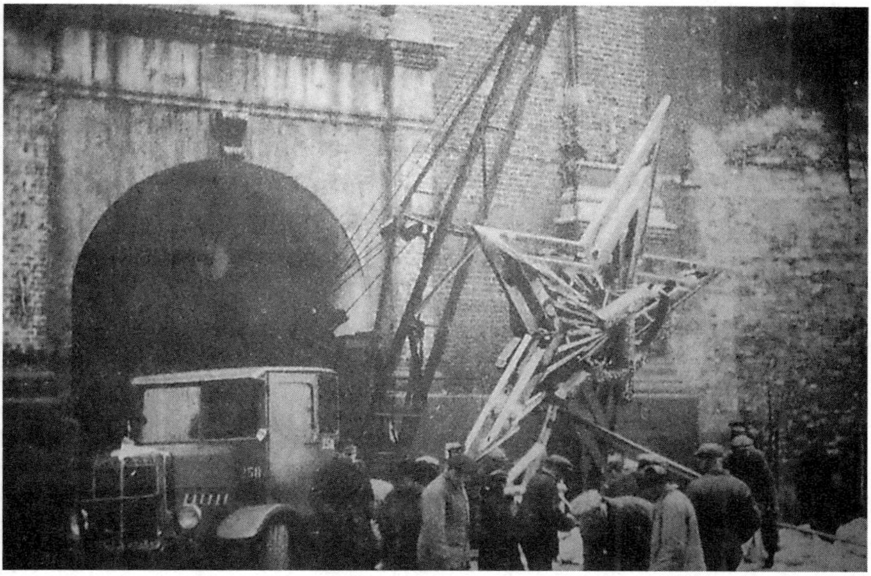

Figure 31. Still from the documentary film *Sotsialisticheskaia derevnia*, November 1935.

over the Kremlin, taking its place in "the ruby constellation." They had just opened an inspection hatch in the star to look inside, when a thunderstorm suddenly broke out. Suspended more than 250 feet above the ground, the workers clung to the star as bolts of lightning flashed, rain poured down, and the gale force of the wind made it impossible to close the hatch. To prevent the wind and water from harming the fragile interior, the men embraced the star, "shielding the opening with their bodies."[68]

Why did the workers risk life and limb to protect these stars? True, they were guided by an imperative from above to preserve the splendor and visibility of the Soviet symbols; yet Topolin's description seems driven by a genuine feeling for those glowing glass constructions. Glass lit from within can appeal to the emotions and sway hearts and minds. If, following Lenin's formula, communism is Soviet power plus electrification, one might say that in the case of the Kremlin stars, Soviet power is electrification plus glass.

The Kremlin stars were originally made not of glass but of metal and semiprecious stones.[69] Early in September 1935, the Council of People's Commissars and the Central Committee of the Communist Party ordered the removal of the double-headed eagles that had perched upon the Kremlin towers since the middle of the seventeenth century. The leadership fur-

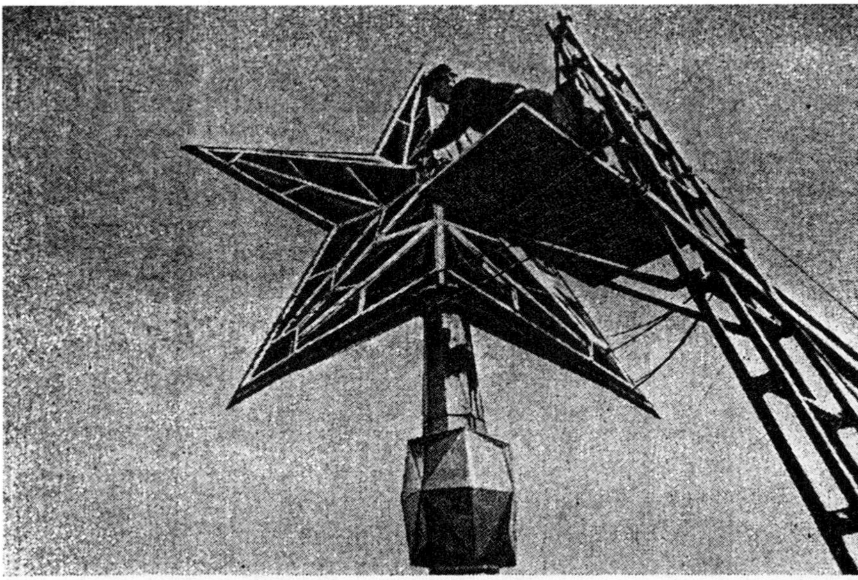

Figure 32. 1937 Kremlin star under repair.

ther decreed that the eagles be replaced by five-pointed stars bearing the hammer-and-sickle emblem.[70] (See figure 31.) The stars were to be "artistically designed" and made of a material that would last "for centuries." Two Moscow factories as well as the Institute of Aero-Hydrodynamics were charged with the task, to be completed in time for the anniversary of the October Revolution.[71]

An article in *Pravda* from October 10, 1935, celebrates the "acrobatic" feats of the six steeplejacks who scrambled up the towers in order to inspect the doomed eagles and their pedestals. As *Pravda* reported, the wings and crowns of the eagles were "shot through with bullets from the October battles." This is a striking detail: eighteen years later, the "heroic" period of the revolution lives on. More to the point, the battle is now being fought on the iconographical front.

Models of the stars destined to replace the eagles were designed at the studio of the Bolshoi Theater (underscoring the theatrical nature of the spectacle). Once installed on the towers, these massive emblems of revolution would indeed revolve on their axes, withstanding the strongest of winds. Meteorological considerations were not the whole story, however. As Topolin recounts, when Soviet officials came to examine the model stars, they approved the design "on the indispensable condition that they would be made to revolve, so that Muscovites and guests of the capital could admire them [*liubovat'sia imi*] from anywhere."[72] In the verb Topolin uses, *liubovat'sia*, the aesthetic dimension is intertwined with emotion, affect, love. Here we see that their ability to revolve has not only a functional but also an aesthetic-ideological basis. The stars are more than simply emblems—they are emblems-in-the-round.

On October 24, the first of the stars was installed atop the Spasskaya tower. The next day's *Pravda* emphasized the efforts of the workers who struggled under its weight to carefully screw the star in place.[73] Many Muscovites were reported to have gathered on Red Square to watch the installation; at 1:47 p.m., they heard a "joyous shout" from above: "All right, it's in place!" The steeplejacks shook hands with one another, and the sound of applause (not yet the stormy kind) rang out "on the Square and in the Kremlin." From the latter detail we can infer that Stalin was watching, as always.[74]

Yet these stars stayed up for less than two years before the government demanded new stars of ruby-red glass. In the space of a year, the semi-precious stones adorning the stars had grown dim from air pollution. The stars also turned out to be too large and looked ungainly atop the Kremlin towers.[75] Most important, while these original stars were illuminated by floodlights, their replacements were to glow from within—it was essential that they not merely reflect but emanate light. These new stars had to be designed to remain untarnished and clean; powerful new lamps had to be created, new technologies invented and tested; and all the work had to be finished in just a few months.[76] Engineers, glassmakers, and untold others labored at the requisite accelerated pace, and on September 29, 1937, *Pravda* announced that "five new ruby stars" would be installed on the Kremlin towers for the twentieth anniversary of the October Revolution: "Unlike the former ones, these will be clearly visible night and day. At night, the stars will be a bright red ruby color, and in the day—a beautiful combination of a gold frame and ruby glass." The repeated invocations of "ruby" suggested that the new stars were made of a more precious, loftier material than mere glass.

These new, improved stars were created through an elaborate feat of electrical engineering and construction.[77] Made of layered glass, they contained lamps as well as hidden mirrors to ensure even lighting throughout the star.[78] Burned-out lightbulbs would be changed "by mechanical means through the spire of the tower." The largest of the stars measured twelve feet across and weighed one and a half tons. Inside were three-, five-, and seven-kilowatt bulbs (sizes that were unprecedented at the time); the stars would be lit up around the clock. As a result, the interior could become extremely hot, and a complex cooling system was installed to keep each star from cracking. What is more, at five-day intervals, jets of water and warm air would shoot out of pipes placed along each star, keeping the surface clear of snow, ice, dust, and dirt at all times. In effect, the stars were subjected to a perpetual purge so that no "alien elements" would obscure their bright glow (eerily appropriate for 1937).[79] The equipment for keeping the stars clean was concealed in the towers below along with air filters, ventilators, pumps, and other machinery.[80] Now it becomes clear why Topolin and his colleagues were kept so busy maintaining the stars. (See figure 32.) To provide workers access to the stars, ladders "invisible to the eye" were placed alongside the roofs of the towers. The emphasis on the stars' visibility combined with the hidden machinery and undetectable ladders typified the paradoxical Stalinist culture of spectacle and concealment.

The first glass star was installed on the Vodovoznaya tower on September 29, and on the following day, *Pravda* reported that Muscovites had "marveled at the astounding sight" (*liubovalis' izumitel'nym zrelishchem*)—not of the workers raising the star, but of the star itself as it "lit up" and "slowly revolved on its axis, standing out boldly against the night sky."[81] This effacement of the worker is appropriate when we consider that while the first set of stars featured the hammer and sickle—the symbol of the workers and peasants in whose name the revolution took place—the second set of stars did not. There was thus a shift in emphasis away from the human labor involved; now all eyes were on the light source that stood for "Soviet power," more specifically, the charismatic power of Stalin, the deity in the Kremlin.[82] Subsequent articles dwell in detail on the changeable appearance of each star.[83] Such descriptions, just like the references to their revolving, endow the stars with dynamism. Initial press accounts depicted the first metal star being installed by a worker. Now that agency was transferred from the human actor to the emblem-in-the-round.

The Kremlin stars combine light and height, two symbolically charged attributes. In traditional symbolism, light is linked with divinity "and, by association, the qualities of knowledge and wisdom, truth and goodness."[84] Light imagery takes on even more explicitly religious connotations when it is combined with that of elevation (evocative of the gods' typically lofty abode). Christel Lane suggests that the tendency to combine light and height in Soviet ritual from the earliest post-revolutionary period was intended to invoke "the qualities and perspectives usually associated with a divine presence."[85] When the five glass stars were finally installed in October 1937, on the very eve of the revolution's anniversary, it seemed as if the state had seized control of nature and timed the stars to rise to mark the most important event in the history of the world. It could not have been a more transparent allusion to the biblical sign of the birth of a new era: the Star of Bethlehem, multiplied by five.

In this way, such physical manifestations of emblems contributed to the sacralization of Soviet power. These gigantic star-shaped lamps evoked

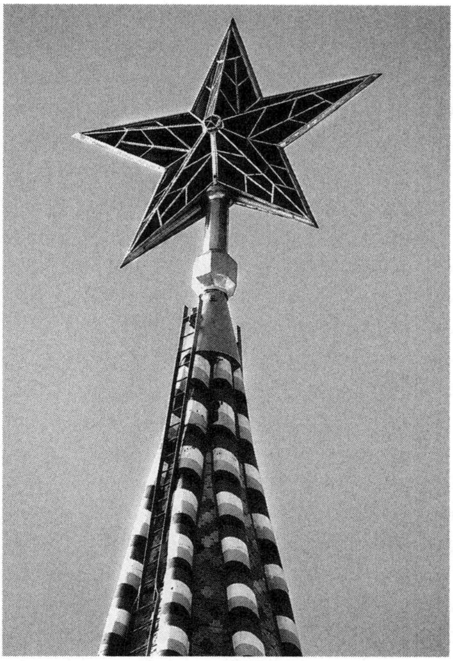

Figure 33. Kremlin star today. Photograph by Serge Freeman.

the official coat of arms, but they also brought to mind the stars' biblical associations. Moreover, through the combination of their lofty position and brilliant glow, they suggested that the state had the godlike ability to refurnish the heavens. Light held captive in glass was what allowed for such an illusion to be created and sustained.[86] (See figure 33.)

The Kremlin stars were built in preparation for the celebration of the October Revolution's anniversary, but they outlasted the festivities and became a permanent fixture in the Soviet sky. Imbued with dynamism both by the engineers who made them and the press accounts that described them, the stars were created to bring about a gradual revolution in the minds of their viewers. These stars were important cultural "texts." Indeed, the first set of stars had to undergo revision, just like the literary texts considered here. The second time around, however, the leadership took great care to guide Soviet citizens in reading the stars.

A poem by A. Kovalenkov called "The Star" appeared in *Pravda* as the glass stars were being raised over the Kremlin. The narrator of the poem bids his comrade to recall the heroic days of the revolution when the Red

Army star led them through war and devastation and inspired the speaker in battle: "it blinded and burned the enemy, and [my] hand gripped [my] rifle more tightly." Nowadays, "the very same star still shines over us," but now, the symbol has become real. The star, "visible to everyone," twinkles, growing ever brighter and more beautiful.[87] The final stanza introduces the idea that the symbol has become embodied in red glass. Here, the poet uses a biblical allusion to legitimize his hyperbolic claims about what the star can do: "Stretching its rays into the seas and the fields, it burns without burning up on the tower of the Kremlin" (*Gorit, ne sgoraia, / Na bashne Kremlia*). This description recalls the famous image from Exodus 3:2: "And the angel of the Lord appeared unto him in a flame of fire out of the midst of a bush: and he looked, and, behold, the bush burned with fire, and the bush was not consumed [*gorit ognem, no kust ne sgoraet*]."[88] Thus, in comparing the star to the burning bush whose form God's angel takes, Kovalenkov appropriates the image and the very wording from scripture. This poem is about the power of symbols; it tells readers what the red star represents, but also, that this symbol has the power to work miracles: to lead one to victory in battle, to "blind and burn" the enemy, to be visible to everyone, and to become embodied in an earthly material, yet perpetually increase in brightness and beauty, transcending all known scientific laws.[89]

On November 6, 1937—the day before the anniversary of the revolution was celebrated—*Pravda* published a letter from Spanish communist leader Dolores Ibárruri under the heading "The Stars of the Kremlin Light the Way for Us." This letter also serves as a caption to ensure that the stars will be "read" correctly by those who view them.[90] Ibárruri praises the red stars that have replaced "the predatory two-headed eagles" as "the symbol of a new world that has been created from the ruins of the old one through the great efforts of a great people." She invokes religious imagery, appropriating its symbolic power even as she condemns religion itself: "Biblical legends tell of stars that appeared and led the ancient Magi. The stars of the Kremlin shine through the gloom of the capitalist hell, dispersing the deceitful fairy tales of the church. They show to the already free Soviet peoples the path of socialism, the path of peace, prosperity, and progress. They show to all of humanity the path of Lenin and Stalin, the path to victory and happiness."[91] Ibárruri's letter draws on a traditional view of stars as heavenly lights that guide weary travelers through the darkness toward a longed-for destination. This association appears in Kovalenkov's poem as well.[92]

The revolutionary "solar myth" continued to be promoted by such works as a 1938 song by Vasilii Lebedev-Kumach that tells of Moscow "bravely conquering all powers of darkness [*sily mraka*], lit up by the blaze of scarlet stars, eight centuries old but eternally young."[93] This paradoxical image of Moscow suggests the ability to transcend chronological time—to overcome nature. An article from the late Soviet period calls the glassworkers of the Red May factory, where the glass stars were rebuilt after World War II, "the creators of the Kremlin constellation." The essay closes with the following description of these stars' ascent and illumination: "The old heavenly bodies had to make room, to make way, to leave their long-occupied places in order to let in stars made by human hands—the youngest stars in the universe that would blaze, never dimming, at its most important intersection."[94]

Ibárruri's letter, Kovalenkov's poem, and other such texts provide a gloss on these new objects on the horizon, helping Soviet citizens derive the correct message from these spectacular constructions. They are reminiscent of the explanations that Peter I would provide to spectators to explain the allegorical meaning of an illumination.[95] In both the Petrine and the Soviet cases we can detect an anxiety about ambiguity—the explanations are there to assign a specific meaning to the luminous spectacle in the sky.

Official discourse around both the Kremlin stars and "Lenin's little lamps" invokes the conquest of unruly nature and even the attainment of divine power by means of technology produced by the triumphant socialist state; and the image of light contained in glass serves as an emblem of this exercise of power. When refracted through a consciously or subconsciously uncooperative imagination, however, as in the case of Olesha, Zoshchenko, or Platonov, these symbols of the nascent regime are far from benevolent and unwavering. Instead, Zoshchenko and Platonov give us the depiction of light as something that blinds and harasses; in *Envy*, Olesha favors the short-lived flash of the imperiled lightbulb to the illusory immortality of a lamp-like leader. Against the state's insistence that its radiance will last forever, "like the eternal memory of our great leader," we see that there are some who, blinking in the panoptic glare, have started to yearn instead for someone to release the flame from its prison and restore, with the darkness, the actual stars.

GLASS, ILLUSION, AND IDEOLOGY

The question of how our material surroundings correspond to and shape the world of ideas is particularly interesting to ask about the Soviet period, from the 1920s through the beginning of the Thaw. As Katerina Clark has shown, such rhetorical constructions as "building socialism" and "living in communism" were once prevalent ways to imagine the goal for which the Party was striving. And fittingly, architecture played a prominent role in the culture of that time.[96] When we consider glass as a specific type of building material, it is revealing to explore how it was used, for both pragmatic and symbolic ends, by those who strove to *literally* build communism.

In the years of Stalin's ascendancy and rule, the Soviet state put glass to rhetorical use in settings from the sublime to the subterranean. The Kremlin stars are a key example of the former; another is the spire of Moscow State University—a mirror made of yellow glass and aluminum that looks like gold when it catches the sun. After a brief excursion to the dizzying heights of the spire, we shall descend into the underworld to consider strategic uses of glass in two subterranean interiors—Lenin's mausoleum, and Avtovo station in the Leningrad metro. The optical qualities of glass are essential for creating the interplay of light and darkness needed to set the proper tone in these ideologically freighted spaces.

In preceding chapters we have explored how the physical properties of glass combined with the magical associations around this material gave rise to the image of the glass house that would transform the consciousness of those dwelling within and gazing upon it from without. Constructivist architects championed glass architecture and embraced the idea of engineering the human psyche through the (re)built environment. Thus, in his influential work *Style and Epoch* (1924), Moisei Ginzburg declared that "from the moment man takes his first steps, form exerts a spontaneous influence, which becomes increasingly more clear, distinct, and concrete"; and in 1927, he designated the task of architecture to be that of "life-building, of organizing the forms of the new life."[97]

The Constructivists were suppressed in Stalin's time;[98] as for the idea of the all-glass house, it was transformed in the mid-1920s from a transparent communal dwelling into a domicile for one when Lenin's body was placed on display in a glass sarcophagus, a container designed to evoke associations with saintly relics and Sleeping Beauty. In what follows, I juxtapose the myths that the Lenin exhibition was meant to propagate with the meanings and discourses that it generated in reality. The emphasis on Lenin's visibility led to his body being placed in a glass case, which rendered him, and the symbolic order he represented, both powerful and vulnerable; and I will document how (and why) his crystal coffin repeatedly came under attack.

I conclude by examining another spectacular use of glass in an underground interior—the Avtovo metro station, the final stop on the first line of the Leningrad metro. It was planned in the early 1950s as a resplendent "underground Crystal Palace," but when Stalin's regime came to an end, so did the construction of the glittering glass interior. Today it remains in its strange half-finished state, its visual style marking the end of Stalinism and the beginning of the Thaw. Lenin's coffin was built in 1924; Avtovo station was unveiled in 1955. These spaces are at opposite ends of a thirty-year time line that traces Stalinist illusion-making from its beginnings to its end.

We can likewise trace a historical trajectory from glass for the masses to glass for the elite in the symbolism around glass objects, both real (the lightbulb as a mass commodity) and imaginary (the utopian glass house), as it evolved from the 1920s to the 1930s.[99] Works of glass including the chandeliers in the exclusive high-rise buildings, the Kremlin stars, and the spire of Moscow State University helped to create and sustain the mystique of Soviet power. The appearance of these objects marked a transition from democratic glass—the utopian dream of a communal glass house in which workers would live together, bathed in natural light thanks to the endless expanses of windows, and with all the other benefits of transparent living spaces—to glass that underscored the hierarchical nature of Soviet society.[100] This evolution is a reversal of the nineteenth-century transition from elite (imperial) glass to democratic (phalanstery) glass. Avtovo station heralds the return of the "democratic" trend, insofar as the press coverage, including letters from the public, stressed that these were "palaces" for everyone. These palaces, however, were underground; and hence, authorities such as Lazar Kaganovich, the overseer of the metro project, took pains to reassure the public that these stations emphatically did *not* resemble crypts. A close look at how the Soviet state attempted to tap the ideological potential of spectacular spaces reveals how fraught with anxiety and contradictions this endeavor turned out to be.

The MGU Spire: From Windows to Window-Dressing

In January 1947 (the year in which the Tsentrosoiuz building was denounced as "the music of architecture dissected like a corpse") the Soviet press published a Resolution of the Council of Ministers of the USSR declaring the government's decision to build eight high-rise buildings (*vysotnye zdaniia*) in Moscow. The style of the buildings was to be "linked to the historical development of Moscow and to the silhouette of the future Palace of Soviets. These new buildings should not, therefore, be copies of the multi-storeyed structures already familiar abroad."[101] A Soviet commentator writes: "The government demanded that architects create buildings whose form and content would reflect the grandeur of socialist culture, the creative powers of our people, the might of the Soviet state." These ferro-concrete palaces, whose style came to be designated as "Stalinist Gothic," were designed expressly not to resemble the glass-covered skyscrapers of America. A majority of these buildings, most prominently the largest, most imposing one of all, Moscow State University (MGU), were topped by a glass spire at Stalin's behest.[102] The spire of MGU was to be made of glass in order to catch the sun and become transformed, through a trick of light, into blazing gold.

In Stalin's time, the Constructivist dream of light, airy, easily transportable, and utterly transparent living spaces, of all-glass buildings whose windows would overtake the function of walls, gave way to buildings that constituted a triumph of heavy opacity, an apparent rejection of the Constructivists' celebration of the crystalline aesthetic.[103] Yet glass reasserted itself in the form of the spire, which became the distinctive feature, one could say the trademark, of these still-standing monuments to Stalin. Thus, when the Constructivists disappeared from the architectural scene, glass did not; instead, its role shifted from walls and windows to exterior decoration, that is, glass not as window but as window-dressing, architecture for the outsider's gaze (glass to be looked at), not for those living within (glass to be looked through). As Bowlt formulates it, transparency fell out of favor in the 1930s because Stalinist culture privileged facades in "a desperate attempt to present surface appearance as the absolute form."[104]

The spire of MGU and the Kremlin stars are decorative elements that draw attention to the monumental height of these structures. MGU was constructed to be the tallest building in Europe;[105] its spire was designed to evoke the architecture of the Kremlin (hence architecture that was "national in form"), in particular the spire of the Spasskaya tower. The Kremlin was appropriated as a symbol by the Soviet state; it metonymically stood for the power within (just as the United States "White House" stands for the executive branch of government). The Kremlin stars in turn metonymically represent the Kremlin, and imbue that architectural structure, and the power structure it houses, with an undeniable mystique.

Glass in the service of ideology can take the form of a lightbulb as the humble human-scale embodiment of Lenin's boundless radiance, a kind of secular icon; it can also be as grandiose as the Kremlin stars or the spire of MGU. This spire constitutes an optical illusion. It is made of orange-yellow glass covering an aluminum backing that, when the sun strikes it, resembles gold.[106] The same kind of glass embellishes the sides of the clock face. During the perestroika period, journalist Dmitry Semyonov described it as follows: "Sheets of glass with an aluminum backing are attached to the steel girders—it's like a mirror, only an orange one. Nowadays hardly anyone knows about that, even among the students, but at one time the designers were very proud of their unusual solution—it was both cheap and beautiful [*i deshevo, i krasivo*]."[107]

The falsification of the MGU spire is double: it is made of glass masquerading as gold, and it conceals a high-frequency radio transmitter.[108] In an article on MGU written in May 1991, Semyonov reported that it was possible to climb up into the very star at the top of the spire, but he and his crew chose not to do so because "it's dangerous there right now—too slippery." Yet in a follow-up article written just five months later, the author admitted that he had not been permitted to climb up into the star because it housed a top-secret radio: "We were prohibited from mentioning the high-frequency radio (by whose fault we could not climb up to the star), although the antennae may be easily seen from ground level with a telescopic lens or ordinary binoculars. Phrases that seemed 'slippery' were removed from the article.'"[109] (Indeed, the word "slippery" is the only sign that the original article ever contained any politically sensitive material!) In the follow-up article, however, Semyonov is more open about whose operations the star conceals: the deep sub-basement of the building houses "the headquarters of what appears to be the Moscow directorate of the KGB," and the agents employed therein were the ones who forbade him to investigate further.[110]

The MGU spire is a mirror reflecting not human features but the sky—recalling the early eighteenth-century mirrors placed, because of church prohibitions, high enough to reflect nothing but the ceiling. This anti-mirror represents the effacement of the human subject in another way as well, in that the spire acts as a substitute for a human figure: originally, a statue of Lomonosov, then of Lenin was to crown the building. In a sense, the radiance of the spire stands in for the radiance of Lenin.[111]

In the craft of illusion, the Soviet state had greater success with glass as a container for captive light than with light allowed to dance and play. The spire of MGU was an attempt to play a trick by using, literally, a trick of light. Yet the plan backfired when the fragility of the glass asserted itself. The glass pieces began to break off, and sharp fragments showered the observation platform at the base of the spire, which had to be closed as a result.[112]

In 1947, the same year that Stalin issued the decree about the "tall buildings," Soviet scientists invented a tempered glass called "Stalinite" (*Stalinit*) and began to produce it in mass quantities. This protective glass, used for windshields of cars and trains as well as other technical applications, had an increased durability and heat resistance; when it shattered, it broke into small rounded fragments without sharp cutting edges. (See figure 34.) Yet it also turned out to possess some undesirable qualities. In 1953 a scholar of the Soviet glass industry described the volatile personality of Stalinite: "There are times when the internal stresses are unevenly distributed and a sheet of Stalinite glass spontaneously self-destructs [*samoproizvol'no razrushaetsia*]. Therefore, Stalinite glass is not used in certain cases when absolutely reliable protection is required."[113] The glass was obviously named after Stalin at the height of his power; it drew attention to the meaning of the leader's pseudonym, "man of steel." The intention was to honor Stalin by naming a new, technologically superior substance after him (recall his own words from the "great oath" speech at the Second Congress of the Soviets on January 26, 1924—two days after Lenin's death: "We [communists] are made of a special material"),[114] yet the irony was that the material turned out to have not-so-flattering characteristics. That is the essence of glass—it is a mischievous material that can never be completely appropriated.

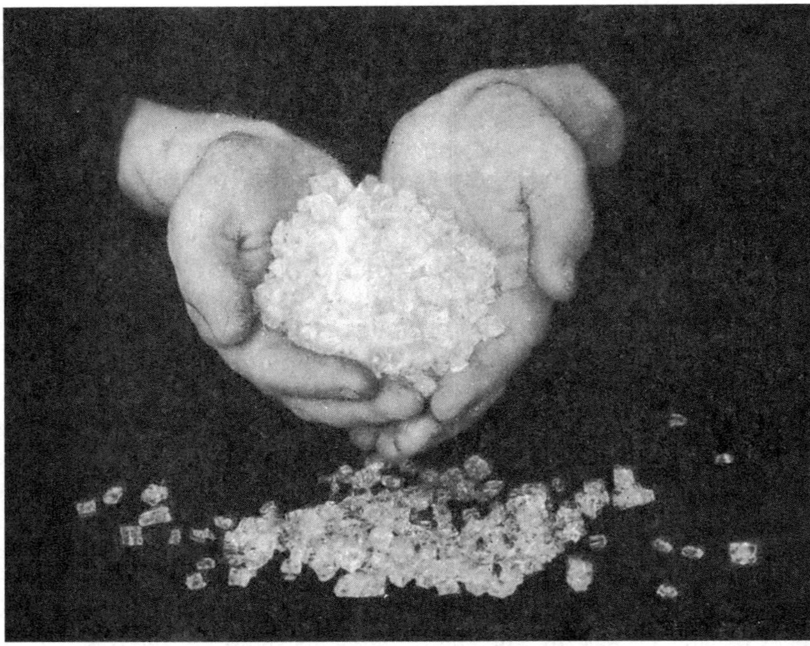

Figure 34. Hands full of broken Stalinite.

Lenin as Sleeping Beauty: The Crystal Coffin

In the past decade, a debate has raged in Russia about what to do with Lenin's body. In September 2005, one of Putin's top officials, Gyorgy Poltavchenko, raised the idea of removing Lenin from the mausoleum on Red Square: "Our country has been shaken by strife, but only a few people were held accountable for that in our lifetime. I do not think that it is right that those who initiated the strife remain in the center of our state near the Kremlin." Filmmaker Nikita Mikhalkov seconded the idea: "Vast funds are being squandered on a pagan show. If we advocate Christian ideals, we must fulfill the will of the deceased." In response, Communist leader Gennady Zyuganov said at a press conference that burying Lenin would be "an attack on our history and culture" and "warned about huge civil disobedience action if authorities tried to bury Lenin." Valeriya Novodvorskaya, head of the Democratic Union (a small reform party), argued: "It is time to get rid of this horrible mummy. One cannot talk about any kind of democracy or civilization in Russia when Lenin is still in the country's main square." Svetlana

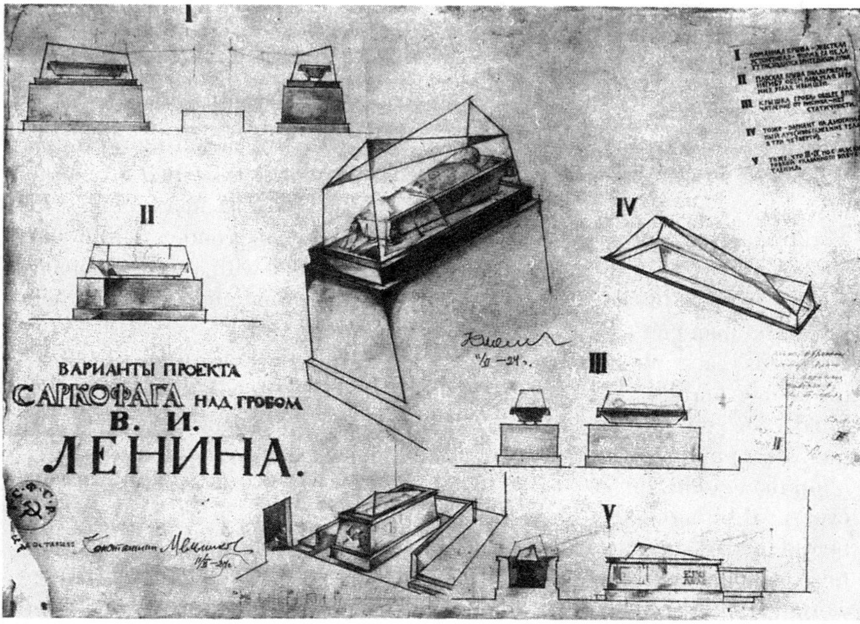

Figure 35. Designs for Lenin's glass sarcophagus, Konstantin Mel'nikov.

Orlova, a deputy speaker of the upper house of the Duma, took a more sympathetic stance in appealing to Lenin's followers to consider "Lenin's soul, which has been searching for peace for nearly a century."[115]

How, then, did Lenin come to be put on display in the first place? Let us turn now to Lenin's display case, the glass heart of the mausoleum, designed by Konstantin Mel'nikov in the form of a crystal. (See figure 35.)

In 1924, while embalmers hurried to preserve Lenin's body, workers dismantled the plate glass window of a restaurant called The Ravine and using this glass of dubious social origin, they cobbled together a sarcophagus.[116] In August 1924, Lenin's body was placed on display in this glass coffin, housed underground in a stone mausoleum on Red Square, his incorruptible remains an allusion to the immortality of Soviet power. The visibility of Lenin's unchanged image was crucial to maintaining the Lenin cult that developed in the years that followed. Glass was the essential element in this ideological spectacle. (See figure 36.)

The decision to place Lenin's body on permanent exhibition stemmed in part from "the overwhelming popular response to Lenin's lying-in-state."[117] On January 21, 1924, the temperature outside was 40 degrees below zero. The Hall of Columns at the Trade Union House was decorated with palm trees; both the trees and Lenin's body were covered with frost. Despite the bitter cold, visitors flooded in from Russia and abroad to bid farewell to Lenin. A *Pravda* correspondent depicted various such pilgrims, from a little old man from a pharmaceutical factory to a worker from a printing press with his six-year-old son in tow. The last visitor described is a young man who went blind in 1921 when he burned his eyes in an accident at his workplace—a glass factory. He wears blue-tinted glasses and carefully steps forward, supported by two coworkers, feeling his way with a cane. Someone asks him why he has come—he won't be able to see anything, so why bother? The blind man pauses to gather his thoughts, then speaks breathlessly, uttering words that could have come from Platonov's pen: "Don't worry, I will see the silence and feel Il'ich. After all, he is my own kin, and though I may be blind I recognize all my kin. Even a blind man can recognize Il'ich." As the mourners crowd around Lenin, hungrily seeking out a glimpse of him, the blind man circles the coffin and tries to pull apart the scar tissue around his eyes, as if trying to see. The correspondent concludes his article thus: "But he did manage to say goodbye to Il'ich. The blind man saw Lenin."[118] In this mythmaking reportage, the body of Lenin has already become a wonder-working relic—it restores the blind man's vision, if only for a moment. Even so soon after Lenin's death, the official coverage already makes him a saint. We can also take note of the multiple layers of irony: the worker is wearing glasses, but not to help him see; glass helps us to see, but an accident at a glass factory robbed the worker of his sight. This vignette turns on its head the notion of glass as a material that improves vision.

As Nina Tumarkin shows, the focal point of the Lenin cult was the leader's preserved body, which "made him simultaneously a proven saint with visibly incorruptible remains and an immortal."[119] Even before Lenin had died, Stalin voiced the idea of putting the leader's body on display to fellow members of the Politburo. He suggested that "certain comrades in the provinces" would see cremation as an insult to Lenin's memory, and that it would be better to embalm Lenin's body and make him accessible to visitors for a time. This suggestion infuriated Trotsky, for whom the idea of embalming Lenin evoked the practices of "the Russian Orthodox Church, that makes relics out of its saints. . . . Earlier there were the relics of Sergius of Radonezh and Serafim of Saratov; now they want to replace these with the relics of Vladimir Ilich."[120]

Just a day after Lenin's death, three suspiciously similar letters appeared in the Moscow daily *Rabochaya Moskva* under the headline, "Lenin's Body Must Be Preserved!" Each one called for Lenin's body to be embalmed and displayed under glass. One letter said, "Under no circumstances can we give to the earth such a great and intensely beloved leader as Il'ich.

We suggest his remains be embalmed and left under glass for hundreds of years. . . . Let him be with us always."[121] It later became a commonplace of Soviet historiography that the "immortalization" of Lenin was a response to a groundswell of popular support. According to the official version of events, the Burial Commission received thousands of telegrams from workers on the subject of what was to be done with Lenin's body, and it was this outpouring of emotion from the populace that led to the decision to preserve Lenin's body in a crypt on Red Square, by the Kremlin wall, that would be made accessible to visitors. One such telegram from a group of Donbass coal miners reads: "The chance to see our beloved leader, even if [he is] immobile, will partially alleviate the grief of losing him and will inspire us to further battles and victories."[122] When the crypt was made accessible to visitors in mid-February 1924, the glass windows installed in the roof of the coffin foreshadowed the sarcophagus that would eventually be built: "The coffin with the body of Vladimir Il'ich was in the center of the room, on a raised pedestal. In the lid of the coffin glass panes were installed through which one could see Lenin's face, illuminated by two chandeliers suspended from the ceiling."[123]

Boris Zbarsky, one of Lenin's original embalmers, wrote in 1946 about the miraculous preservation of Lenin's features: "After the many years that have passed since the day that Vladimir Il'ich died, in the Mausoleum one can see him just at he was in the moments after death. Vast numbers of people have flooded, are flooding, and will flood [*stekalis', stekaiutsia, i budut stekat'sia*] to this place."[124] The repetition of the verb *stekat'sia*, literally "to flow together," evokes the noun *steklo*, "glass," which covers the beloved leader and whose presence manifests itself in Zbarsky's language. Both words, *stekat'sia* and *steklo*, contain the notion of flow, and at the same time, the word *steklo* literally means "that which has flowed together" as if evoking the merging of melted particles and freezing the very moment at which this has happened. The features of Lenin "just at he was in the moments after death" are likewise frozen forever in the crystal coffin.[125]

If Lenin were to be eternally visible, by analogy the Party and philosophy he founded would last forever. Lenin's embalmers insisted that there was "nothing miraculous" about what they had done;[126] yet it certainly appeared that way to those inclined to believe in miracles. Scholars have cited such sources of inspiration for the Lenin display as the Russian Orthodox belief about incorruptible remains as proof of sanctity and the "educational exhibit" inaugurated by Peter the Great and his Kunstkamera.[127] As long as Lenin's features remained unchanged, and visitors to the mausoleum could attest that this was so, the preserved leader would serve as a symbol of both the sanctity and the scientific might of the Soviet state.

New York Times reporter Walter Duranty visited the mausoleum (or as he called it, the "shrine") days after it was first opened. He described his descent down red-carpeted steps into the tomb's interior, and he reported that a gallery ran "around the room on the exact level of the couch upon which Lenin's body lies. . . . From the gallery one looks down upon Lenin, lying as if asleep in a hermetically sealed pyramid of cut glass so transparent that one knows it's there only by the flash, along the surface, of the shaded lights above. . . . His face is serene."[128] Thus transparency was a critical feature of the sarcophagus: visitors would see the unchanging Lenin and even seem to have direct access to him. But the glass container did not only make Lenin visible; it also made him radiant.

As we have seen, an important strategy of the Lenin cult was the association of Lenin with light, a traditional attribute of the divine. This was done by emphasizing his role as the one who brought light to the Soviet people through the electrification campaign and his "little lamps"; furthermore, poems and works of visual art often portrayed Lenin as a literal source of heavenly light. In a written testimony by Nikolai Tkachev, a worker from the Diatkovo glass factory, the appearance of Lenin coincides with a dazzling light show. Tkachev came to Moscow in 1919 with his fellow glassmakers, bearing gifts for Lenin: a crystal version of the Soviet Constitution as well as pitchers, inkwells, and vases engraved with portraits of Marx, Liebknecht, and Lenin himself. In Tkachev's account, the anticipated speech from the great man is somewhat of a letdown, but it is more than compensated by the display of radiant light that appears as Lenin's inevitable attribute:

> We spread out the gifts on a desk. The sun pouring through the big window lit up our crystal, making it sparkle with different-colored lights and reflect the sun beautifully in every direction. It looked like there *was* no crystal on the desk, just a shimmering golden radiance. At that very moment Vladimir Il'ich steps out of his office, glances at the desk, and declares in a jolly sort of way, "Oho, those whiny aesthetes should get a load of these fantastic thingamajigs!" I never forgot those words. Later on, people explained to me about the aesthetes . . .[129]

Katerina Clark notes that Socialist Realist art has used the image of a sudden bright, blinding flash of light to confer sacred qualities upon political figures. Such a flash of light typically accompanied the moment at which the positive hero encountered the Great Leader or found himself in a sacred space.[130] Tkachev's account certainly adheres to this convention. As for the words "whiny aesthetes," they refer to those members of the intelligentsia who claimed that the revolution had brought nothing but destruction, that workers were capable of creating only utilitarian objects, not things of beauty. Practical Lenin thus sees the aurora borealis on his desk as the perfect opportunity to attack his ideological foes.

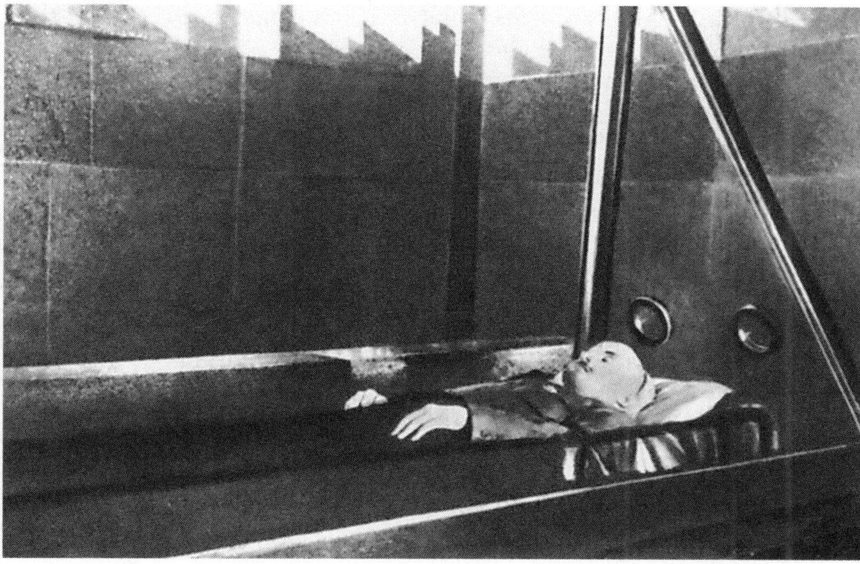

Figure 36. Lenin's embalmed body in the first version of the glass sarcophagus.

A variation on the techno-hagiographical discourse in Tkachev's narrative appears in Nikolai Bukharin's obituary for Lenin on the front page of *Pravda* on January 24, 1924. The text begins: "Lenin has died. Never again will we see that colossal brow, that wondrous head radiating revolutionary energy in every direction."[131] Bukharin creates a descriptive link between Lenin's legendary head[132] (whose phenomenal frontal lobe already suggests the dome of a lightbulb) and the "lamps" for whose creation he was (mythically) responsible.

Fittingly, Konstantin Mel'nikov's design for Lenin's sarcophagus presents the leader as a light source. Mel'nikov's initial plan called for a purely glass construction, with no metal frame: S. Frederick Starr describes the design as a four-sided pyramid bisected by two planes of glass tilting in opposite directions whose intersection "formed a strict horizontal diagonal, thus breaking up the static rectangle of the casket into two lively acute triangles."[133] The result would be, in Mel'nikov's words, "a crystal with a radiant play of light in the interior."[134] In the early 1920s Mel'nikov was intrigued by the German Expressionist celebration of crystals as "symbols of an eternal and perfect order." Mel'nikov owned a Russian translation of a poem by Expressionist Paul Scheerbart whose final image was that of light that "suffuses the Universe / And comes alive in the crystal." Starr concludes that

Mel'nikov designed a crystalline coffin as an apt container for Lenin, "the light that illuminated the Revolutionary order."[135]

The form of Lenin's mausoleum as a dark passageway in which Lenin serves as the source of guiding light was echoed in Mel'nikov's design of the Soviet pavilion at the 1937 Paris Exposition. Here, the visitor moves through the dark into "a light-filled sanctuary . . . The building is thus transformed into an ancient temple, in which the public would undergo a rite of purification so as to emerge in the end into the dazzling light of Soviet life."[136] Progression through a dark passageway is a key component of Masonic rites, which had enjoyed popularity in tsarist Russia for centuries; in particular, the ritual of "hoodwinking" requires the initiate to make his way, blindfolded, through a sacred space toward the revelation of a secret truth.

Lenin's sarcophagus underwent several reconstructions, and each time, designers paid great attention to the lighting of the body. In the most recent version, forty-four projectors with incandescent lamps are installed inside the roof of the sarcophagus. As a Soviet scholar describes, the lamps "illuminate Lenin's face with a soft, even light. . . . The sarcophagus is lit from beneath with special lamps that are invisible to visitors."[137] Reflector lamps concealed in the ceiling contribute to the overall effect.[138]

A 1963 poem by Andrei Voznesensky responds to this version of the sarcophagus, the model that brought to technical perfection the "radiant" idea that was already present in the first version. In the poem, visitors seeking solace emerge from the darkness toward the light that Lenin embodies. But Voznesensky then compares the leader to an X-ray machine, laying bare the oppressive nature of the spectacle: Lenin sees right through his viewers, and the architectural ideal of see-through buildings from decades past is revived in a demand for personal transparency: "We are X-rayed by Lenin. . . . With a sunny and passionate light, his transparent brow blazes like a lamp."[139]

Glass was also instrumental *behind the scenes* in keeping Lenin's body on display, in hidden lamps and various climate-control devices constructed from glass; for example, the light fixtures had special protective glass filters to absorb heat energy.[140] According to one of Lenin's embalmers, the leader's body underwent periodic chemical treatments in special glass tubs—unlike metal, glass is non-reactive.[141] Thus Lenin's body was perpetually transferred from one glass case to another.[142] The interior of Lenin's tomb, then, was the site of public rituals of political veneration, but also of other rituals that took place under the cover of night. As we will see below, these secret rituals of preservation had a negative counterpart in anti-rituals of destruction that were hidden from the public for decades.

Displaying Lenin under glass made sense from several perspectives. The transparency of the glass made Lenin visible and seemingly accessible to visitors; at the same time, the capacity of this material to capture light was used to illuminate the dead leader, creating continuity with his image as propagated by the myth of "radiance." But glass has other characteristics that interfered with the transmission of the message that the Lenin spectacle was meant to convey. In a curious counterpart to the proliferation of Lenin's images in the years following his death, visitors to the mausoleum would see three Lenins: the man himself, and two reflections, thanks to the unusual tilt of the glass walls.[143] By 1939, a new sarcophagus with walls that were virtually invisible was in the works; completed in 1945 at the Red Proletarian factory, it took the form of "a rectangular prism whose sides are made of crystalline glass that does not create reflections. The absolute transparency of the glass panes is achieved thanks to the angle at which they tilt."[144] During the war, Lenin's body had been secretly evacuated to the Urals and returned to Moscow in April 1945; on September 16 of that year, the mausoleum was again opened to the public. Boris Zbarsky wrote on the occasion: "The Soviet people once again see the beloved face of Vladimir Il'ich, whose every dear little feature is familiar [*rodnoe kazhdoi svoei chertochkoi*]. . . . There is something wondrous about Lenin's new sarcophagus: when you look at Lenin, you forget that Lenin's bed [*leninskoe lozhe*] is under a crystal dome."[145] Glass allows for the "wondrous" way in which the new sarcophagus seems to disappear, giving visitors the illusion of direct access to Lenin.

The body of Lenin on display was a spectacle that demanded reverence but generated ambivalent responses. Some, like Stalin, intended it to evoke saintly relics under glass.[146] To others, though, the displayed body called forth folkloric associations that invited mockery, not veneration. Thus, when the mausoleum was first opened to the public, the secret police took note of a certain clerk Antipov joking that "Lenin will lie in his coffin like a 'Sleeping Beauty.'"[147] To complicate the matter, the designer of Lenin's sarcophagus meant this association in earnest. In addition to Scheerbart's adoration of the crystal, Mel'nikov was inspired by the glass coffin of Sleeping Beauty when he designed Lenin's resting place.[148] When interviewed in 1967, the architect affirmed that "he intended this comparison to be taken literally."[149]

Olesha picked up on this fairy-tale allusion in a poem he wrote in 1926 as his alter ego, Zubilo ("The Chisel"), for *Gudok*, the proletarian newspaper where he worked for six years as a "poet-agitator." Throughout the poem, Olesha repeats the familiar platitudes: he insists that while Lenin was mortal, his deeds and influence live on, and he claims that Lenin's posthumous fate is more wondrous than any fairy tale. In an image recalling the "blind man who saw" the leader at his lying-in-state, the poem claims that the very word "Lenin" is powerful enough to make the blind see ("With that word, with that name—every blind man has gained sight and strength"). Lenin's name can melt the "Samoyed sadness" of Russia; it has ascended over the country "for ever and ever" and outshines the polar rainbows; it inspires the folk (*narod*) and calls them to battle. These lines elevate Lenin to the status of a divinity. Yet at the same time, Olesha dwells obsessively on the mortal body on display. The poem begins: "His earthly envelope lies in a glass coffin, as if in a fairy tale"[150] and returns thrice, spellbound, to contemplate Lenin's "earthly envelope" (*zemnaia obolochka*) that itself lies enveloped in an invisible crystalline skin.

There is something not quite right about the poem's repetition of "*zemnaia obolochka*" in reference to Lenin's body. The feminine noun unsettles the gender of the corpse, and again reminds us of the female Sleeping Beauty; it seems part of a strategy to point out the inappropriateness of the spectacle, the discontinuity between the displayed "earthly envelope" and the transcendent deeds and spirit of Lenin. The artists Vitaly Komar and Alexander Melamid recall that when they were children, fairy tales and poems about princesses in crystal coffins colored their viewing of Lenin's body; and that the gender confusion that the exhibit induced in them was exacerbated when Stalin's body was placed next to that of Lenin: "the two sarcophagi resembled those displayed in the Gothic wing of the Pushkin museum . . . In that murky hall, a king lay in his glass coffin, with the queen on his left-hand side . . . A crazy question entered our minds: was Stalin a woman? After all, he was also placed on Lenin's left. Then again, Lenin resembled a princess long before Stalin's arrival."[151] In "Zubilo's" ostensibly panegyric poem, we can glimpse Olesha's veiled dismay over Lenin's display. When Duranty first saw Lenin in his sarcophagus, the leader seemed smaller-than-life: "The body is in a perfect state of preservation, its lineaments as natural as life, but now shrunken and small." *Obolochka* is a feminine word and a diminutive one—thus Lenin is twice diminished by being put on display.[152]

In the third reference to the glass coffin, Olesha puts the word "glass" in the rhyme position, thereby emphasizing the material. The next stanza again returns to glass, now depicting Lenin as "buried" in it (*V steklo pokhoronennyi Lenin*). The choice of the ominous word "buried" emphasizes the leader's mortality, and in doing so, it contradicts the rhetoric customary for the time (and reproduced in the same poem) proclaiming that Lenin "is more alive than the living." Olesha draws our attention to the glass surrounding Lenin's body, and the material, with its unpredictable behavior, makes us see Lenin in a new, defamiliarized way. Olesha's poem thus becomes irreverent in spite of itself, turning from ritual to anti-ritual.

Olesha's novel, *Envy*, published a year after his pseudonymous poem appeared, offers another unsettling portrayal of Lenin's crystal coffin in the image of a glass cube with a body inside. This image also holds a potential explanation for antihero Kavalerov's estranged way of seeing; as he recounts:

> When I was a schoolboy, I was taken to a wax museum. There, in a glass cube, was a handsome man in evening clothes, a still-smoking wound in his chest, dying in someone's arms. My father explained: "That's the French President Carnot. He was shot by an anarchist." . . . A splendid man, his beard thrust upward, was lying in a greenish cube. . . . I swallowed ecstatic tears. I decided to become famous, so that one day my wax double, filled with the drone of time that only a few can hear, would be just as elegantly poised in a greenish cube.[153]

In the wax museum, the young Kavalerov simultaneously becomes aware of his own mortality and comes to see spectacular display as the way to triumph over death. An impressionable youth, he sees an edifying exhibition that shapes him irrevocably—thus testifying, it would seem, to the power of visual propaganda. Yet the effect of this wordless spectacle is unpredictable, and in *Envy*, it has a sinister outcome: Kavalerov imagines that the sign accompanying his wax double will proclaim his notoriety for an unspecified "despicable crime" (Olesha, *Zavist'*, 21).

The description of the waxworks display in Olesha's novel bears a number of allusions to the displayed body of Lenin, hinting that that the figure in the mausoleum is, by analogy, not the authentic body of the leader but a wax copy. Such a suggestion is scandalous in itself: after all, the miraculous preservation of Lenin's body was touted as yet another scientific triumph that could only be possible under Soviet power. Olesha's subtle iconoclasm can be seen as a discursive counterpart to the attacks and other forms of irreverence aimed at Lenin in his tomb.

Not long after Lenin's body was put on display, a folktale titled "Sly Lenin" was published "along with two other allegedly authentic folktales about the Civil War" in the journal *Novyi mir*.[154] It was said to have "circulated in 1925 among the peasants of the Viatka countryside," but was apparently fabricated by writer Rodion Akul'shin. Lenin worries about how his country would fare without him, so he "asks 'the chief Soviet physician' to render him dead 'not completely, but just for appearances.'"[155] That way he can travel around incognito and see how Soviet Russia is doing. The doctor tells Lenin, "We will put you not in a grave . . . but in a spacious room, and we will cover you with glass so that no one can poke you with his fingers."[156] In addition to the hint at how Doubting Thomas digitally verified Christ's divinity, there is in this narrative some ambiguity about why a visitor would try to reach out and touch Lenin—with good or not-so-good intentions. The folktale foreshadows the actual attempted violations that were to take place in the mausoleum in the decades to come. These acts were a subversive response to the officially sanctioned ritual behavior that was meant to take place in that sacred space—visitors paying their *dis*respects, as it were.

The glass around Lenin paradoxically both protected him and made him more vulnerable. There were a series of attacks on the sarcophagus, one as early as 1934. In March of that year, collective farmer Mitrofan Nikitin entered the mausoleum and aimed a revolver at Lenin's corpse. When guards prevented him from shooting, he turned the gun on himself. A search at his house turned up "a letter he had written about atrocities connected with the famine of 1933. . . . 'Our rulers, entrenched inside the walls of the Kremlin, will not see that the people do not want this sort of life . . . Rulers, where are you leading the nation? We are on the slippery slope to the abyss.'"[157] The reference to the Kremlin walls is notable here. Nikitin is trying to shoot through the sarcophagus which becomes a metonymic stand-in for the Kremlin. The leaders in the Kremlin are alive, but unresponsive, as if dead. The display of Lenin's body thus generated another unintentional effect—in this case, a dangerous misreading.

The attacks continued. In 1959, a man whose name is lost to us flung a hammer—one half of the omnipresent Soviet emblem symbolizing the union of workers and peasants—at the sarcophagus; it smashed through the glass and landed on Lenin's chest, covering the leader with slivers and shards.[158] Here, not for the first time or the last, the material revealed its menacing side. In July of the following year, a certain K. N. Minibaev pulled a stunt of the sort that Kavalerov could only dream about as a passport to eternal notoriety. He leapt up on the barrier adjacent to the sarcophagus and shattered the glass with a kick. Once again, Lenin's face and hands became covered with numerous glass fragments. Those charged with maintaining Lenin's appearance had to repair a centimeter-long tear above his right eyebrow.[159] Il'ia Zbarsky (the son of Boris Zbarsky, who carried on his father's job) reports a case of someone setting off an explosion inside the mausoleum; a guard was injured, but Lenin's body remained intact. In the wake of this incident, stronger security measures were taken, including the installation of bulletproof glass and electronic devices for the detection of weapons and explosives. Still, in 1987 on two separate occasions a visitor threw a bottle of gasoline at the base of the sarcophagus and set the gasoline on fire.[160]

What could account for all these attacks on something so sacrosanct, at such obvious risk to oneself? One must consider not only political convictions but also the motivation, visual, tactile, and auditory, for breaking glass, and in particular, a light source encased in glass. Wolfgang Schivelbusch writes about the anarchic ritual of lantern-smashing in seventeenth- and eighteenth-century Paris, which offered the disenfranchised a symbolic way to smash the authority that these lights represented, as well as a more visceral thrill:

> The sound of breaking glass is like an explosion. Something that a moment ago was solid, an object with a highly symbolic significance, is suddenly wiped

out. The desire to wreak such destruction and also to experience a symbolic sexual release in the loud splintering of breaking glass were probably the deeper motives behind lantern smashing.[161]

Recalling the mythical image of Lenin as a light source can further help to explicate the behavior of those visitors who lashed out at the ideological spectacle before them, placing their hopes in the destructive potential of the very material that protected and deified the leader.

Avtovo Station: The Underground Crystal Palace

Anxiety about breaking glass manifested itself in press descriptions of Avtovo station, the showcase stop on the first line of the Leningrad metro that was dubbed an "underground Crystal Palace" when it was opened in November 1955 as one of the first seven metro stations in the city. (See figure 37.) Glass is the main material in the ornamentation of the interior, in mosaics, bas-reliefs, and stately columns covered with cut glass that newspapers assured

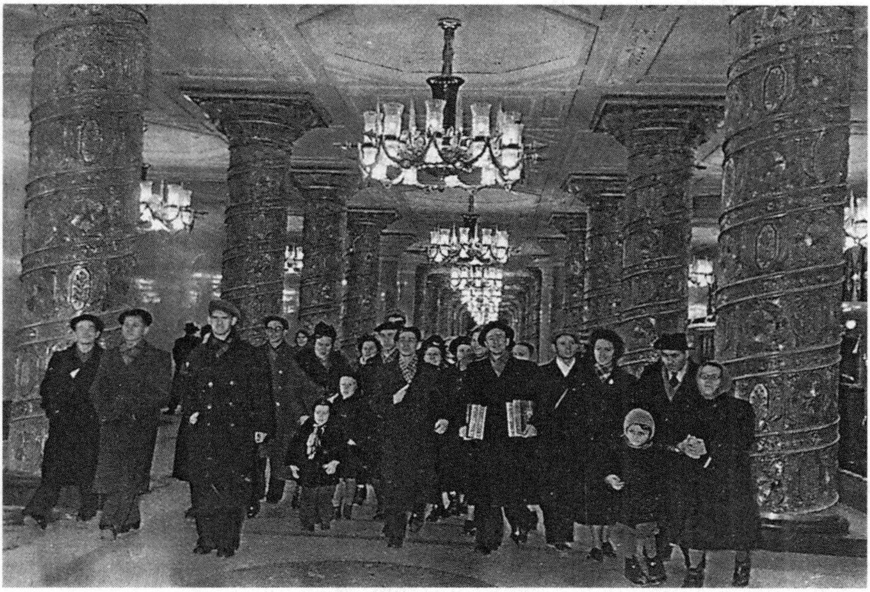

Figure 37. Visitors (by special invitation) to Avtovo station on November 6, 1955, the day when the first train departed from the station. Photograph by I. Baranov and V. Kapustin.

readers was "stronger than marble."[162] These columns, featuring images of five-pointed stars, banners, and sheaves of wheat, were lit by small projector lamps discreetly concealed in the ornamental ceiling.[163] Glass barriers and a colored glass floor were also in the works. Eventually, however, only 16 of the 46 Avtovo columns ended up being covered in glass[164]—work on them ceased when Stalin died, and the rest of the station was executed in a plain, unadorned style.

Like its Moscow cousin, the Leningrad metro was an ideologically charged space. The first train departed from Avtovo station on November 6, 1955, the eve of the anniversary of the October Revolution (a connection that was emphasized in the press coverage). On November 15, the day when the metro was opened to the public, the front-page editorial in *Leningradskaia Pravda*, titled "For the Good of the People," called the metro a "wondrous gift" (*chudesnyi podarok*) to the city from the Communist Party and the Soviet government: "The stern, genuinely artistic beauty of these underground palaces is lit up and warmed by a great love for mankind." It was concern for "the workers of the city" that guided the "architects, sculptors, and artists who adorned the metro stations in marble, bronze, and crystal, illuminating the subterranean darkness with the light of electric suns." These images of light and heat present the Party in a victorious struggle against the darkness and cold of the underground. Glass is still being used to create an ideological spectacle of light, but the discourse around that spectacle has subtly changed; in Lenin's tomb, the light served to denote the leader-tyrant's divinity and appeared to issue from his body, whereas now the light, identified as nurturing and life-giving, is dispersed throughout a space that has been appropriated, sanctified, and transformed into an embodiment of the radiant future.

The crystal columns in Avtovo station were themselves designed to be light sources—the original plan called for them to glow from within. So much glass was used to decorate Avtovo station to convey the feeling of light—this time, not the "sacred light" of Lenin, but rather the conquest or denial of darkness. The interior of the deepest subway in the world was designed to look like a bright sunny day.[165] In a speech before the grand opening of the Moscow metro (the stylistic model for the first line of the Leningrad metro) in May 1935, Lazar Kaganovich contrasted the subways in capitalist nations, whose dirty and dim interiors were "crypt-like," with the Soviet metro, which would be not only convenient but "palatial," "creating feelings of joy and happiness, or *zhizneradost'*." In order to convey this impression, "architects of the metro's first line were required to create brightly lit, high-ceilinged halls . . . Soviet planners made mathematical calculations to ensure that the light would reflect from the marble with the desired brilliance."[166] As Karen Kettering points out, Avtovo station constituted the culmination of attempts to create "an interior that would seem airy and 'sunny.'"[167] Glass is not only spectacular, but also man-made, thus capable of imitating the works of nature, from marble to ice, but totally under human control (or so it would seem). As such it appeared to fit perfectly into the promethean thinking that informed the grand Soviet schemes for the transformation of the natural world.[168]

The call for a bright environment in the metro was a matter of creating continuity with the ideal of the "bright future" toward which Soviet citizens were striving. After all, the metro interiors frequently presented idealized images of communist paradise achieved. As Catherine Cooke explains, "In the standard phrase which encapsulated Stalin's promise to his people, their labor would deliver a *svetloe budushchee*: a radiant future. . . . In the society working for this [future], a *svetloe* [radiant] material environment was both the ideological activator and the ultimate reward."[169]

Another meaning of the well-lit interior of the Avtovo station can be glimpsed in the press coverage of the grand opening: here, the metro becomes a place for romantic trysts, and we catch a glimpse of everyday surveillance, an act in which all are invited to participate (in contrast with the subterranean space of Lenin's tomb, where the dead leader alone has the gift to "see through" people): "The above-ground vestibule keeps growing more populated and more animated. All the public telephone booths are occupied and—let's listen in! hear that?—someone is already designating a rendezvous in the metro. Where, where? Ah, by the second chandelier on the left in the central hall of the Technological Institute station." In this voyeur society, light makes everyone visible. As Gaston Bachelard observes, "Everything that casts a light sees."[170] Moreover, Avtovo station serves as a meeting place in a number of ways; akin to Lenin's tomb, to which visitors "flood" from all points on the globe, the metro brings disparate people together, a fact underscored by the official description of the materials used in the construction of the interior: "The crystal chandeliers illuminate the warm red and glistening gray marble of the Caucasus, the sunny-yellow and white, delicately veined marble from the Urals, and the pink and black granite from Ukraine."

In the press coverage following the launch of the metro, photographs of Avtovo station appeared more frequently than those of the others. A front-page image in *Leningradskaia Pravda* shows the glass column at center stage, flanked by smiling passengers on one side and a speeding train on the other. These glass-covered columns were indeed the focal point of the station. They were a modern reply to tsarist-era columns for which that city was famous, such as the massive malachite columns in the Winter Palace.[171] These crystal columns were the Soviet version, and they were "stronger than marble."[172] The columns also conferred on the station interior the aura of classical antiquity. Andrew Jenks writes apropos the use of columns in the first lines of the Moscow metro (which, we recall, was the stylistic model for the first line of its Leningrad counterpart): passengers entering the Kirov or Sokolniki stations would pass through "pavilions supported by massive columns reminiscent of Greek temples . . . marking the division between sacred and profane spaces."[173]

The designers of the Avtovo crystal columns mounted the glass elements inside a spiral armature winding vertically along the column from top to bottom. The spiral design was informed by that of the great Trajan column of Rome as well as the column in the Place Vendôme in Paris (itself modeled on the Trajan column).[174] It is appropriate that in a period when Neoclassicism dominated the decorative arts, the designers of the Avtovo station would emulate the Trajan column, a monument of classical antiquity, and furthermore, a war monument: the original design of the Avtovo columns included images commemorating the defense of Leningrad during the Second World War.[175] Yet the spiral design suggests another comparison, or rather contrast, with a construction from more recent times—the iron-and-glass double spiral of Tatlin's Monument to the Third International. Let us note the progression from one ideological use of glass to another. The glass chambers of the Tatlin monument, had it been built, would have served as material embodiments of the ideal of transparency in politics and social life—openness, access to information, and an end to secrecy. The glass of the Avtovo columns was not used to embody or encourage transparency; on the contrary, the construction embodied the ideals of showiness, sham, and secrecy that were intrinsic to the High Stalinist style. Both the Avtovo station and Lenin's crystal coffin were designed to be seen by throngs of spectators every day, using spectacular glass and a subterranean setting to instill awe and mystery.

A stylistic disparity within the station serves as an emblem of the end of High Stalinism and the start of the Thaw. During construction, the ornate glass decor was abandoned less than halfway through when the Lomonosov factory in Leningrad could not fulfill the order in time; fewer than half of the Avtovo columns ended up being covered in glass, and the unfinished station was left that way when the opulent ("monumental-pompous") style associated with Stalinism became politically incorrect. There is a curious tension in the press accounts between praising the lavish decor of the new metro stations and the campaign against "excesses" in building being trumpeted in the same pages.[176] This discrepancy attests to the complexity of the situation: Soviet citizens were not uniformly willing to assimilate the rhetoric of de-Stalinization and give up the fairy-tale dream of the previous era.[177]

On November 5, 1955, the Leningrad metro was given a trial run. "Hundreds of Leningraders, mostly schoolchildren" received tickets inviting them to ride the first trains. The press reported how "schoolchildren filled the underground palaces of the metro"; the children sat in the sky-blue train cars "as if enchanted" (note the color of the cars—another example of celestial brightness in the underground setting); they got out at each stop to admire the "stateliness and unique beauty" of the stations. This phrasing raises two important points: Soviet citizens were to think of these metro stations as "palaces," thereby appropriating palatial architecture from the aristocracy of old, an especially important strategy in a city such as Leningrad, the former tsarist capital bursting with palaces (in this connection it is important to recall Anna's Ice House as well). Thus, a letter to the *Leningradskaia Pravda* in praise of the new metro betrays a palpable anxiety about measuring up to the West and to Russia's own tsarist past: "I had the chance to travel abroad, and I saw the foreign subways with my own eyes. Our subways—both the Moscow and the Leningrad ones—are immeasurably better and more beautiful." But also, the formula "underground palace"—an epithet that would be repeated in subsequent press coverage, including letters to the editor—brings to mind the "underground kingdom" (*podzemnoe tsarsvo*) of Russian fairy tales, turning the metro into an otherworldly, folkloric space. Indeed, the first visitors (children—the predominant consumers of fairy tales) appear to be "enchanted" as they take in the sights and sounds of the metro.

The "fairy-tale" idea recurs in press coverage of the Leningrad metro from subsequent days. This magical motif is intertwined with references to how brightly lit the metro is inside. Thus, a first-time visitor wrote: "One underground palace after another rose up before us, *as if by magic*. When we descended into the metro, it was cloudy outside, but underground at every station there is so much light and air that it seems as if the sun is shining brightly. It's all just like in a fairy tale!"[178] More popular reactions to the Leningrad metro were recorded in the comment books at every station, and they reiterated the folkloric motifs of palaces and magic.[179] L. Parfil'eva proclaimed: "The Leningrad metro is beautiful! You can't help but feel moved when you look at its palaces. This is far better than the best fairy tale." The Zelenko family wrote: "We Leningraders, who have lived through the blockade, thank the Party and the government wholeheartedly for their gift to our hero-city." And an elderly woman with the last name Chevleva testified that the subterranean space resembled its polar opposite: "I've been to the metro—it's like being in heaven [*kak v raiu*]. Now I'm not even afraid to die."[180]

An article by architect L. Shimakovsky written soon after the grand opening claims that the Avtovo interior creates an "impression of extraordinary spaciousness . . . You cannot help but forget that you are underground."[181] The designers of the Avtovo interior likewise extolled the craft of illusion in describing their work. When they drew up a list of essential criteria for the construction of the columns' glass facing, the very first item emphasized that the ferroconcrete shaft at the center of the column must not be visible under any circumstances in order to convince the viewer that it was made of crystal through and through. The designers claimed that using an ingenious faceting technique allowed them to optically "disguise" the shafts at the center of each column, making them seem to dissolve in the crystal "monolith."[182] Glass is often at the center of these behind-the-scenes scenarios of power, ingenuity, and illusion: we recall the monumental glass spire of MGU that masquerades as gold.[183]

Shimakovsky's article states that the Avtovo station has quickly become known as the "Crystal Palace." Readers would doubtless pick up on the utopian associations of this image; but how many would also remember Dostoevsky's attack in *Notes from Underground* on the utopianism of Chernyshevsky, who dreamt up a Crystal Palace for Russia and who served as such an inspiration for Lenin? Notably, in Dostoevsky's novel, his antihero launched his attack on the Crystal Palace and all that it represented—the denial of free will, the advent of industrial capitalism, false unity, and the triumph of materialism over spirituality—from the *underground*; that space of rebellion was quickly usurped with the advent of Soviet power.[184]

The Avtovo station, like the Lenin mausoleum, was created to inspire wonder and otherworldly associations, as attested by the religious and folkloric rhetoric that proliferates in descriptions of these spaces. Both sites served as conduits of visual propaganda, but also as venues for human activity and performance, places where events unfolded, both ongoing processes (as in the case of visitors viewing Lenin's body and commuters traveling through the metro) and discrete, one-time-only rituals—the grand openings of both sites and other ceremonies (and anti-rituals) that took place there. Lenin's mausoleum was a reliquary, a pilgrimage site, a place to become indoctrinated or strengthen one's faith, and a tribune for the living leaders; the tomb intentionally resembles the tombs of the pharaohs, while Lenin himself is both man and monument. The Avtovo metro station is not only a means of travel but also a historical monument to the hero-city surviving the siege; as in the case of the mausoleum, the design of the station alludes to overcoming nature, defying mortality; and it "transports" people in several different ways.[185]

Both subterranean spaces are spectacular sites that ritualize human activity. In the fixed ritual of mausoleum-going, visitors have to keep on moving, and reflection is not allowed. In the words of architectural historian Selim Khan-Magomedov, "A person does not simply go to the Mausoleum as to a museum, and does not stand before the sarcophagus, but seems to participate in a funeral procession in which people walk in mournful silence to bid farewell to the great leader. . . . Nowadays we cannot even imagine any other ritual of attending the Mausoleum."[186] Khan-Magomedov underscores the intention behind the Lenin display to recall the leader's lying-in-state that took place in January 1924—the memorable and moving spectacle at which "the blind man saw Lenin"—and to reenact that ritual time and time again.

The enforced movement within the space of Lenin's tomb echoes the flow of commuters inside the metro: it is a society on the march, always moving forward. A. M. Sokolov's 1957 study of the Leningrad metro speaks to this idea: noting that each station features "works of monumental painting and sculpture" created by "a large collective of artists and sculptors," the author is quick to add: "It stands to reason that one could not get too absorbed in looking at such elements of decor. After all, metro stations are railway stations situated underground, and by no means museum halls or art galleries."[187] The author's words reinforce the notion of perpetual motion that is meant to take place in Lenin's tomb and Avtovo station.

The interior of both Lenin's tomb and Avtovo station can be characterized as the decor of denial: denial of death (Lenin is made to look as if he is alive, and furthermore, he is a light source just as he was in life), and denial of depth (the bright lighting and impression of spaciousness belies the fact that the visitor is deep underground). Both spaces rely on the conjunction of light and glass to create visual effects that underscore their respective functions.[188] At the same time, the delicate glass decor of both spaces draws attention to the instability of the ideological messages embodied in spectacular objects; the possibility of multiple interpretations and unfettered actions arises by virtue of the physical properties of glass—its fragility and unpredictable play of light.

Conclusion

> The vessel of faith is filled with the invisible—
> not with the hidden, but on the contrary,
> with the transparent. God's invisibility is His
> perfect transparency . . . In antiquity, heaven
> was understood as a piece of glassware worked
> by the greatest Master, and this was not a
> metaphor for heaven but a fact about glass
> itself, which is nothing but the bowl of heaven,
> charged in holy hands with pouring forth divine
> light and illuminating the frame of things.
> —The Glaziers' manifesto

> [In the near future,] trains will race along
> glass rails, glass chairs will come into use, glass
> pavements will be built and you will be able to
> stroll along them with a glass walking stick in
> your hand, and if anyone takes it into his head
> to get rid of a glass object, he will have to bury
> it in the ground because it will be impossible to
> break it.
> —Nikolai Kachalov

IN A 1931 LYRIC set in Moscow, Osip Mandelstam declares that he is out of step with his age, predicts that he will not live to see the bright future, and paints a portrait of architectural eclecticism taken to a grotesque extreme: "Not even as a light shadow / Will I enter glass palaces on chicken legs."[1] As an Acmeist, Mandelstam saw the word as a building material, and "chose architecture, the art with the most concrete material, as a model" for his verse.[2] If in Mandelstam's symbolic system, stone metonymically stands for the cathedral of world culture, what sort of edifice does glass represent? In what follows, I will use Mandelstam's poetic treatment of glass to foreground the dual function of this material—as a key ingredient of the ideological spectacle and as a source of artistic inspiration—that

I have traced through a series of case studies in the preceding pages. I will then take a broader view of the overarching themes in my study and suggest directions for further exploration of the ways in which literature reveals how glass, and the material world more broadly, resonates with meaning far beyond the utilitarian.

Before turning to Mandelstam, let us recap a number of central points in this study. As I have argued, Russians have a unique relationship with glass for a variety of reasons, from the visual orientation of Russian culture to the material's association with Westernization and modernization, both of which are processes that are crucial to the debates around Russian self-identity. I have sought to illustrate how glass in Russia was a means to both realize and symbolize modernity. Glass in the form of windows, optical lenses, mirrors, and spectacular constructions transformed how and what Russians saw; moreover, the physical (optical and other) qualities inherent to glass gave rise to symbolic associations, which generated discourses (whether by rhetoricians employed by the state or by independent visionaries) that appealed to the popular imagination and transfigured the ways in which people thought and dreamed. The latter set of considerations resonates particularly with Mandelstam's use of glass.

The significance of glass in the cityscape in Mandelstam's poetry changes over time. In "Peterburg strophes" (1913), Mandelstam uses the reflective capacity of glass to help set the scene: a solar ray ignites the thick glass of a porthole of a steamship.[3] In the later "Stanzas" (1935), glass struck by the sun appears again, and the St. Petersburg cityscape is invoked through a reference to the Admiralty spire, but now the image is a disturbing one: Russia "took notice of me, and suddenly, like a lens, ignited me with the Admiralty's ray [*kak chechevitsa, Admiralteiskim luchikom zazhgla*]" (Mandel'shtam, *Izbrannoe*, 319). The glass surface that is Russia becomes a burning lens, and the poet himself is its target.

The ominous treatment of glass in the cityscape applies to Moscow as well. The lyric in which Mandelstam states that he will never enter "glass palaces on chicken legs" ("Today one can make decals") alludes, as Vladimir Papernyi points out, to the controversial Tsentrosoiuz building designed by Le Corbusier, "the only crystal palace in Moscow."[4] The edifice, then, that Mandelstam conjures up in his poem is a composite of utopian fiction and contemporary architecture—the Tsentrosoiuz building, a crystal palace in which ideals collided with reality. Mandelstam wrote this poem at a time when, according to Nadezhda Mandelstam, the poet "came to believe in the future for the first time but understood that he would not be a part of it. He envisioned 'the new' in the form of sports festivals. . . . and 'glass palaces'—doubtless alluding to Dostoevsky's 'crystal palace' as well as the abominably constructed house on Miasnitskaia Street."[5] The fact that the building was balanced on stilts (Le Corbusier's *pilotis*) earned it the nickname "hut on chicken legs"—Baba Yaga's domicile.[6] Mandelstam appropriates the epithet and conflates it with Chernyshevsky's dream-edifice, and in so doing, he turns the architectural symbol of socialist utopia into a site of folkloric evil; in addition, his formulation recalls the demotion of the Crystal Palace into a "chicken coop" in *Notes from Underground* and thus breathes new life into the Underground Man's rebellion.

In the later "Stanzas" (1935), Mandelstam again associates glass with the Moscow cityscape: he describes the city as "more tender than the sea, more mixed-up than a salad of wood, glass, and milk" (Mandel'shtam, *Izbrannoe*, 319). With this image Mandelstam not only evokes the chaos of the socialist metropolis but suggests that there are irreconcilable contradictions at the heart of it. Milk stands for nourishment of the sort that "Mother Moscow" ought to provide, while wood and glass are architectural components (of "old" and "new" Moscow, respectively); but the three ingredients do not make for a salad that is tasty or even safe to eat. By this time, Mandelstam was barred from Moscow and living in exile in Voronezh, a year after his arrest for reciting his infamous Stalin epigram. Physically far from the capital city, the poet kept revisiting it in his verse and treading over the glass that inevitably lay at its center; and thus, a poem from two years later alluding to a military demonstration on Red Square presents Moscow in the guise of a burning glass heart: "the glass of Moscow blazes between faceted ribs [*steklo Moskvy gorit mezh rebrami granenymi*]" (Mandel'shtam, *Izbrannoe*, 361).[7] Red Square featured a key example of monumental glass lit from within—Lenin's sarcophagus, which had been in existence for over ten years by this time. The poet was keenly aware of the link between spectacular glass and Soviet power. Indeed, the line in question ushers in the voice of Stalin ("indispensable words from the Kremlin") as well as his composite portrait[8] in subsequent stanzas, accompanied by the tolling of the Kremlin bells.[9]

In the poems cited above, glass appears to collude with the totalitarian regime. But other references to glass in Mandelstam's oeuvre are of a quite different tonality. As an Acmeist, Mandelstam celebrated the materiality of the word as Logos. The title of his first collection of poetry, *Stone*, alludes to the image of the poet as a master craftsman who transforms resisting stone into lacy and lofty cathedrals. Yet glass—another architectural requisite—also makes numerous appearances in Mandelstam's poetry. How then did Mandelstam envision the relationship between glass and Logos?

Some answers to that question can be found in an intertextual dialogue between Mandelstam and Khlebnikov. Among the twentieth-century artists we have considered, Khlebnikov stands out as the greatest glass enthusiast. Yet, paradoxically, in a late work by Khlebnikov, the long poem *Zangezi* (1922), the window is an unsettling, ambivalent presence. The eponymous hero, the author's stand-in, introduces himself as follows:

> I, a butterfly that has flown / into the room of human life, / am to leave the handwriting of my dusty coat / across the stern windows [*po surovym oknam*], / in the signature of a prisoner, / upon the austere windowpanes of fate. / How tedious and gray / is the wallpaper of human life! / The transparent "no" of windows! / I have already rubbed off my blue glow, the patterns of dots, / the first freshness of my wing's sky-blue storm, / the pollen has been removed, my wings have faded and become transparent and stiff, / I throw myself exhaustedly against humanity's window.[10]

In this passage, the glass expanse of the window takes the form of a word, an utterance: "The transparent 'no' of windows [*Okon prozrachnoe 'net'*]." Glass constitutes an objection: it stands in opposition to the opaque construction material that surrounds it. We recall that Khlebnikov's City of the Future featured "glass vowels and iron consonants." In both cases, Khlebnikov presents glass in terms of language; in the later work, however, the glass carries an aura of negation.[11] The word emerges out of the glass as if by magic; and the glass-word, as if it were an incantation, has a magical effect: the narrator's "wings have faded and become transparent and stiff" as he beats against the window—in other words, they take on the physical attributes of that window. The artist-butterfly sacrifices himself to transparency, undergoing a fatal metamorphosis.

Khlebnikov's image of "the windowpanes of fate [*steklakh roka*]" resonates with that of "the windowpanes of eternity" in an earlier poem by Mandelstam, "A body has been given to me" (1909), a famous work that Khlebnikov would have known. The two poets shared an interest in the connection between architecture and verbal art.[12] Both were highly attuned to the materiality of language and strove to build eternal cathedrals from it.[13] Their intertextual dialogue reveals the way in which an everyday artifact made of glass—the windowpane—can provoke a meditation on the nature of artistic creation:

> A body has been given to me; what shall I do with it,
> So indivisible and so my own?
> Tell me, whom am I to thank
> For the quiet joy of breathing and being alive?
> I am the gardener, and I am also the flower;
> In the dungeon of the world, I am not alone.
> My breath, my warmth has already settled
> Upon the windowpanes of eternity.
> A pattern, unrecognizable of late,
> Shall be imprinted upon it.
> Let the dregs of the moment flow down—
> The dear pattern cannot be crossed out.[14]

A windowpane serves as a figure for eternity in Mandelstam, and for fate in Khlebnikov. Both artists take abstract concepts and make them palpable; and for both, the otherworldly quality of glass allows it to embody abstract, metaphysical conceptions.

Mandelstam's image of warm condensed breath on a glass surface suggests a person at an intimate proximity to a window; thus is the "windowpane of eternity," a potentially lofty Symbolist metaphor, domesticated. In his essay "About the Nature of the Word" (1922, reworked in 1928) Mandelstam states that the task of the poet is to domesticate the material world. He wishes to foster the "Hellenism" of Russian poetry, which he defines as the metamorphosis of "indifferent objects . . . into the utensil, the humanization of the surrounding world; the environment heated with the most delicate teleological warmth."[15] The original Russian text reveals an interplay between the sounds of the word *telo*, *teplo*, and *teleologicheskii*.[16] A similar play with sound appears in "A body has been given to me (Dano mne telo) . . ." when Mandelstam makes the reader aware that the word *steklo* (glass) has the word *telo* (body) in it, as does *teplo* (warmth). Thus he creates a network of associations bringing the three words together. The "dear pattern," then, can refer to a line drawing traced by a finger in the condensed vapor, which disappears when the vapor fades, but in fact remains indelible. When the glass steams up again, the pattern reappears. "A body has been given to me"—Mandelstam's own "exegi monumentum"—evokes precisely this phenomenon.

Mandelstam's oeuvre has other examples of the creative act taking the form of an inscription on glass: thus, in the early lyric, "On the pale blue enamel" (1909) God is a "dear artist" who "neatly traces" a pattern of tree branches "on the firmament of glass" (Mandel'shtam, *Izbrannoe*, 33).[17] The modifier for "artist" in this poem is "*milyi*," the same word as in the "dear pattern" (*uzora milogo*) in "A body has been given to me." This echo underscores the godlike way in which Mandelstam sees the work of the artist. Mandelstam draws our attention to the transparency of the sky, and to the fact that glass is the earthly, material way in which human beings can grasp something so otherworldly and divine. In the words of the mystical Glaziers: "Heaven, mounted in a setting of stone or iron, becomes a magnifying glass, a precious splinter of transparency . . . what we are holding in our hands is a visible image of the invisible."[18] Moreover, in "A body has been given to me," it is the artist's breathing that creates the immortal work of art; the artist, then, does God one better: while the Deity breathed life into mortal man, the breath of the artist creates a work of life that shall never be "erased"!

A number of Mandelstam's poems, including the monumental "Slate Ode" of 1923 and his 1937 ode to Stalin, reveal a fascination with the materiality, and hence the potential demise, of inscription. Mandelstam's repeated references to inscription on glass can be read as a response to Odoevsky's utopia in letters (discussed in chapter 4) in which writings on glass have survived when all others have fallen prey to the ravages of time. Odoevsky's work is obsessed with the perishability of the written text; in Mandelstam's time, the survival of the text had a poignant meaning the likes of which Odoevsky could not have imagined.

In his later poetry, Mandelstam moves from glass as surface for inscription to glass as a figure for language itself. The resulting image of language is an alarming one: it is something of which you are not aware until you struggle with it, and then it resists and wounds you. Mandelstam's *Second Moscow Notebook* contains a poem about the perils of translation. The poem was written in May 1933, during a time when translation was the only literary work that Mandelstam could obtain.[19] The Eulenspiegel affair of 1928–29, when he had been wrongly accused of plagiarizing another's translation, was also a recent and painful memory. The opening lines liken the act of translation to biting through glass: "Do not tempt [*ne iskushai*] foreign dialects, but try to forget them: after all, you still won't manage to sink your teeth into glass!" (Mandel'shtam, *Izbrannoe*, 283).[20] The language of the poem is puzzling. It would seem to make more sense to say "do not be tempted by foreign dialects"; by invoking incorrect usage, Mandelstam appears to be purposely creating the impression of a bad translation. The word *iskushat'* means to tempt, but *iskusit'* also means to taste, to try; thus, the suggested meaning is "do not taste foreign dialects."

Mandelstam is playing here on the common verbal root *-kus-* of *iskusit'*, to tempt/taste, and *ukusit'*, to bite. In both cases he is calling attention to the mouth, the site where the sounds of language are produced;[21] he then draws an analogy between the foreign language and glass, which has the potential to inflict a wound upon the speaking subject. (We recall that in "Stanzas," written two years after "Do not tempt foreign dialects," Mandelstam compares Moscow to a salad with glass as one of the ingredients, again with an implication of "biting into glass" and injury inflicted upon the mouth.) Thus, according to Mandelstam, trying to translate a foreign language, or to speak in a foreign dialect, is akin to trying to bite into glass. The idea of translation has broader implications; at the time when he wrote this poem, Mandelstam was feeling profoundly alienated from "correct" language as a whole.[22] The official Soviet discourse that Mandelstam had been trying to import into his art can be seen as another type of dangerous "foreign dialect."[23] In Mandelstam's earlier work, glass stands for art and creativity. Yet Mandelstam came to realize the potential of this material to hurt anyone who abused or misapplied it. That is why the early glass images are so hopeful and lovely and the later ones, so painful. Mandelstam's glass imagery in his later verse reveals his anxiety that attempting to speak the obligatory language would do irreparable harm to him as a poet, inflicting a wound onto the very source of poetic speech.

In the foundational "A body has been given to me," glass serves as a surface for layers of inscription. Multiple layers of writing, preserved through the ages, suggest a palimpsest. With its capacity for creating a superimposition of visual planes, glass inspires Mandelstam as a metaphor for poetic language, which itself constitutes a palimpsest of world culture. Mandelstam's early poems "Hagia Sophia" and "Notre Dame" celebrate ancient buildings for the layers of historical time that they embody and preserve, "surviving the attacks of time."[24] In his later poems Mandelstam deconstructs the utopian associations around glass and exposes its capacity for bodily harm; in doing so, he reveals the double-edged nature of language itself, with its potential to preserve or destroy.

Mandelstam's poetic practice provides a vivid illustration of how the material presence of glass can enable literary creation; for some artists, the tangible properties of this material suggest the workings and the potential of language itself. Taking a broader view of how this material has functioned historically demonstrates that the physical qualities of glass made it a perpetual source of inspiration for writers and visual artists alike.

In 1947 the sculptor Vera Mukhina, best known for the monumental *Worker and Collective Farm Girl* (1937), crafted a glass bust of Nikolai Kachalov, the leading Soviet glass scientist; and in 1952 she fashioned a delicate female torso out of glass. Mukhina had worried about the impression that the translucent sculpture would make, given that the back of the figure might be glimpsed from the front; but after an exhibition, she reported proudly that "there was not a single person who didn't caress the torso. It appealed to them."[25] The glass woman proved irresistible to the touch, just as the crystal columns of Avtovo (built in the same decade) invited caresses from passersby; thus, a longtime resident of Leningrad recalls tracing the patterns of stars and other ideological symbols: "As a child I liked to run my fingers over the smooth shapes on those columns."[26] Glass looks like ice but warms to the touch, and this is part of its fascination. Architectural discourse frequently presents glass as a kind of skin; indeed, this material has a sensual potential. On the face of it, glass seems unlikely to have such associations—its appearance evokes coldness, and its potential to break into shards seems to alienate it from any association with the living body. Yet if we look deeper, we discover the corporeality of glass.

Robert Herrick's metaphysical poem "The Lily in a Crystal" (1648) is an early example of such awareness. The poem presents a series of images before spelling out its argument about beauty improved through artifice: a rose covered with fine transparent linen ("a cobweb-lawn"); a lily in crystal;

a strawberry in cream; amber submerged in water; grapes and cherries in a glass. Herrick presents this last image in a way that draws attention to how glass plays with vision: "Put purple grapes or cherries in- / To glass, and they will send / More beauty to commend / Them, from that clean and subtle skin, / Than if they naked stood / And had no other pride at all / But their own flesh and blood / And tinctures naturall." The line break of "in- / To glass" seems to mimic the effect of light refraction, one of the optical effects that glass offers to the keen observer, and reinforces Herrick's point about the importance of optical effects for tantalizing the eye and (thereby) stirring the soul.

"Clean and subtle skin" is a striking metaphor for glass, making the cold and fragile material animate. Khlebnikov described the buildings in his vision of the future as having glass flesh; and we recall how Robert Hughes articulated the appeal of glass to modernist architects: "It suggested a responsive skin, like the sensitive membrane of the eye."[27] In characterizing the veneration of glass shared by twentieth-century architects, Hughes draws an important parallel to stained glass windows as objects of worship. According to Robert Sowers, when gazing at the stained glass windows of the Gothic cathedral of Sainte-Chappelle, the viewer finds himself "possessed by a luminous energy that seems almost animate."[28] The play of light in glass is what makes the material seem alive and can help to account for the glass-body analogies documented above.

Chapter 1 of the present study cited a mysterious inscription on a window made by Catherine II. The image of writing on glass recurs in Odoevsky and Mandelstam, now signifying an indelible trace. How can one reconcile this notion of permanence with the fragility of the material? One reason may be that glass is transparent, and inscribing it creates the illusion of writing on the world. Furthermore, the fact that it is an invisible medium has inspired writers to draw fruitful analogies between glass and language.

The capacity of glass to function as an invisible medium makes scenarios of power possible: it lets in, captures, and manipulates light, creating a spectacle that may be used to serve a dominant ideology. The eighteenth-century glassware that was designed to be looked at demonstrates in miniature the spectacular potential of glass. As larger-scale glass constructions became possible, this spectacular potential was harnessed more and more successfully, as seen in the examples of the nineteenth-century Crystal Bed, and in the twentieth century, the Kremlin stars. Even lightbulbs took on a sacral aura and were implicated into the Lenin cult; "Lenin's little lamp" is on the same continuum as the Kremlin stars as an attempt by the Soviet state to lay claim to the domain of light. In *Envy* Olesha takes note of this appropriation of light and tries to reclaim glass as a liberating material for artists and dreamers. Throughout Olesha's novel, glass is the crucial material to demonstrate Kavalerov's double vision—looking-at and seeing-through: he sees both the familiar, phenomenal reality, and also sees through that reality, catching a glimpse of something fantastic and new, what a character in one of Olesha's stories calls "the invisible land."[29] He reaches out to glass as a potential source of salvation: the display case that stands for posthumous glory; and the source of optical play that transfigures an oppressive reality. Olesha recognizes the power in the conjunction of glass and light, yet his use of glass is markedly different from that of the state that he is meant to serve. He understands that glass is "always in between," not only in Armstrong's sense as an omnipresent medium, but also in the way that it is situated on the border between art and technology, beauty and utility, and holds out the hope of synthesis—conventionally opposed elements "flowing together."

Olesha struggled against the relentless march of history that threatened to relegate him, an imaginative artist, to the margins. For this reason, perhaps, glass functions as a time machine in Olesha's writings: the fragment of glass from the demolished Sukharev Tower through which one could catch sight of Peter the Great; and the street mirror in *Envy* that makes time move backward. In Zhukov's time-travel story (written three years before *Envy*), the young pioneers jump to the year 1957 through a glass-covered aperture. Tellingly, Olesha uses glass to move backward in time, and the official Soviet discourse uses it to move forward. What allows glass to function as a time machine? The material invites a restless movement of the eye, from looking-at to seeing-through and back again; hence it suggests dynamism as well as transportation into another realm.

Looking at and through glass thus fosters the ability to move mentally from one plane to another, to imagine new possibilities. Glass suggests the presence of another reality—and as an extension of this idea, glass can suggest utopia (and anti-utopia), as it did to so many, from Chernyshevsky to Khlebnikov and Zamyatin. Tracing the evolution from the Crystal Bed, which served to glorify the empire, to the Crystal Palace, which fueled the fantasy of social transformation and equality, reveals how glass can embody elite visions as well as democratic ideals.

In the twentieth century, the optical capacity of glass took on explicitly sociopolitical dimensions. Changing how and what we see promised to change not only how we live but also who we are. The fantasy of a New Man suited to live in the New World became embodied in the concept of transforming "human material" (*chelovecheskii material*), thus envisioning the human body in terms of a construction material that can be refashioned into something better.[30] Cement and steel were two well-known examples, as seen in Gladkov's novel *Cement* (1925) and Ostrovsky's novel *How the Steel Was Tempered* (1932–34).[31] A late Soviet documentary tale about glassworkers even proposed glass as a metaphor for "human material" undergoing transformation, presenting the ordeals that glass endures in the process of becoming a splendid work of art (from cutting and fire to acid baths) as analogous to what a person must go through to become "a real somebody" and "filled with light, like the facet of a crystal."[32] We recall, too, Khlebnikov's analogy between glass and body and the Constructivists' characterization of the glass building as a living organism. But, as we have seen, the analogy between glass and the body predates the twentieth century. The perceived "humanness" of glass has to do with the way in which it is created, with an artisan's animating breath, and the forms that it takes, as vessels suggestive of body and skin; as the German Romantic writer Novalis imagined it, "people are crystal vessels for the soul."[33]

A long-standing association between glass and body is found in the literature of the Middle Ages. When light passes through a stained glass window, it takes on the color of the glass. In the writings of the church fathers and medieval poets, this optical phenomenon inspired a simile: the union of light and color was likened to the mystical union of the spirit and the flesh (as manifested in Christ, who possessed both a human and a divine essence).[34] This mystical association may be at the root of Scheerbart's adoration of colored glass and his insistence that it will transform those who dwell within it.

These parallels must be seen in the context of the protean potential of glass that has served as a major source of inspiration for artists, yet has also been a deeply troubling attribute of the material. The theatricality of glass lends itself to deception as well as to liberating play. Lomonosov reveled in the lifelike pliability of glass, which invested him with the power of original creation. At the same time, because glass excels at imitation, it gives rise to anxieties about authenticity. In Lomonosov's case, the authenticity that was questioned was that of Lomonosov himself. For Eisenstein, the playfulness of glass, manifested both in the "plasmaticness" of the material and its capacity for optical illusion-making, resonated with his ideal of a body that is capable of endless metamorphosis. Yet his films, through self-reflexive glass imagery, exhibit some doubt about the optical playfulness of glass, now reconfigured as deceptiveness. He uses glass to tell his stories, and wonders whether he is really telling the truth.

Using his experiments in the glassmaking workshop as a model, Lomonosov strove to create a simultaneously transparent and sparkling poetic language out of humble materials. Mandelstam cherished the material's fragility and defiantly reenvisioned that frailty as strength, presenting glass as an indestructible surface for an artist's inscription (just as he reenvisioned "tongue-tiedness" as eloquence). Artists who are drawn to glass have a particular obsession with the epistemological value of vision. The presence of glass in our environment makes us conscious of the extent to which we rely on the sense of sight to make sense of the world, as well as the vulnerability of the truth that eyesight conveys. While those who control the means of production may manufacture glass objects with the intention of creating and nurturing a self-image, once these objects become a part of the visual environment, they take on another function in the eye of the individual beholder as a model and a catalyst for the imagination.

Notes

INTRODUCTION

The chapter epigraph is a folk speculation on the fate that had befallen Peter I during his trip abroad, cited in S. M. Solov'ev, *Istoriia Rossii s drevneishikh vremen v piatnadtsati knigakh*, book 8 (Moscow: Izdatel'stvo Sotsial'no Ekonomicheskoi literatury, 1962), 100; see also the variants on 109 and 111. Solov'ev cites as his source *Dela Preobrazhenskogo prikaza* (the files of a government office charged with investigating and prosecuting political crimes) for 1704 (ibid., 306).

1. Elena Frolova, "Ne ochen' prozrachnaia istoriia," *Material* 2 (2002).

2. The method was invented by British engineer Alastair Pilkington in 1959. See William S. Ellis, *Glass: From the First Mirror to Fiber Optics, the Story of the Substance That Changed the World* (New York: Avon, 1998), 57.

3. For a recent overview, see Alan Macfarlane and Gerry Martin, *Glass: A World History* (Chicago: University of Chicago Press, 2002). The authors argue that "glass was absolutely crucial to western development" (208) in part because of the instrumental role of glass in transforming visual culture during the Renaissance, and in part because of the role that the microscope, the telescope, and the barometer played in revolutionizing biology, medicine, astronomy, and chemistry.

4. Marco Beretta, *When Glass Matters: Studies in the History of Science and Art from Graeco-Roman Antiquity to Early Modern Era* (Florence: Leo S. Olschki, 2004), x–xi.

5. Armstrong writes of "the beginning of an avidly scopic culture" in the nineteenth century: "glass, in the endless multiplicity of forms capable of being generated from just four elements, prefabricated panels, the lens, windows, containers, was always in between." She argues that as the use of this material became more widespread, it provoked in people an "anxiety of mediation" as they became aware "that, in the movement between one state and another, there is a third term. The world is triangulated." See Isobel Armstrong, "Transparency: Towards a Poetics of Glass in the Nineteenth Century," in *Cultural Babbage: Technology, Time and Invention*, ed. Francis Spufford and Jenny Uglow (London: Faber and Faber, 1996), 125 and 131.

6. Research on visual categories in Russian shows the close kinship between seeing and knowing in the language itself. Thus vision has an added dimension of significance in the Russian context. See Edna Andrews, "Seeing Is Believing: Visual Categories in the Russian Lexicon," in *Meaning as Explanation: Advances in Linguistic Sign Theory*, ed. Ellen Contini-Morava and Barbara Sussman Goldberg (Berlin: Mouton, 1995), 361–77. I am grateful to Alfred Sproede for bringing this article to my attention.

7. Iu. M. Lotman, *Besedy o russkoi kul'ture: Byt i traditsii russkogo dvorianstva XVIII–nachalo XIX veka* (St. Petersburg: Iskusstvo-SPB, 1994), 6 (emphasis in the original).

8. Armstrong, "Transparency," 140.

9. Daniel Miller, "Artefacts and the Meaning of Things," in *Companion Encyclopedia of Anthropology*, ed. Tim Ingold (London: Routledge, 1994), 399.

10. Jules David Prown, "The Truth of Material Culture: History or Fiction?," in *History through Things: Essays on Material Culture*, ed. Steven Lubar and W. David Kingery (Washington, D.C.: Smithsonian Institution, 1993), 5.

11. Miller, "Artefacts and the Meaning of Things," 407.

12. Krisztina Fehervary, "From Socialist Modern to Super Natural Organicism: Political Affect and the Materialities of the Home," 6–7 (paper delivered at the "Objects of Affection: Towards a Materiology of Emotion" conference, Princeton, N.J., May 4–6, 2012). I am grateful to Dr. Fehervary for introducing me to the concept of qualisigns.

13. Anne Meneley, "Oleo-Signs and Quali-Signs: The Qualities of Olive Oil," *Ethnos* 73, no. 3 (September 2008): 307.

14. Ibid., 321.

15. Mikhail Epstein, "Thing and Word: On the Lyrical Museum," in *After the Future: The Paradoxes of Postmodernism and Contemporary Russian Culture*, trans. Anesa Miller-Pogacar (Amherst: University of Massachusetts Press, 1995), 254–55.

16. Jane Bennett, *Vibrant Matter: A Political Ecology of Things* (Durham, N.C.: Duke University Press, 2010), 3. Bennett borrows the term "actant" from Bruno Latour.

17. Ibid., 9.

18. See Michel Foucault, *Discipline and Punish: The Birth of the Prison*, trans. Alan Sheridan (New York: Penguin, 1977).

19. Richard S. Wortman, *Scenarios of Power: Myth and Ceremony in Russian Monarchy*, vol. 1 (Princeton, N.J.: Princeton University Press, 1995).

20. For two examples of Russian literary texts in which a doppelganger emerges from a magical mirror, see Valery Bryusov's "In the Mirror" (1901) and Alexander Chayanov's "The Venetian Mirror, or the Remarkable Adventures of a Glass Man" (1922).

21. Cited in V. V. Kamenskii, *Zhizn' s Maiakovskim* (Munich: Wilhelm Fink Verlag, 1974), 31–32.

22. Armstrong, "Transparency," 124.

23. Cited in Wolfgang Schivelbusch, *Disenchanted Night: The Industrialization of Light in the Nineteenth Century*, trans. Angela Davies (Berkeley: University of California Press), 146–47.

24. Jean Baudrillard, *The System of Objects*, trans. James Benedict (London: Verso, 1996), 41–42.

25. The idea of glass as an ideal model for human beings can be found as far back as Cervantes's story "El Licenciado Vidriera" ("The Lawyer of Glass," 1613). I am grateful to Svetlana Boym for this reference.

26. See Rosemarie Haag Bletter, "The Interpretation of the Glass Dream—Expressionist Architecture and the History of the Crystal Metaphor," *Journal of the Society of Architectural Historians* 49 (March 1981): 20–43.

27. This is a slightly abbreviated version of the passage from the Book of Revelation, 21:10–21:23.

28. Grigorii Revzin, "Khram kuptsa-spasitelia," *Kommersant"-Vlast'*, March 27, 2001.

29. Papernyi contrasts the dynamic culture of the revolutionary period, "Culture One," with the Stalinist "Culture Two," which privileged stasis and monumentality. See his *Kul'tura "Dva"* (Ann Arbor, Mich.: Ardis, 1985), translated as *Architecture in the Age of Stalin: Culture Two*, trans. John Hill and Roann Barris (Cambridge, Eng.: Cambridge University Press, 2002).

30. Walter Benjamin, "Paris: The Capital of the Nineteenth Century," in *Reflections: Essays, Aphorisms, Autobiographical Writings*, trans. Edmund Jephcott (New York: Schocken, 1978), 146–47.

31. For example, see Maryse Fauvel on the peculiar timelessness of the Louvre pyramid in "From Iron to Glass: Transparency and Pluralism," *Studies in Twentieth-Century Literature* 20 (1996): 341.

32. Benjamin, "Paris: The Capital of the Nineteenth Century," 147.

33. The circumstances under which the Crystal Palace came into being further shed light on the link between accelerated time and the "modern" materials of iron and glass: "Because the [exhibition] commission was on a tight schedule, the building had to be composed of prefabricated material—iron and glass rather than brick and mortar—that would be ready at once to house exhibits." See Thomas Richards, *The Commodity Culture of Victorian England: Advertising and Spectacle 1851–1914* (Stanford, Calif.: Stanford University Press, 1990), 22.

34. Mikhaïl Iampolski, "Le cinéma de l'architecture utopique," *Iris* (1991): 39.

35. I am grateful to Vivek Chadaga for this insight.

36. While working independently of one another, Isobel Armstrong and I each arrived at the term "glass consciousness" as a way to designate phenomena of perception peculiar to the times and places that serve as the respective objects of our study. See Armstrong, "Technology and Text: Glass Consciousness and Nineteenth-Century Culture," in *Culture, Landscape and Environment:*

The Linacre Lectures 1997, ed. Kate Flint and Howard Morphy (Oxford: Oxford University Press, 2000).

37. Katerina Clark documents this phenomenon thoroughly in *Petersburg, Crucible of Cultural Revolution* (Cambridge, Mass.: Harvard University Press, 1995).

38. Marcus Levitt draws a parallel between the "radical cultural reorientations" of the eighteenth century and the Soviet period in *The Visual Dominant in Eighteenth-Century Russia* (DeKalb: Northern Illinois University Press, 2011), 16. Levitt analyzes the visual orientation of the former period within the framework of a continuity between "Orthodox and Enlightenment paradigms of vision" (ibid., 21).

39. Valerie A. Kivelson and Joan Neuberger, eds., *Picturing Russia: Explorations in Visual Culture* (New Haven, Conn.: Yale University Press, 2010), 6.

40. Thomas Noonan et al., "The Development and Diffusion of Glassmaking in Pre-Mongol Russia," in *The Prehistory and History of Glassmaking Technology*, ed. Patrick McGray (Westerville, Ohio: American Ceramic Society, 1998), 294 and 299.

41. T. I. Dul'kina and N. A. Asharina, *Russkaia keramika i steklo 18–19 vekov: Sobranie gosudarstvennogo istoricheskogo muzeia* (Moscow: Izobrazil-tel'noe iskusstvo, 1978), 12.

42. Ekaterina I. Batanova and N. Voronov, *Sovetskoe khudozhestvennoe steklo* (Moscow: Iskusstvo, 1964), 11.

43. E. A. Levinson et al., *Khudozhestvennoe steklo i ego primemenie v arkhitekture* (Leningrad: Gosudarstvennoe izdatel'stvo literatury po stroitel'stvu i arkhitekture, 1953), 89.

44. Cited in Nikolai Kachalov, *Steklo* (Moscow: Izdatel'stvo Akademii Nauk SSSR, 1959), 207.

45. According to Noonan et al., "Ladoga's central role in the fur-bead trade was probably the reason why glassmaking arose at the site: glass beads have traditionally been key goods exchanged for fur" ("Development and Diffusion of Glassmaking," 299).

46. See Andrei Chernov, "Tak vot gde tailas' Rossiia moia . . . ," *Ogonek* 29 (July 1998): 53–54.

47. Kachalov, *Steklo*, 212. According to Ellis (*Glass*, 4), mourners in ancient Egypt "caught their tears in small glass vials."

48. Batanova and Voronov, *Sovetskoe khudozhestvennoe steklo*, 10.

49. Ibid., 9. According to Dal''s dictionary, *sleznitsa* (or *sleznik*) also referred to vessels in which mourners collected their tears; the vessels were then buried together with the deceased.

50. The fish egg sacks were sewn together and used as window coverings. See Richard Hellie, *The Economy and Material Culture of Russia, 1600–1725* (Chicago: University of Chicago Press, 1999), 134.

51. Levinson et al., *Khudozhstvennoe steklo*, 52. In the seventeenth century, the tsar's palace featured windows glazed with mica that was at times painted with images of people, animals, birds, or flowers. See M. G. Volkhovskoi, comp., *Domashnii byt russkikh tsarei v XVI-XVII vv. po Zabelinu, Kliuchevskomu, Karnovichu i drugim* (1904; Moscow: Panorama, 1992), 21–22.

52. James Cracraft, *The Petrine Revolution in Russian Imagery* (Chicago: University of Chicago Press, 1997), 179. In 1713, the tsar ordered 40 poods of mica, and in 1715, 150 crates of glass windowpanes to be purchased abroad and shipped to St. Petersburg. See S. P. Luppov, *Istoriia stroitel'stva Peterburga v pervoi chetverti XVIII veka* (Moscow: Izdatel'stvo Akademii nauk SSSR, 1957), 106–7.

53. Kachalov, *Steklo*, 213.

54. "Okno," in *Entsiklopedicheskii slovar'*, ed. I. E. Andreevskii, 43 vols. (St. Petersburg: F. A. Brokgauz and I. A. Efron, 1897), 824.

55. Volkhovskoi, *Domashnii byt russkikh tsarei*, 31.

56. Ibid., 25.

57. Hellie, *Economy and Material Culture*, 221.

58. Ibid., 592. For detailed descriptions of Muscovy mirrors, see I. E. Zabelin, *Domashnii byt russkikh tsarei v XVI i XVII stoletiiakh*, book 1 (Moscow: Kniga, 1990), 193–95.

59. Batanova and Voronov, *Sovetskoe khudozhestvennoe steklo*, 8; see also Noonan et al., "Development and Diffusion of Glassmaking," 304.

60. Volkhovskoi, *Domashnii byt russkikh tsarei*, 13.

61. Evgenii P. Prokof'ev, *Russkii khrustal': Gusevskii khrustal'nyi zavod* (Leningrad: Khudozhnik RSFSR, 1970), 6.

62. A. Oreshnikov, "Aptekarskaia posuda vremeni Petra Velikago," *Starye gody* (February 1908): 89.

63. Kachalov, *Steklo*, 223.

64. See, for example, the discussion of aesthetic enjoyment using the metaphor of looking through versus at a glass windowpane in José Ortega y Gasset, "The Dehumanization of Art," in *The Dehumanization of Art, and Other Writings on Art and Culture* (Garden City, N.Y., Doubleday, 1956), 9–10.

65. See the collection of decrees in *Opis' imennym vysochaishim ukazam tsaria-imperatora Petra Velikago 1704–1725*, comp. P. Baranov (St. Petersburg, 1872).

66. See Will Grohmann, *Wassily Kandinsky: Life and Work* (New York: Harry N. Abrams, 1958), 112; and Hans Konrad Röthel, introduction to *Vasily Kandinsky: Painting on Glass (Hinterglasmalerei); Anniversary Exhibition* (New York: Solomon R. Guggenheim Museum, 1966).

67. Calvin Tomkins, *Duchamp: A Biography* (New York: H. Holt, 1998), 125.

68. Velimir Khlebnikov, *Tvoreniia*, ed. M. Ia. Poliakov (Moscow: Sovetskii pisatel', 1986).

69. Scheerbart was a German poet and visionary best known for his influential 1914 treatise *Glass Architecture*. See the discussion of Scheerbart in chapter 5.

70. Robert Hughes, *The Shock of the New: Art and the Century of Change*, rev. ed. (New York: Knopf, 1991), 178.

71. B. I. Zbarskii, *Mavzolei Lenina* (Leningrad: Gosudarstvennoe izdatel'stvo politicheskoi literatury, 1946), 22.

72. For a discussion of how glass is used to invoke "an all-seeing Bolshevik state" in the stage set for Sergei Tret'iakov's 1926 play *I Want a Child!*, as well as Tret'iakov's film script based upon the play, see Christina Kiaer, *Imagine No Possessions: The Socialist Objects of Russian Constructivism* (Cambridge, Mass.: MIT Press, 2005), 246 and 259.

73. Space constraints prevent me from addressing such striking examples of optical glass in nineteenth-century literature as Pierre's spectacles in Tolstoy's *War and Peace* through which he fails to see his wife's infidelity, and Anna's lorgnette in Chekhov's "Lady with a Lapdog" that she loses just before her adulterous "fall" (both examples are linked with transgressive sexuality, as is the case with the nineteenth-century literary references to windows that I consider in chapter 1). Especially because the nineteenth century saw the proliferation of glass vision aids in Russia, this is a rich topic that awaits further scholarly exploration.

74. I am grateful to Sean Pollock for this information.

75. Mikhail Epstein, "On the Stature of Things in Russian Thought," *Symposion: A Journal of Russian Thought* 2 (1997), http://www.emory.edu/INTELNET/sympo_epstein_things.html.

76. See Mikhail Epstein, *Cries in the New Wilderness: From the Files of the Moscow Institute of Atheism*, trans. and intro. Eve Adler (Philadelphia: Paul Dry, 2002). The original title is *Novoe sektantstvo: Tipy religiozno-filosofkikh umonastroenii v Rossii (1970–1980 gg)*.

77. In his "comedy of ideas," Epstein draws upon both the worldviews expressed by fellow Soviet intellectuals and on popular religious beliefs he encountered during fieldwork in southern Russia and Ukraine. See *Cries in the New Wilderness*, 6–7.

78. Ibid., 146 (translation slightly modified).

79. Ibid., 148 (translation slightly modified).

80. Ibid., 149.

CHAPTER ONE

The chapter epigraph is quoted in Aleksei Erofeev, "Chto otkryvaetsia v Evropu?," *Smena—Informatsionnaia gazeta,* April 6, 2002, http://www.smena.ru/arc/22654-log.html.

1. See the entry on *okno* in I. I. Shangina, *Russkii traditsionnyi byt: Entsik-*

lopedicheskii slovar' (St. Petersburg: Azbuka-klassika, 2003), 105–6 and http://www.slavya.ru/trad/afan/II.htm.

2. See my article "No Mere Reflection: Mirrors as Windows on Russian Culture," *Studies in Twentieth- and Twenty-First Century Literature* 34, no. 2 (Summer 2010): 170–206. This article also provides additional illustrations of Russian mirrors and discusses contemporary Russian architecture in which windows take on the function of mirrors.

3. See Stephen Lessing Baehr, "Sacred into Secular," in *The Paradise Myth in Eighteenth-Century Russia: Utopian Patterns in Early Secular Russian Literature and Culture* (Stanford, Calif.: Stanford University Press, 1991).

4. Jurij M. Lotman and B. A. Uspenskij, "Echoes of the Notion 'Moscow as the Third Rome' in Peter the Great's Ideology," in *The Semiotics of Russian Culture*, ed. Ann Shukman, Michigan Slavic Contributions 11 (Ann Arbor: University of Michigan Press, 1984), 62.

5. V. K. Makarov, *Khudozhestvennoe nasledie M. V. Lomonosova: Mozaiki* (Moscow: Izdatel'stvo Akademii nauk SSSR, 1950), 21–22.

6. E. V. Dolgikh, *Russkoe steklo XVIII veka: Sobranie Gosudarstvennogo muzeia keramiki i "Usad'ba Kuskovo XVIII veka"* (Moscow: Iskusstvo, 1985), 10.

7. William Craft Brumfield, *A History of Russian Architecture* (Cambridge, Eng.: Cambridge University Press, 1993), 217.

8. James Cracraft, *The Petrine Revolution in Russian Architecture* (Chicago: University of Chicago Press, 1988).

9. M. A. Tseitlin, "Kazennye (imperatorskie) 'stekliannyi' i zerkal'nyi zavody v S.-Peterburge," in *Sbornik nauchnykh trudov Leningradskogo finansovo-ekonomicheskogo instituta* (Leningrad: Institut, 1948), 155.

10. N. V. Voronov and M. M. Dubova, *Nevskii khrustal': Ocherki osnovnykh etapov razvitiia* (Leningrad: Khudozhnik RSFSR, 1984), 10. Light fixtures such as sconces were attached to mirrors so that every lit candle would be reflected in them. See also A. I. Leonov, ed., *Russkoe dekorativnoe iskusstvo, 18-i vek*, vol. 2 (Moscow: Izdatel'stvo Akademii Khudozhestv, 1963), 344–47.

11. In some lanterns, mica was used instead of glass (Kachalov, *Steklo*, 228).

12. Leonov, *Russkoe dekorativnoe iskusstvo*, 346. On the Baroque fascination with glass, see Peter N. Skrine, *The Baroque: Literature and Culture in Seventeenth-Century Europe* (London: Methuen, 1978), 147.

13. Another way in which glass was used in interiors peculiar to the eighteenth century was in the interior decoration of grottoes, artificial caves placed in formal gardens. Two such grottoes, built in 1755–61, can be found on the estate of Kuskovo.

14. E. Poz'e, "Zapiski pridvornogo brilliantshchika o prebyvanii v Rossii s 1729–64 gg.," in *Russkaia starina 1870 g.*, reprinted in P. E. Mel'gunova-Stepanova, *Russkii byt vo vospominaniiakh sovremennikov: XVIII vek: Sbornik otryvkov iz zapisok, vospominanii i pisem* (Moscow: Zadruga, 1914), 328.

15. N. M. Karamzin, "Moia ispoved'," vol. 1 of *Sochineniia v dvukh tomakh*, ed. G. P. Makogonenko (Leningrad: Khudozhestvennaia literatura, 1984), 534 (emphasis in the original).

16. Natal'ia Borisovna Dolgorukaia, *The Memoirs of Princess Natal'ja Borisovna Dolgorukaia*, ed. and trans. Charles E. Townsend (Columbus, Ohio: Slavica, 1977), 44.

17. Ibid., 46.

18. Ibid., 66.

19. Lewis Mumford, *Technics and Civilization* (New York: Harcourt, Brace, 1934), 125–26.

20. Wortman, *Scenarios of Power*, 95.

21. Dolgorukaia, *Memoirs*, 60.

22. Ibid., 74.

23. Lutz Koepnick, *Framing Attention: Windows on Modern German Culture* (Baltimore: Johns Hopkins University Press, 2007), 10.

24. An influential discussion of the relationship between possession and the gaze is found in John Berger, *Ways of Seeing* (New York: Penguin 1990 [reprint from 1972]).

25. The question of how writers working in other time periods employ the image of the window is beyond the scope of this study. For a rich analysis of how windows in the poems of Boris Pasternak serve to express two of his central themes ("'unity, or contact' between the small-scale, everyday manifestations of life and the universe" and "[the] 'maginificent intensity' of existence"), see Alexander Zholkovsky, "'Window' in the Poetic World of Boris Pasternak," *Themes and Texts: Toward a Poetics of Expressiveness* (Ithaca, N.Y.: Cornell University Press, 1984), especially 138 and 150.

26. A. S. Pushkin, "Pikovaia dama," in *Stikhotvoreniia, Poemy, Proza* (Moscow: Panorama, 1995), 663.

27. Ibid., 665.

28. Early on in the story, the Countess is surprised to hear that Russian novels even exist; such a scarcity suggests that Liza reads foreign novels too.

29. Nathan Rosen links the story's presentation of the Countess within several rectangular frames, including a window, with her final manifestation as the Queen of Spades in Hermann's imagination. See his article "The Magic Cards in *The Queen of Spades*," *SEEJ* 19, no. 3 (Autumn 1975): 268.

30. I. S. Turgenev, *Ottsy i deti*, in *Polnoe sobranie sochinenii i pisem v dvadtsati vos'mi tomakh*, Sochineniia, vol. 8 (Moscow: Nauka, 1964), 291 (ellipsis in the original).

31. For example, see Jane T. Costlow, *Worlds within Worlds: The Novels of Ivan Turgenev* (Princeton, N.J.: Princeton University Press, 1990).

32. Ibid., 299 (ellipsis in the original).

33. L. N. Tolstoi, *Anna Karenina*, in *Sobranie sochinenii v dvadtsati tomakh*

(Moscow: Gosudarstvennoe Izdatel'stvo Khudozhestvennoi literatury, 1963), 8:121.

34. See Amy Mandelker, *Framing Anna Karenina: Tolstoy, the Woman Question, and the Victorian Novel* (Columbus: Ohio State University Press, 1993), 132 and 135.

35. Tolstoi, *Anna Karenina*, 122.

36. Ibid., 131 and 136.

37. See Armstrong, "Technology and Text," 168.

38. M. I. Pyliaev, *Zabytoe proshloe okrestnostei Peterburga* (St. Petersburg: Izdatel'stvo A.S. Suvorina, 1889), 457.

39. Ibid., 529.

40. See Ramie Targoff, *John Donne, Body and Soul* (Chicago: University of Chicago Press, 2008), 67–68. Elizabeth's window inscription is cited from John Foxe's *Acts and Monuments*.

41. Natal'ia Kochetkova, "Zhal', chto ego bol'she net s nami," *Izvestiia*, July 18, 2009.

42. Targoff reads the name inscribed on the glass as "a metonymic substitution for Donne's own presence. For his purpose is to create not a spiritual bond, but a physical union" (*John Donne, Body and Soul*, 68).

43. T. V. Volobaeva, "Vitrazh v russkoi kul'ture: Sankt-Peterburg i ego pamiatniki," diss., St. Petersburg State University, 1999, http://www.nature.ru/db/msg.html?mid=1156475&uri=general.htm. Volobaeva is citing B. Kirikov and A. Zorina, "Vitrazhi Peterburga," *Nashe nasledie* no. 4 (1991): 156.

44. Shonquis Moreno, "Through the Looking Glass," in *Forefront: The Culture of Shop Window Design* (Amsterdam: Birkhäuser, 2005), 8.

45. Peter N. Stearns, *Consumerism in World History* (London: Routledge, 2001), 76.

46. As Christine Ruane documents, the "sartorial revolution" instigated by Peter the Great helped to bring about this change in fashion merchandising. By mid-century, the large number of foreign names among Moscow shopkeepers "suggests the preponderance of foreign capital at the beginnings of Russian commercial development." See Ruane, *The Empire's New Clothes: A History of the Russian Fashion Industry, 1700–1917* (New Haven, Conn.: Yale University Press, 2009), 116.

47. The shop window began life as a regular window, but by the middle of the eighteenth century (in Western Europe) it had become "a glassed-in stage on which an advertising show was presented." See Schivelbusch, *Disenchanted Night*, 146–47.

48. The original text reads: "Ну, уж эти французы! Что и говорить, уж ежели захотят что-нибудь того, так уж точно того . . ." See N. V. Gogol', *Shinel'*, in *Sobranie sochinenii* (Moscow: Gosudarstvennoe Izdatel'stvo khudozhestvennoi literatury, 1959), 3:145.

49. Elizabeth Outka, *Consuming Traditions: Modernity, Modernism, and the Commodified Authentic* (New York: Oxford University Press, 2009), 137 and 147.

50. Qtd. in Christina Lodder, *Russian Constructivism* (New Haven, Conn.: Yale University Press, 1983), 202. There were numerous other attempts to transform vision at this time, such as Mikhail Matiushin's *Zorved* project of 1923, whose goal was a physiological transformation that would extend the human field of vision to a full 360 degrees.

51. A. S. Boldyrev, ed., "Stekol'naia promyshlennost'," in *Promyshlennost' stroitel'nykh materialov SSSR 1917–1967* (Moscow: Izdatel'stvo literatury po stroitel'stvu, 1967), 223–24.

52. Stephen White, *The Bolshevik Poster* (New Haven, Conn.: Yale University Press, 1988), 67.

53. E. V. Barkhatova, ed., *Iz istorii russkogo plakata: "Okna" ROSTA i Glavolit prosveta 1919–1922: Katalog vystavki* (St. Petersburg: Rossiiskaia natsional'naia biblioteka, 2000), 5.

54. Ibid., 4. Examples include "the dead of the Paris Commune have been resurrected beneath the red banner of the Soviets" and "Peasants, you were given soil, but you cannot eat it. You must cultivate it. The soil will yield crops. Give the city grain. The city will give you all that you need."

55. White, *The Bolshevik Poster*, 68.

56. Outka, *Consuming Traditions*, 153.

57. Sheila Fitzpatrick discusses this phenomenon in detail in *Tear Off the Masks! Identity and Imposture in Twentieth-Century Russia* (Princeton, N.J.: Princeton University Press, 2005).

58. Fedor Gladkov, *Tsement* (Moscow: n.p., 1927), 205.

59. Barkhatova, *Iz istorii russkogo plakata*, 4.

60. Ibid., 8.

61. This connection is most obviously manifested in the notion of eyes as the windows of the soul—a proverb dating from the mid-sixteenth century; one variant has "the eyes . . . are the wyndowes of the mynde, for both ioye and anger . . . are seene . . . through them" (*Oxford Concise Dictionary of Proverbs*, comp. John Simpson and Jennifer Speake, 3rd ed. [New York: Oxford University Press, 1998], 90).

62. A related word is *zenki*, "eyes." *Zenki nalit'*, "to fill one's eyes to the top," means to become intoxicated.

63. As Armstrong ("Transparency," 131) points out, "window" comes from an Old Norse word meaning "wind's eye.'"

64. Ian Frazier takes note of this tendency of Russian to animate the material world in his essay "On the Prison Highway," *The New Yorker*, August 30, 2010.

CHAPTER TWO

The chapter epigraph is taken from P. Baiburova, "Russkii usadebnyi dom serediny XVIII veka kak element razvlekatel'noi kul'tury barokko," in *U istokov razvlekatel'noi kul'tury Rossii novogo vremeni, XVIII–XIX veka*, ed. E. V. Dukov (Moscow: Gosudarstvennyi in-t iskusstvoznaniia, 1996), 84.

1. Iu. M. Lotman, *Besedy o russkoi kul'ture*, 7.

2. Note this ecstatic Soviet-era description: "These light fixtures were transformed into fantastic constructions, shimmering and glimmering, iridescent, sparkling, and suddenly blazing with blinding white, green, red, fiery beams when the onlooker shifted in place or when one of the crystal pendants was accidentally set in motion by an air current, or when the building shook." See Batanova and Voronov, *Sovetskoe khudozhestvennoe steklo*, 21.

3. The Russian custom of clinking wineglasses following a toast calls for holding the vessels close to the base of the stem so that the sound is amplified as much as possible.

4. N. V. Voronov and M. M. Dubova, *Nevskii khrustal': Ocherki osnovnykh etapov razvitiia* (Leningrad: Khudozhnik RSFSR, 1984), 12. See also Batanova and Voronov, *Sovetskoe khudozhestvennoe steklo*, 16. According to St. Petersburg historian Pyliaev, the bells produced a variety of tunes, and the soft, harmonious sounds issuing from them were very pleasant (*Zabytoe proshloe okrestnostei Peterburga*, 307).

5. Batanova and Voronov, *Sovetskoe khudozhestvennoe steklo*, 13.

6. N. A. Asharina, "Russkoe khudozhestvennoe steklo," in *Na rubezhe dvukh vekov: Iz istorii preobrazovanii Petrovskogo vremeni*, ed. L. G. Beskrovnyi (Moscow: Sovetskaia Rossiia, 1978), 67–68.

7. The reasons for this ranged from the demand for more window glass to suit the new style of architecture, to the use of glass to imitate the forms of metallic, porcelain, and even wooden dishes, to purely aesthetic considerations. See Asharina, "Russkoe khudozhestvennoe steklo," 79.

8. Ibid., 74. Many discoveries in Russian glassmaking, such as the first Russian crystal (lead ruby), were made at the privately owned Mal'tsev factories. Prokof'ev, *Russkii khrustal'*, 7. In 1745 the College of Manufacturing declared the works from the Mozhaisk factory (one of the largest privately owned glass factories in Russia, owned by Vasilii Mal'tsev, the founder of the Mal'tsev glass dynasty) to be "superior to foreign glass." See Dul'kina and Asharina, *Russkaia keramika i steklo*, 13.

9. Dul'kina and Asharina, *Russkaia keramika i steklo*, 12.

10. Asharina, "Russkoe khudozhestvennoe steklo," 87.

11. N. A. Asharina, "Russkie zavody khudozhestvennogo stekla XVII–XVIIIvv.," in *Iz istorii russkoi keramiki i stekla XVII–XIX vekov: sbornik trudov*,

ed. N. A. Asharina (Moscow: Gosudarstvennyi ordena Lenina Istoricheskii muzei, 1986), 15.

12. For example, the system of versification that he introduced in the first half of the eighteenth century has remained virtually unchanged to the present day.

13. Soviet academician Nikolai Kachalov claims that Lomonosov laid the first truly scientific foundation for glassmaking, thus outpacing Europe, which was still confined to an "alchemical" understanding of the world. See E. A. Levinson et al., *Khudozhestvennoe steklo*, 11. Kachalov was writing in a time when it was mandatory to make such claims for Russian priority in scientific achievements.

14. Batanova and Voronov, *Sovetskoe khudozhestvennoe steklo*, 19–20.

15. Makarov, *Khudozhestvennoe nasledie M. V. Lomonosova*, 43. Elsewhere Lomonosov writes that he conducted "over four thousand experiments." Cited in M. V. Lomonosov, *Polnoe sobranie sochinenii* (Moscow: Akademiia nauk SSSR, 1959), 8:1004.

16. It was not until the mid-nineteenth century that other scientists would make the same discovery. See M. A. Bezborodov, "Issledovatel'skaia rabota Lomonosova po tsvetnym steklam," *Nauka* 1 (1947): 80.

17. Ibid., 63.

18. Ibid., 43.

19. Asharina, "Russkie zavody khudozhestvennogo stekla XVII–XVIII vv.," 13.

20. Makarov, *Khudozhestvennoe nasledie M. V. Lomonosova*, 69.

21. Batanova and Voronov, *Sovetskoe khudozhestvennoe steklo*, 21–23.

22. By the time that Lomonosov wrote the poem, the Senate had already issued a decree (December 14, 1752) granting him permission to open the factory; however, he still needed a plot of land where he could situate the factory, villages that only the empress could provide. Shuvalov was planning to make an appeal to the empress on behalf of Lomonosov, and it is most likely that Lomonosov addressed the "Letter" to him with this in mind. See Aleksandr Morozov, commentary to "Pis'mo o pol'ze stekla" by Lomonosov, *Polnoe sobranie sochinenii*, 8:1004. According to a 1752 deed, Lomonosov received "a total of 211 souls, with all the land attached to them." Cited in V. V. Danilevskii and N. P. Tikhonov, "Restavratsiia mozaiki Lomonosova 'Poltavskaia bataliia,'" *Problemy istoriii dokapitalisticheskikh obshchestv* 9 (1935): 183.

23. M. V. Lomonosov, *Stikhotvoreniia*, Biblioteka poeta, Malaia Seriia, 3rd ed., ed. A. Morozov (Leningrad: Sovetskii pisatel', 1954), 267. The original text reads: Неправо о вещах те думают, Шувалов, / Которые Стекло чтут ниже Минералов, / Приманчивым лучом блистающих в глаза: / Не меньше польза в нём, не меньше в нём краса.

24. Ibid., 268.

25. There is, in fact, a connection between drinking and scientific discovery.

According to Macfarlane and Martin, "the fine glass needed for the earliest microscopes was made from fragments of Venetian wine 'cristallo'" (*Glass: A World History*, 183). The authors connect technical improvements in glassmaking and eventually the creation of test tubes, measuring flasks, thermometers, and barometers with the development of glass containers.

26. In 1701 Peter I ordered a set of inscribed apothecary vessels of clear glass to be made in Holland for pharmacies being set up in Moscow. Up until then, Russian pharmacies only served the tsar's family and a few select others, not broad masses of the population, who self-medicated with herbs bought at a special market (*Zeleinyi Riad*). The death by poisoning of boyar Petr Saltykov after he had taken one such herb served as an impetus for Peter to shut down the herb market and set up eight public pharmacies in Moscow. See A. Oreshnikov, "Aptekarskaia posuda vremeni Petra Velikago," *Starye gody*, February 1908: 89.

27. In a petition to the empress in 1757, Lomonosov writes that he wishes to create in his factories "sacred images for churches and, for public buildings, the faces and deeds of your great ancestors, and particularly your most precious parents of immortal memory, as well as the ascent of your heroic majesty upon your paternal throne . . . based on originals or drawings . . . for an appropriate sum." Cited in Danilevskii and Tikhonov, "Restavratsiia mozaiki Lomonosova," 183.

28. Morozov notes that this address to peasant women was quite unusual for the literature of the time ("Commentary," 1007).

29. M. V. Lomonosov, "Pis'mo o pol'ze stekla," in *Stikhotvoreniia*, 273.

30. Ibid., 276.

31. Ibid., 280.

32. Lomonosov, *Polnoe sobranie sochinenii*, 8:1006–7.

33. See Stählin on Lomonosov's mosaics, qtd. in Makarov, *Khudozhestvennoe nasledie M. V. Lomonosova*, 12.

34. Levinson et al., *Khudozhestvennoe steklo*, 99–100.

35. Qtd. in Makarov, *Khudozhestvennoe nasledie M. V. Lomonosova*, 46.

36. M. A. Bezborodov, *M. V. Lomonosov—Osnovopolozhnik nauchnogo steklodeliia* (Moscow: Gosudarstvennoe izdatel'stvo literatury po stroitel'nym materialam, 1956), 42–43.

37. The poem is not a true ode, because it is not in the high style, to follow Lomonosov's own classification. It is a natural-philosophical poem in the guise of a familiar letter, as defined by Morozov (Lomonosov, *Stikhotvoreniia*, 32).

38. Bezborodov, *M. V. Lomonosov*, 78.

39. Qtd. in Lomonosov, *Stikhotvoreniia*, 45.

40. Ibid.

41. Qtd. in A. I. Efimov, *M. V. Lomonosov i russkii iazyk* (Moscow: Izdatel'stvo Moskovskogo universiteta, 1961), 7.

42. Qtd. in Aleksandr Morozov, "Lomonosov i barokko," *Russkaia literatura* 2 (1965): 79.

43. Ibid., 40–41.

44. Roland Barthes, *Mythologies*, trans. Annette Lavers (London: Paladin, 1972), 97–98.

45. Morozov writes: "All the colors in [Lomonosov's] odes are intensified. They glow like mosaic pieces [*smal'ty*] and their artificiality is not at all troubling" ("Lomonosov i barokko," 78). Morozov's article does not address Lomonosov's glassmaking activity, however.

46. Makarov, *Khudozhestvennoe nasledie M. V. Lomonosova*, 45.

47. Ibid. 129.

48. See Lomonosov, *Stikhotvoreniia*, 40.

49. This mosaic is on display in the Academy of Sciences building in St. Petersburg.

50. Makarov, *Khudozhestvennoe nasledie M. V. Lomonosova*, 10.

51. Ibid., 11.

52. Ibid., 80.

53. According to a legend published in *The Muscovite* (*Moskvitianin*), no. 1 (1845), 17–18, Lomonosov once came to a dinner party at Shuvalov's dressed in a caftan with glass buttons. One of the guests remarked that glass buttons had gone out of fashion, provoking an indignant speech from Lomonosov, who defended the merits of the material. The legend has it that Shuvalov was so enthralled by this outpouring that he asked Lomonosov to write a poem on the topic. (Cited in Lomonosov, *Polnoe sobranie sochinenii* 8:1004.)

54. Batanova and Voronov, *Sovetskoe khudozhestvennoe steklo*, 34.

55. Makarov, *Khudozhestvennoe nasledie M. V. Lomonosova*, 282–85.

56. Nikolai Gogol, "The Tale of How Ivan Ivanovich Quarreled with Ivan Nikiforovich," in *The Complete Tales of Nikolai Gogol*, ed. Leonard J. Kent, vol. 2 (Chicago: University of Chicago Press, 1985), 188. I have slightly revised this translation. For the original, see N. V. Gogol', "Povest' o tom, kak possorilsia Ivan Ivanovich s Ivanom Nikiforovichem," in *Sobranie khudozhestvennykh proizvedenii v piati tomakh* (Moscow: Izdatel'stvo Akademii Nauk SSSR, 1951), 2:292.

57. See Wortman, *Scenarios of Power*, for a detailed discussion of how the Russian ruling classes made use of myth and ritual to perpetuate their power by ceremonial means.

58. In addition, in 1767 the Senate decreed that copies of Catherine's Instruction (*Nakaz*) must be kept next to the *zertsalo* in every judicial office. Cited in S. M. Solov'ev, *Istoriia Rossii s drevneishikh vremen*, book 14 of vol. 27–28 (Moscow: Mysl', 1965), 119.

59. The metal collection in the History Museum in Moscow has a bronze *zertsalo* with a dark blue color scheme on a gilded wood pedestal, from the second half of the nineteenth century. The decrees, now lost, were placed behind glass plates on each side. This *zertsalo* is about two feet tall. The wood collection in the History Museum has two *zertsala* from the turn of the nineteenth century,

one of which can turn on its axis. These massive *zertsala* (about three feet tall) feature volutes at the sides, columns, and stylized leaf designs. Lions with teeth bared crouch among flowers at the foot of the gilded wood pedestal. The decrees are mounted inside glass doors. Another *zertsalo* has a doorknob providing access inside.

60. This *zertsalo* is described in Leonov, *Russkoe dekorativnoe iskusstvo*, 426–27.

61. A. G. Man'kov, ed., *Zakonodatel'stvo perioda stanovleniia absoliutizma: Rossiiskoe zakonodatel'stvo X–XX vekov v deviati tomakh*, vol. 4 (Moscow: Iuridicheskaia literatura, 1986), 186 (April 17, 1722, emphasis added). See also V. M. Zhivov, "Istoriia russkogo prava kak lingvo-semioticheskaia problema," in *Semiotics and the History of Culture: In Honor of Jurij Lotman; Studies in Russian*, ed. Morris Halle et al. (Columbus, Ohio: Slavica, 1988), 78.

62. As Morozov (93) observes, Petrine utilitarianism found emblems and allegory well suited to its goals; he characterizes this fusion as the "rhetorical rationalism of the baroque." ("Lomonosov i barokko," 93).

63. This handbook "served as a main source of imagery for Peter and his entourage when naming ships built for the Russian fleet, mounting their elaborate fireworks, and designing triumphal arches for Moscow and St. Petersburg. Indeed, the handbook is a remarkable document in the diffusion to Russia of European symbolic imagery." Cracraft, *Petrine Revolution in Russian Imagery*, 177.

64. I use this term to mean a visible symbol that represents an abstract idea and/or contains a veiled moral meaning.

65. See the text of the February 7, 1723 decree, in B. I. Syromiatnikov, ed., *Zakonodatel'nye akty Petra I*, vol. 1, *Akty o vysshikh gosudarstvennykh ustanovleniiakh* (Moscow: Izdatel'stvo akademii nauk Soiuza SSR, 1945), 124.

66. Liudmila A. Aksenova, a curator at the Museum of the City of Petersburg at the Peter and Paul Fortress, arguing that Peter would not have come up with the design himself, characterizes him as "not an artist but a craftsman"; yet this point is debatable, especially when one considers all the objects that Peter is known to have designed, including a fancy wood-frame mirror in Peter's Summer Palace dating from 1710–11, an unusual chair in the study of the Little House (Domik), and the ornate candelabrum of walrus ivory and wood, over whose carving Peter presided, that is displayed in the Hermitage.

67. Liudmila Aksenova refers to the *zertsalo* as not only a symbol of autocracy but also a conduit of ideology.

68. I am grateful to Elena Aleksandrovna Ivanova of the Russian Museum for this insight.

69. Batanova and Voronov, *Sovetskoe khudozhestvennoe steklo*, 21.

70. See Leonov, *Russkoe dekorativnoe iskusstvo*, 359. Such mirror placement can be found in the ballroom of the Menshikov Palace in St. Petersburg: the mirrors are situated near the ceiling, above the glass doors.

71. Peter himself had four early eighteenth-century English rosewood mirrors in his Summer Palace bedroom, while his wife Catherine I had six mirrors in hers.

72. To cite one example, the Vorob'ev factory was producing mirrors in the eighteenth century that were of significant size for the time: some were as large as nine feet in length and four and a half in width. Many were in glass frames. See Asharina, "Russkie zavody khudozhestvennogo stekla XVII–XVIIIvv," 6.

73. For a guide to this phenomenon, see Herbert Grabes, *The Mutable Glass: Mirror-Imagery in Titles and Texts of the Middle Ages and English Renaissance*, trans. Gordon Collier (Cambridge, Eng.: Cambridge University Press, 1982). See also James I. Wimsatt: "Works called mirrors generally aim in some way both at inclusiveness and the presentation of ideals; they are either compendiums of exemplars or compendiums of more or less corrupted entities in which exemplars are implicit." *Allegory and Mirror: Tradition and Structure in Middle English Literature* (New York: Pegasus, 1970), 139.

74. A typical title: "A true mirror of love, or a manual on the proper way to love or to hate, in which is depicted the lofty soaring of philosophical thoughts, by means of which the Author convincingly argues the material presented in the present book, having combined the keenness of his reason with utility and pleasure for the readers" (Moscow, 1783).

75. As a symbol, the mirror has had a range of often-conflicting associations, but here I will focus on the attributes that are helpful for understanding the genesis of the *zertsalo* itself. Starting in the Middle Ages, the duality of mirror symbolism can be seen in the coexistence of the notion of Virgin Mary as the "spotless mirror" who perfectly reflects divine truth with the iconographic association of Venus with a mirror, a symbol of the search for truth but also self-absorption and sinful pride. Seemingly opposing attributes (vanity vs. spiritual enlightenment) were at times intertwined: thus, in the twelfth-century Latin manuscript *Speculum Virginium*, the author "explains the term *speculum*: maidens look into mirrors . . . to see whether there is any increase or decrease of their adornment, but Scripture is a mirror from which they can learn how they can please the eternal spouse." See Benjamin Goldberg, *The Mirror and Man* (Charlottesville: University Press of Virginia, 1985), 127. On the "split personality" of reflection, see also Goldberg, *The Mirror and Man*, 121; and Hope B. Werness, *The Symbolism of Mirrors in Art from Ancient Times to the Present* (Lewiston, N.Y.: Edwin Mellen, 1999), 9.

76. Theodore Ziolkowski, *Disenchanted Images: A Literary Iconology* (Princeton, N.J.: Princeton University Press, 1977), 152.

77. Goldberg, *The Mirror and Man*, 118.

78. Ibid., 127.

79. One reason that compendia were identified with mirrors had to do with the physical aspect of mirrors at the time: up until the seventeenth century, mir-

rors were convex, "thus allowing reflection and reduction. The printed book, which makes its appearance in the second half of the fifteenth century—and in which pre-existing material is re-presented in a condensed form—is declared to have the same function as a mirror." See Anna Torti, *The Glass of Form: Mirroring Structures from Chaucer to Skelton* (Cambridge, Eng.: D. S. Brewer, 1991), 24–25.

80. See *The Lubok: Russian Folk Pictures 17th–19th c.*, selected and intro. Alla Sytova, trans. Alex Miller (Leningrad: Avrora, 1984).

81. A similar combination of the empirical and the mystical is found in a Russian oral legend about a mirror that once belonged to Pyotr Tchaikovsky. This mirror still hangs in the hall of his former residence in Klin; witnesses attest to having seen the late composer in the mirror. It is believed that the silver amalgam in the backing of the mirror acted as a daguerreotype to capture Tchaikovsky's repeatedly reflected image. I am grateful to L. A. Aksenova for this information.

82. See Richard Wortman, *The Development of a Russian Legal Consciousness* (Chicago: University of Chicago Press, 1976), 17.

83. Cited in V. I. Lebedev, comp., *Reformy Petra I. Sbornik dokumentov* (Moscow: Gosudarstvennoe sotsial'no-ekonomicheskoe izdatel'stvo, 1937), 108.

84. In *Chicanery*, Kapnist describes procurator Khvataiko as having "an all-seeing eye" in that he grabs everything he sees, i.e., takes any opportunity for collecting a bribe. See V. V. Kapnist, *Sobranie sochinenii v dvukh tomakh*, ed. D. S. Babkin (Moscow: Izdatel'stvo Akademii nauk SSSR, 1960), 1:541.

85. The latter two images are reproduced in A. S. Chistiakov, *Istoriia Petra Velikogo* (Moscow: Buklet, 1992), on the frontispiece and p. 413, respectively.

86. Cited in V. M. Zhivov and B. A. Uspenskii, "Tsar' i bog: Semioticheskie aspekty sakralizatsii monarkha v Rossii," in *Iazyki kul'tury i problemy perevodimosti*, ed. B. A. Uspenskii (Moscow: Nauka, 1987), 70n18. The image is reproduced in Lotman, *Besedy*, between pp. 336 and 337.

87. See Dolgikh, *Russkoe steklo XVIII veka*, 196.

88. See Asharina, "Russkoe khudozhestvennoe steklo," 86.

89. See Baehr, *Paradise Myth in Eighteenth-Century Russia*. For a detailed history of the sacralization of the tsar in texts and images, the Byzantine and western European sources of this phenomenon, and its Russian manifestations before, during, and after the Petrine period, see Zhivov and Uspenskii, *Tsar' i bog*, in particular 73, 79, 85, 95, 104, 120, and 133n88.

90. See Zhivov, *Istoriia russkogo prava*.

91. The sacral associations around the *zertsalo* persisted into the late nineteenth century, as evidenced in an autobiographical work by V. G. Korolenko (written 1904–18, published 1922) that covers the period from 1853 to 1884. In a description of a provincial courthouse, the religious aura of the *zertsalo* stands out in stark relief. The author's father, the local judge, treats the *prisutstvie*—

the room where the *zertsalo* stands on a long table covered with a green cloth with gold tassels—as a sacred space: "He always entered this sanctuary with a grand and solemn expression, as if it were a church, and that set the tone for the others." The *zertsalo* "seemed to us some kind of magical tabernacle [*skiniia*]." V. G. Korolenko, "Istoriia moego sovremennika," in *Sobranie sochinenii v 10-i tomakh* (Moscow: Gosudarstvennoe izdatel'stvo khudozh. literatury, 1954), 5:156.

92. See Claes Peterson, *Peter the Great's Administrative and Judicial Reforms: Swedish Antecedents and the Process of Reception* (Stockholm: Bloms Boktryckeri AB, 1979).

93. G. J. Snoek, *Medieval Piety from Relics to the Eucharist: A Process of Mutual Interaction* (Leiden: E. J. Brill, 1995), 137, 288–89.

94. See Cracraft, *The Petrine Revolution in Russian Imagery*, 144.

95. On the importance of iconography for consolidating and propagating autocratic authority as well as the self-image of the privileged sectors of society in Petrine and post-Petrine Russia through "certain visual representations of [official] status and power" in the form of seals, medals, coins, flags, etc., see Cracraft, *Petrine Revolution in Russian Imagery*, 258. See also Wortman, *Scenarios of Power*.

96. T. N. Muntian describes a glass embellished with silver and gold made at the Bakhmet'ev factory in the 1780s: "the shimmering design" of garlands, bows, butterflies, bees, wild strawberries, and wheat sheaves "hovers in an immaterial fairy-tale space. Such decoration was typical for the time, when the vivid effects of lavish fireworks and unusual theatrical spectacles were particularly popular." See "Izdeliia Nikol'sko-Bakhmet'evskogo stekol'nogo zavoda v sobranii muzeev Kremlia," in *Dekorativnoe i prikladnoe iskusstvo: Materialy i issledovaniia*, ed. Aida Nasibova (Moscow: Moskovskii Kreml', 1993), 140. We recall the Petrine-era goblet whose allegorical military design reproduced that of an illumination, described above.

97. I am grateful to Annette Pein for this insight.

98. The curator of the Lomonosov Museum at the Kunstkamera in St. Petersburg generously provided me with the texts of the decrees.

99. One exception is Leonid Pasternak's painting *A Court of Law in the Seventies* (1909), from a series of historical illustrations for the journal *From the History of Russian Culture*. See William E. Butler, "On the Formation of a Russian Legal Consciousness: The Zertsalo," in *Russia and the Law of Nations in Historical Perspective: Collected Essays* (London: Wildy, Simmonds and Hill, 2009), 96–97. This essay provides information on the ceremonial uses of the *zertsalo* and describes *zertsala* preserved in such towns as Perm, Tver, and Irkutsk, in addition to the ones listed in the present study. For an illuminating analysis of the *zertsalo* within a legal context, see Butler, "The Zertsalo: Further Reflection" (forthcoming).

100. See Wortman, *Development of a Russian Legal Consciousness*, 22. The

legal clerk Skobeev was the scheming rogue hero of a tale dating to circa the late seventeenth century that is widely considered one of the first Russian examples of secular literature. See Gitta Hammarberg, "Eighteenth Century Narrative Variations on 'Frol Skobeev,'" *Slavic Review* 46, no. 3/4 (Autumn-Winter, 1987): 529–39.

101. Cited in A. Matsai, *"Iabeda" V. V. Kapnista* (Kiev: Izdatel'stvo Kievskogo gosudarstvennogo universiteta im. T. Shevchenko, 1958), 102. An earlier version of the scene clarifies the meaning behind the reference to the *zertsalo* being "hidden away": ordered by Khvataiko to "put a night cap" onto the *zertsalo*, the servants cover the object with a cloth case, whereupon it slips out of their hands, and Anna remarks ominously, "Soon the whole lot of you will keel over, too" (cited in *Russkaia komediia i komicheskaia opera XVIII veka*, ed. P. N. Berkov [Moscow: Iskusstvo, 1950], 711). For a detailed discussion of *"Iabeda"* as well as the decrees displayed upon the *zertsalo*, see my article "Mirror Writing: The Literary Traces of the *Zertsalo*" in *The Russian Review* 61 (January 2002): 73–93. This article also contains additional images of the *zertsalo* and the *Iabeda* frontispiece described in this chapter.

102. Kapnist, *Iabeda*, 296. The original reads: "В Зерцало взглянь судов: Петра черты священны / Безмездно там велят по истине судить." Here, *zertsalo* refers not only to the artifact itself but also to the entire body of law.

103. Ibid., 104.

104. The protagonist of V. I. Lukin's didactic comedy, *Shchepetil'nik* (1765), calls his time "an age of trifles."

105. I. A. Krylov, *P'esy*, vol. 1 of *Polnoe sobranie sochinenii v dvukh tomakh* (Moscow: Iskusstvo, 1944), 250.

106. P. A. Plavil'shchikov, *Sochineniia* (St. Petersburg, 1816), 71.

107. O. B. Lebedeva, *Russkaia vysokaia komediia XVIII veka: Genezis i poetika zhanra* (Tomsk: Izdatel'stvo Tomskogo universiteta, 1996), shows how *Iabeda* is the culmination of the sacral "metasiuzhet" of Russian eighteenth-century high comedy and identifies the ways in which *Revizor* is indebted to this complex play.

108. For a discussion of the *zertsalo* in Gogol's *Dead Souls*, Dostoevsky's *Notes from the Dead House*, and Tolstoy's *Anna Karenina*, see my "Mirror Writing."

109. Lebedeva (*Russkaia vysokaia komediia XVIII veka*, 314 and 327) argues that the code of laws itself was seen as embodying a rupture between corrupt reality and ideal justice.

110. For example, during a fireworks display on April 25, 1754, a "fiery fountain" was placed into a grotto containing four statues, one of which consisted of a lavishly attired female figure signifying "pleasure" with a mirror and the inscription "in excess" [с избытком]. Described in Morozov, "Lomonosov i barokko," 92.

111. Lotman, *Besedy o russkoi kul'ture*, 11–12 (emphasis in original).

112. See Iu. M. Lotman, commentaries to A. S. Pushkin, *Evgenii Onegin* (Moscow: Atrium, 1991), 361.

113. Lotman, *Besedy o russkoi kul'ture*, 129.

114. See Kirill Rets, "Teatral'nye binokli i lornety," http://goodcoins.narod.ru/antic/raznoe/teatral.htm.

115. Lotman, *Besedy o russkoi kul'ture*, 129.

116. Cited in Richard Corson, *Fashions in Eyeglasses*, 2nd rev. ed. (London: Peter Owen, 1980), 125–26.

117. Lorgnettes, especially popular at the turn of the nineteenth century, were an attribute of upper-crust women of all ages. See Ia. N. Rivosh, *Vremia i veshchi: Ocherki po istorii material'noi kul'tury v Rossii nachala XX veka* (Moscow: Iskusstvo, 1990), 118.

118. Pierre Marly, "Spectacles through the Ages, from the *Clouants* of the 13th Century to the Modern Day," in *Spectacles & Spyglasses*, trans. Barry Tulett (Liguge, Poitiers: Editions Hoebeke, 1988), 13.

119. Lotman, *Besedy o russkoi kul'ture*, 130.

120. See Iu. M. Lotman, "The Poetics of Everyday Behavior in Russian Eighteenth-Century Culture," in *The Semiotics of Russian Culture*, ed. Ann Shukman (Ann Arbor: Michigan Slavic Contributions, 1984).

121. V. I. Lukin, *Shchepetil'nik*, in *Russkaia komediia i komicheskaia opera XVIII veka*, ed. P. N. Berkov (Moscow: Iskusstvo, 1950), 99.

122. Robert Dodsley, *The Toy-Shop* (1735), Augustan Reprint Society (Los Angeles: William Andrews Clark Memorial Library, University of California, 1983), 218–19. See Hugh McLean, "The Adventures of an English Comedy in Eighteenth-Century Russia: Dodsley's *Toy Shop* and Lukin's *Ščepetil'nik*," in *American Contributions to the Fifth International Congress of Slavists, Sofia, September 1963* (The Hague: Mouton, 1963).

123. See Vladimir Gurikov, "Obrabotka i shlifovka linz v epokhu Petra I," http:/www.optika.ru/pressa/history/5–2001/index.php.

124. Cited in G. A. Printseva, *Pamiatniki russkoi kul'tury vremeni M. V. Lomonosova v Gosudarstvennom Ermitazhe* (Leningrad: Izdatel'stvo Gosudarstvennogo Ermitazha, 1961), 21.

125. Dodsley, *The Toy-Shop*, 15.

126. Lukin, *Shchepetil'nik*, 118.

127. Ibid., 119.

128. Daniel J. Boorstin, *The Discoverers* (New York: Random, 1983), 312–13.

129. Ibid.

130. Vincent Ilardi, *Renaissance Vision from Spectacles to Telescopes* (Philadelphia: American Philosophical Society, 2007), 321.

131. E. Rosen, "The Invention of Eyeglasses," *Journal of the History of*

Medicine and Allied Sciences 11 (1956): 13–46, 183–218. As MacFarlane and Martin point out, "The invention of spectacles increased the intellectual life of professional workers by fifteen years or more" (*Glass: A World History*, 145).

132. Ilardi, *Renaissance Vision*, 263–64.

133. Iu. Olesha, *Zavist'*, in *Ni dnia bez strochki* (Minsk: Izdatel'stvo BGU im. V. I. Lenina, 1982), 32.

134. Evgenii Zamiatin, *Ostrovitiane, in Izbrannoe* (Moscow: Pravda, 1989), 99.

135. See Rivosh, *Vremia i veshchi*, 118–19.

136. Cited in Richard Stites, *Revolutionary Dreams: Utopian Vision and Experimental Life in the Russian Revolution* (New York: Oxford University Press, 1989), 75.

137. I. Babel', "Moi pervyi gus'," in *Odesskie Rasskazy: Konarmiia* (Moscow: Izvestiia, 1994), 111.

138. Eisenstein's last films, *Ivan the Terrible I* and *II* (1944, 1946), feature the character of a foreign ambassador who wears dark glasses that are always lifted over his eyes. This is the final manifestation of the self-referential lenses seen in Eisenstein's earliest films.

139. See David Bordwell, *The Cinema of Eisenstein* (Cambridge, Mass: Harvard University Press, 1993), 69–71, for an analysis of the motif of eyeglasses in this film and a discussion of how glass vision aids intensify the visceral impact of specific scenes.

140. Anne Nesbet reads this sequence in light of the Medusa motif that she identifies in the film. See Nesbet, *Savage Junctures: Sergei Eisenstein and the Shape of Thinking* (London: I. B. Tauris, 2003), 67.

CHAPTER THREE

The chapter epigraph is cited in Fred Anderes and Ann Agranoff, *Ice Palaces* (New York: Abbeville, 1983), 11.

1. Anna Novak, "Ice Palace Unveiled in St. Petersburg," RIA Novosti, February 8, 2006.

2. The palace was 56 feet long, 17.5 feet wide, and over 21 feet high; see Anderes and Agranoff, *Ice Palaces*, 15.

3. This information about the interior of the ice palace is cited in I. de la Shepard, "V Rossii," in *Russkii byt vo vospominaniiakh sovremennikov: XVIII vek*, ed. A. V. Butorov (Moscow: AST, 2012), 304–5. Another ice palace was built in Russia in 1754, during the reign of Empress Elizabeth (Anderes and Agranoff, *Ice Palaces*, 15).

4. Vladimir Sedov contests the historical accuracy of Lazhechnikov's novel, citing Krafft's text to argue that there was no jester's wedding in reality. See Sedov, "Koshmar shuta," at www.projectclassica.ru. (Sedov does not, however,

mention the 1740 engraving that depicts the jester's wedding with the ice house in the background.) What is important for my purposes is the persistence of this legend and its resonance in Russian cultural memory.

5. In the account of M. Nechkina, "the old-timers could not recall such a brutal winter" as that of 1740 (in I . I. Lazhechnikov, *Ledianoi dom* [Moscow: Izdatel'stvo "Sovetskaia Rossiia," 1977], 15.

6. The martial symbolism around Anna's Ice House, as well as the spectacular play of light in and around this construction, set the tone for later such palaces built in the United States and Canada. As Anderes and Agranoff recount, ice palaces frequently served as settings for "a mock battle . . . climaxed by a dramatic display of fireworks" (*Ice Palaces*, 10). Anderes and Agranoff trace the origin of this ritual to a "sham battle" (documented by G. W. Krafft) taking place in 1734 when a fortress on the Neva, made of snow and ice, "was attacked and defended according to all the rules of war, and finally taken, 'sword in hand' " (ibid., 15).

7. Lazhechnikov, *Ledianoi dom*, 61. All subsequent references to this source will be cited in parentheses in the text.

8. Krafft's description details how the ice house was built: "Using the purest ice available, workers chopped it into large square tiles, decorated it with architectural ornaments, measured it with a compass and a ruler, then placed one tile on top of another by means of levers and poured water over each row; the water would immediately freeze and serve as a strong cement." See G. W. Kraft, *Podlinnoe i obstoiatel'noe opisanie postroennogo v Sankt-Peterburge, v Genvare 1740 goda, ledianogo doma* . . . (Pechatano pri Imperatorskoi Akademii nauk, 1741), cited in Lazhechnikov, *Ledianoi dom*, 174.

9. Kraft, *Podlinnoe i obstoiatel'noe opisanie*, 174.

10. Ibid., 175.

11. Ibid., 311.

12. For a detailed discussion of the *raek*, see Catriona Kelly, "Territories of the Eye: The Russian Peep Show (Raek) and Pre-Revolutionary Visual Culture," *Journal of Popular Culture* 31, no. 4, (1998): 49–74.

13. Ibid., 49–51.

14. Cited ibid., 57; the original text by P. Vitengof appeared in *Moskovskie ocherki* (Moscow, 1842), reprinted in *Moskva v ee proshlom i nastoiashchem*, vol. 10 (1911): 39.

15. Kelly, "Territories of the Eye," 57–59.

16. Lotman, *Besedy of russkoi kul'ture*, 10–11 (emphasis in original).

17. This goblet was displayed at the Kuskovo estate in Moscow in the summer of 1998 as part of the exhibition titled "The Art of Ceramics and Glass," organized by the State Ceramics Museum.

18. Their factories frequently operated at a loss, because their goal was not profit but the creation of objects of great artistic value (Asharina, "Russkie zavody khudozhestvennogo stekla XVII-XVIIIvv," 13–15).

19. Pyliaev, *Zabytoe proshloe okrestnostei Peterburga*, 68.

20. Tseitlin, "Kazennye (imperatorskie) 'stekliannyi', 155.

21. Asharina, "Russkie zavody khudozhestvennogo stekla," 14.

22. Voronov and Dubova, *Nevskii khrustal'*, 22–25. The water pipes were manufactured for export to Persia.

23. E. V. Dolgikh, *Russkoe steklo XVIII veka*, 9.

24. The floral designs developed out of a style of ornamentation known as "English engraving," which became widespread in the late eighteenth century at the factories of Potemkin and Orlov. These engravings, applied to vodka flasks, goblets, and wineglasses featured the large blossom and supple stem of a tulip, a daisy, or a rose (Dul'kina and Asharina, *Russkaia keramika i steklo*, 15). These flower motifs originated in the English system of royal flower symbolism.

25. For other examples of inscribed drinking vessels made for provincial consumers, see Asharina, "Kubki s emblematami," *Nauka i zhizn'* 6 (1972): 69–71.

26. Voronov and Dubova, *Nevskii khrustal'*, 78.

27. Dolgikh, *Russkoe steklo XVIII veka*, 22.

28. The items described in this paragraph belong to the State History Museum.

29. These items were displayed at the Jubilee exhibition of the State Ceramics Museum at Kuskovo in 1998.

30. These vessels belong to the State History Museum.

31. This item belongs to the Museum of Applied and Folk Art (DPI) in Moscow.

32. Dul'kina and Asharina, *Russkaia keramika i steklo*, 12; and N. A. Asharina, "'Shutikhi' sela Izmailova," *Nauka i zhizn'* 11 (1973): 151–53.

33. I am grateful to Inna Ivanovna Sergeenko, the glass curator at the State History Museum, for this information. These vessels were part of a larger "culture of jokes and tricks" (*kul'tura shutikh-obmanok*) in the applied art of the eighteenth and early nineteenth century.

34. This item was displayed at the Jubilee exhibition of the State Ceramics Museum at Kuskovo.

35. Analogous drinking vessels were produced in seventeenth-century Germany (Dul'kina and Asharina, *Russkaia keramika i steklo*, 285). The Corning Museum of Glass has several "trick" glasses on display, including one from late seventeenth–early eighteenth-century Germany.

36. Dul'kina and Asharina, *Russkaia keramika i steklo*, 14–15.

37. Pyliaev (*Zabytoe proshloe okrestnostei Peterburga*, 310–11) has a description of these fountains.

38. See also Brumfield: "Hydraulic engineering created at Peterhof one of the most complex ensembles of fountains, cascades, and decorative ponds in Europe, thus proclaiming the resources and might of Russia's transformed autocracy." The fountain ensemble contains "symbolic references to Peter's triumph not only over his enemies, but also over the natural elements" (*History of Russian Architecture*, 220).

39. For details on these phenomena, see Lindsey Hughes, *Russia in the Age of Peter the Great* (New Haven, Conn.: Yale University Press, 1998), 65 and 249–57.

40. This information is taken from R. I. Onufrieva and E. V. Gil', eds., *Ermitazh: Istoriia i arkhitektura zdanii* (Leningrad: Avrora, 1974), 218. I am grateful to Katia Dianina for bringing the crystal pavilion to my attention.

41. The information about Gonzaga's stage design is in Volobaeva, "Vitrazh v russkoi kul'ture."

42. The original text reads: Не Солнцев ли сей дом? / Он весь блестит огнями! / Нет! храм, светящийся сердцами, / Когда счастлив народ царём.

43. Gavrila Derzhavin, *Sochineniia Derzhavina s ob"iasnitel'nymi primechaniiami I. A. Grota*, 2nd ed., 7 vols. (St. Petersburg: Izdatel'stvo Imperatorskoi Akademii nauk, 1868–78), 336. The grammatical construction of the last line (the word "tsar" is in the instrumental case; thus, the people are happy literally "by means of the tsar") makes explicit the workings of this scenario, whereby the monarch acts as a force that "lights up" the hearts of the populace.

44. As early as 1807, the imperial mirror factory was overhauled according to the English model. For details on the development and overall modernization of the imperial glass factories in the nineteenth century, see Tseitlin, "Kazennye (imperatorskie) 'stekliannyi'."

45. These 16.5-foot-tall light fixtures were manufactured in St. Petersburg for the Hermitage in the second quarter of the nineteenth century (Batanova and Voronov, *Sovetskoe khudozhestvennoe steklo*, 41).

46. For example, a balustrade of crystal was designed in the 1830s for the Smolny Cathedral by architect V. P. Stasov and manufactured at the Diatkovo glassworks. For details, see Levinson et al., *Khudozhestvennoe steklo*, 124–26.

47. The notion of an artifact's "biography" is found in Igor Kopytoff, "The Cultural Biography of Things," in *The Social Life of Things: Commodities in Cultural Perspective*, ed. Arjun Appadurai (Cambridge, Eng.: Cambridge University Press, 1986).

48. J. G. Kohl, *Russia and the Russians in 1842* (London: Henry Colburn, 1842), 1:26.

49. Ibid., 2:12–13. At the time of Kohl's sojourn in Russia, sheet glass was produced through a combination of blowing and melting in a furnace. According to a description of the workings of the Malinovskii factory (characteristic of other glass factories of the time) in 1848, workers blew glass into a cylindrical shape, which was then cut lengthwise. Such cylinders were known as "*kholiavy*" (the word translates as "top of a boot" and has a range of other, frequently comical associations). These were then transported to the dissolving area (*razvodnoe otdelenie*); when a sufficient number of them was collected, they were placed into the furnace. Here the cylinders melted down into flat sheets, then were allowed to cool in a different compartment of the furnace. Over the course of twelve

hours, four workers would create from 1,000 to 2,000 sheets of glass. See K. I. Iurchuk, *Votchinnye manufaktury v stekol'noj promyshlennosti Rossii v kontse XVIII-pervoi polovine XIX veka: K probleme genezisa kapitalizma* (Voronezh: Izdatel'stvo Voronezhskogo universiteta, 1988), 30.

50. Pyliaev, *Zabytoe proshloe okrestnostei Peterburga*, 68. The columns are also mentioned in Kachalov, *Steklo*, 249.

51. Already in the eighteenth century, a predisposition toward monumentalism could be observed in Russian glass. For example, wineglasses reached 25–30 centimeters in height in the 1720s–1740s. "At this scale they produced a surprisingly massive impression and seemed designated for some jolly fairy-tale giants" (Batanova and Voronov, *Sovetskoe khudozhestvennoe steklo*, 17).

52. Ibid.

53. This information comes from V. Parfenov, *Biulleten' "Steklo mira"*, no. 3–2001, http://www.akma.spb.ru/html/articles/gplant.html.

54. See Pyliaev, *Zabytoe proshloe okrestnostei Peterburga*, 68; and Robert Sears, *An Illustrated Description of the Russian Empire* (New York: R. Sears, 1855), 463.

55. Kohl, *Russia and the Russians*, 2:14.

56. The second half of the nineteenth century marked a turning point for the Russian glass industry. With the emancipation of serfs, such unprofitable enterprises as the Imperial and Bakhmet'ev factories suffered great setbacks, while the Mal'tsev dynasty flourished as never before, gaining a virtual monopoly over Russian crystal production (Dul'kina and Asharina, *Russkaia keramika i steklo*, 20). For details on this glass dynasty, see K. A. Bol'sheva, "K istorii Mal'tsevskogo stekol'nogo proizvodstva," in *Izobrazitel'noe iskusstvo* (Leningrad: Akademiia, 1927).

57. Iurii Tynianov's *Smert' Vazir-Mukhtara* (1929) is a fictional treatment of this event; see also Laurence Kelly, *Diplomacy and Murder in Tehran: Alexander Griboyedov and Imperial Russia's Mission to the Shah of Persia* (London: I. B. Tauris, 2002).

58. Prokof'ev, *Russkii khrustal'*, 21.

59. Batanova and Voronov, *Sovetskoe khudozhestvennoe steklo*, 35–36.

60. On the Russo-Persian Wars, see Nicholas V. Riasanovsky, *A History of Russia*, 5th ed. (New York: Oxford University Press, 1993), 308 and 330.

61. Kachalov (251) characterizes this gift-giving as done "in the spirit of the customs of Oriental [*vostochnykh*] peoples."

62. For example, Sears mentions "an enormous mirror sent to the Turkish sultan" (*Description of the Russian Empire*, 463).

63. In the eighteenth century the imperial glass factory in St. Petersburg already began to specialize in diplomatic gifts. A particularly great effort was made to impress the English, who had discovered lead crystal in the middle of the seventeenth century and managed to keep the recipe a secret until the end

of the eighteenth. In the early nineteenth century, Prince William of England was presented with a monogrammed crystal table service and two candelabras (Batanova and Voronov, *Sovetskoe khudozhestvennoe steklo*, 23–24).

64. The following is based on information in Kachalov, *Steklo*, 1959, 251–55; and Noskov's first-person account, "Posol'stvo poruchika Noskova v Persiiu s khrustal'noi krovat'iu," *Istoricheskii Vestnik* 30 (November 1887) (henceforth cited as "Posol'stvo").

65. In the 1820s Ivanov helped to develop a new technique for producing large crystal constructions. See N. A. Asharina, Tamara Malinina, and Liudmila Kazakova, *Russian Glass of the 17th–20th Centuries* (Corning, N.Y.: Corning Museum of Glass, 1990), 45.

66. Armstrong ("Technology and Text," 127) characterizes the 27-foot-high glass fountain exhibited in Paxton's Crystal Palace as a site where "the static transparency formed by technology and the moving transparency of water converged."

67. On the other hand, a bed makes a curious gift to a potential enemy nation, considering the sinister associations of sleep, especially in the martial context (hence, the fallen warriors in the *Igor Tale* are compared to guests at a banquet asleep after a great feast).

68. The first Russo-Persian War had been fought from 1804 to 1813. It ended with the Treaty of Gulistan. The Crystal Bed was part of a diplomatic attempt to uphold this peace treaty. Yet another war broke out between the two countries, lasting from 1826 to 1828.

69. Noskov, "Posol'stvo," 425; see the prefatory note by the editor of *Istoricheskii Vestnik*.

70. Ibid.

71. Ibid., 428.

72. Ibid.

73. Ibid., 431.

74. Kachalov, *Steklo*, 253.

75. Noskov, "Posol'stvo," 431.

76. The bed may have had associations with the gold and jewel-encrusted Peacock Throne, which the Persians plundered from India in 1739.

77. Ibid., 433.

78. A. N. Boldyrev considers "crystal bed" a misnomer, even though that is what it was called at the time: "It was really more of a throne than a bed—a throne for the Persian shah in the form of a wide, low divan [*takhta*]." See "Khrustal'nyi tron," *Zvezda* 5–6 (1945): 153. In a letter to the director of the St. Petersburg factory expressing gratitude for other crystal gifts he had received, the shah refers to the tsar's cabinet as "the chief rulers of the Most August Divan [Avgusteishego Divana]" (Kachalov, *Steklo*, 253). One of the meanings of "divan" is "council of state."

79. Volkhovskoi, *Domashnii byt russkikh tsarei*, 74.

80. The notes of a witness to Griboyedov's reception by the shah in 1828 mention a "glass saloon" in the shah's palace where the ruler sat in state to receive the Russian delegation (cited in Kelly, *Diplomacy and Murder in Tehran*, 184). (The Russian version of these notes has "*zerkal'nyi zal.*") This prestigious placing of mirrors in the royal palace attests to the high esteem with which glass was regarded in Persia at the time.

81. Noskov, "Posol'stvo," 434.

82. See Marcel Mauss, *The Gift: Forms and Functions of Exchange in Archaic Societies*, trans. Ian Cunnison (New York: Norton, 1967) on gift-giving rituals in traditional societies and the resonance of these rituals in the modern world, as well as on the bond of obligation between giver and receiver, the politics of gift exchange, and the relationship between persons and things in the process of such exchanges.

83. Noskov, "Posol'stvo," 434.

84. Kachalov, *Steklo*, 254.

85. Ibid.

86. Ibid. In Soviet times, this tradition was revived when a monumental, 14-foot-tall crystal fountain was built for the USSR pavilion at the 1939 World's Fair in New York. For details, see Levinson et al., *Khudozhestvennoe steklo*, 34–38.

87. Kohl, *Russia and the Russians*, 1:38.

88. The original text reads: "Не удалось тебе переладить нас на свою погудку, попляши же, басурман, под нашу дудку."

89. Batanova and Voronov, *Sovetskoe khudozhestvennoe steklo*, 28. In the 1830s, a series of crystal plates appeared that were engraved with allegorical depictions of the battles of the Napoleonic War based on the wax models of medallist and sculptor Fedor Tolstoy (Dul'kina and Asharina, *Russkaia keramika i steklo*, 17).

90. The drawing was based on a caricature by Terebenev from 1813. Scaevola (Lat., "left-handed") was a legendary Roman hero. Captured while trying to kill the Etruscan king Lars Porsena, who was laying siege to Rome, Scaevola was taken to the king. He held his right hand over a fire until it burned off "to show the Etruscan he would not shrink from torture. This fortitude was so remarkable that Porsena at once ordered his release and made peace with the Romans." See Ebenezer Cobham Brewer, *Brewer's Dictionary of Phrase and Fable*, 14th ed. (New York: HarperCollins, 1989), 985.

91. V. V. Krasheninnikov, ed., *S. I. Mal'tsov i istoriia razvitiia Mal'tsovskogo promyshlennogo raiona* (Briansk: Grani, 1994), 59. The second half of the nineteenth century featured a number of revivals in the applied arts (pseudo-Gothic, second Rococo). Glassware in the "Russian style" was quite popular. It was typified by opaque, enameled dishes made to resemble the carved wood and cast

metal forms of seventeenth-century drinking vessels (Batanova and Voronov, *Sovetskoe khudozhestvennoe steklo*, 35–36).

92. The choice of glass versus porcelain drinking vessel even became a gendered one: "Thus in the petit bourgeois and rural milieu there developed the notion that men should drink from glasses because they frequent taverns, so they would be more used to it, while drinking tea from porcelain cups is the privilege of women. Unfortunately, this ridiculous custom has been preserved in some families to this very day." V. V. Pokhlebkin, *Chai i vodka v istorii Rossii* (Krasnoiarsk: Krasnoiarskoe knizhnoe izdatel'stvo, 1995), 391.

93. The imperial glass factory in St. Petersburg was producing lead crystal of remarkable clarity at the beginning of the nineteenth century; by the middle of the century, however, the factory had made concessions to market demands and begun to produce cheaper soda-lime glass of inferior quality, which, however, "found a ready demand among the new industrial middle class." See Paul Schaffer, "A Survey of Trends in the Russian Decorative Arts in the First Half of the Nineteenth Century," in *Art and Culture in Nineteenth-Century Russia*, ed. T. G. Stavrou (Bloomington: Indiana University Press, 1983), 217–18. Both Soviet and Western sources acknowledge that the quality of Russian glass production went into a decline in the second half of the century.

CHAPTER FOUR

The chapter epigraph is from Fyodor Dostoevsky, *Notes from Underground*, trans. Richard Pevear and Larissa Volokhonsky (New York: Vintage Classics, 1993), 24–25. For the original, see F. M. Dostoevskii, *Zapiski iz podpolia*, vol. 5 of *Polnoe sobranie sochinenii v 30-i tomakh*, ed. V. G. Bazanov (Leningrad: Nauka, 1972), 133.

1. For an overview of the polemic between Chernyshevsky and Dostoevsky, see Irina Paperno, *Chernyshevsky and the Age of Realism: A Study in the Semiotics of Behavior* (Stanford, Calif.: Stanford University Press, 1988), 203.

2. Ibid., 35–36, slightly revised. For the original, see Dostoevskii, *Zapiski iz podpolia*, 120.

3. See Charles Fourier, *Design for Utopia: Selected Writings of Charles Fourier*, trans. Julia Franklin (New York: Schocken Books, 1971), 146–47 and 152.

4. Mikhail Iampolskii's illuminating analysis situates the Crystal Palace in the context of utopian socialist thought and provides an extensive listing of plans for glass buildings that preceded it and followed in its wake. See his *Nabliudatel': Ocherki istorii videniia* (Moscow: Ad Marginem, 2000), 123.

5. N. G. Chernyshevskii, *Chto delat'? Iz rasskazov o novykh liudiakh*, ed. T. I. Ornatskaia and S. A. Reiser (Leningrad: Nauka, 1975), 284.

6. Ruth Eaton, "Architecture and Urbanism: The Faces of Utopia" in *Utopia: The Search for the Ideal Society in the Western World*, ed. Roland Schaer,

Gregory Claeys, and Lyman Tower Sargent (New York: New York Public Library, 2000), 298.

7. This recalls Lomonosov's argument to the Senate in favor of increasing domestic glass production.

8. Faddei Bulgarin, "Plausible Fantasies, or A Journey to the 29th Century," in *Pre-Revolutionary Russian Science Fiction: An Anthology*, ed. and trans. Leland Fetzer (Ann Arbor, Mich.: Ardis, 1982), 30.

9. V. F. Odoevskii, "The Year 4338: Letters from Petersburg," in *Pre-Revolutionary Russian Science Fiction*, 46. Translation slightly revised; for the original Russian text, see V. F. Odoevskii, *4338-i god: Peterburgskie pis'ma*, ed. Orest Tsekhovitser (Moscow: Izdatel'stvo "Ogonek," 1926).

10. In his introduction, Odoevsky speaks of the feasibility of manufacturing the "flexible glass" out of which clothing is made in his utopia and decries the lack of such clothing in his time (Odoevskii, *4338-i god*, 14).

11. Ibid., 40.

12. Ibid., 53.

13. K. Paustovskii, "Stekol'nyi master," in *Sobranie sochinenii v vos'mi tomakh* (Moscow: Khudozhestvennaia literatura, 1969) 6:524.

14. N. V. Gogol, *Taras Bul'ba* (Moscow: Akademiia nauk SSSR, 1963), 73.

15. See Paustovskii, "Stekol'nyi master," 524–27 (emphasis added).

16. Armstrong writes apropos of glassmaking in England, but what she says is quite applicable to the Russian glass industry, which largely took its cues from the English example: "If glass was blown, and in mid-century blown sheet glass, extended to four-foot cylinders, cut and rolled, became the commonest form of manufacture, then the observer would look through the residues of somebody else's breath. Look through in two senses: one would look past, and look by means of, the breath which had distended red-hot glass and which was now sealed within it" ("Transparency," 128). I am indebted to Armstrong for drawing my attention to this essential dimension of glassmaking.

17. When the column was built in 1830–34, it was the tallest modern obelisk in the world.

18. Kohl, *Russia and the Russians*, 2:14–15.

19. Possible sources for Vershinin's style are the method known in Bohemia since the 1730s whereby gilded foil inscribed with designs was placed between two layers of glass, creating an illusion of spatial depth; and the handicrafts typical of "estate culture" (*usadebnaia kul'tura*), such as wax flowers placed under a glass dome (Muntian, "Izdeliia Nikol'sko-Bakhmet'evskogo stekol'nogo zavoda," 140).

20. Batanova and Voronov, *Sovetskoe khudozhestvennoe steklo*, 27.

21. Ibid.

22. Cited in Kachalov, *Steklo*, 264.

23. Prokof'ev, *Russkii khrustal'*, 26.

24. Ibid. Zubanov's statement in the original reads: "До чего ж красив узор! Здорово было бы сделать такой же не стекле."

25. See Viktor Poltoratskii, *Gnezdo khrustal'nogo gusia: Rasskaz o proshlom, nastoiashchem i budushchem rossiiskogo steklograda, o zamechatel'nykh masterakh i khudozhnikakh russkogo khrustalia* (Moscow: Sovetskaia Rossiia, 1959), 13.

26. Volobaeva, "Vitrazh v russkoi kul'ture."

27. Kohl, *Russia and the Russians*, 2:14.

28. By contrast, Batanova and Voronov tell of glassblowers giving their dying breath to create monumental trifles for the idle rich (*Sovetskoe khudozhestvennoe steklo*, 28).

29. N. G. Anisimov, *Ogni nad Volgoi: Ocherk istorii Vasil'evskogo steklozavoda "Pobeda Truda"* (Kazan: Tatknigoizdat, 1967), 8.

30. It took 900,000 square feet of glass to build the Crystal Palace, "and it was all mouth-blown glass that, as cylinders, had to be split and ironed flat" (Ellis, *Glass*, 241).

31. Kachalov, *Steklo*, 379.

32. Benjamin, "Paris, the Capital of the Nineteenth Century," 157.

33. In his *Seven Lamps of Architecture* (London: J. M. Dent, 1928), John Ruskin speaks of light entering a Gothic cathedral through a window as taking the form of a star that hovers over the heads of the worshippers and dematerializes the interior.

34. Between the end of the eighteenth century and the middle of the nineteenth, the number of Russian glass factories increased nearly fivefold. By the time of the reforms of the 1860s, there were 180 glass factories in all; two of these manufactured mirrors, around twenty made crystal, while the others were split evenly between window and bottle glass (Kachalov, *Steklo*, 267).

35. The latter word derives from Old French *estui*, "prison," from *estuier*, "to keep."

36. Richards articulates how display under glass enabled the spectacular presentation of commodities: they became "a sensual feast for the eye of the spectator, and they [took] on the ceremonial trappings of the dominant institutions and vested interests of mid-Victorian England" (*Commodity Culture of Victorian England*, 21). As Fauvel notes, Pei's pyramid "puts the Louvre under glass, protects it, enhances the value of its contents, as do bell jars, shop windows, glass coffins" ("From Iron to Glass," 341).

37. Chernyshevskii, *Chto Delat'?*, 344.

38. Akin to the Crystal Palace, the Passage bathed its visitors in natural light while offering protection from heat and cold. Ruane traces the development of arcades in Moscow and St. Petersburg, a response to the increasing scarcity of space in the upscale shopping districts. The Passage was the first arcade to be built in St. Petersburg (in 1848). In Moscow, the Golitsynskii arcade was built

between 1835 and 1839, and by the beginning of the twentieth century, it was one of at least ten such arcades in Moscow (*The Empire's New Clothes*, 122).

39. In such representations, the future yet to come is ultimately "wedded to elements from prehistory" (Benjamin, "Paris, the Capital of the Nineteenth Century," 148).

40. Rastrelli's design for the Grand Palace in Peterhof included this use of mirrors.

41. Chernyshevsky did not actually see the Palace until 1859; here he was relying on the compiled accounts of western European journalists.

42. N. G. Chernyshevskii, "Novosti literatury, iskusstv, nauk i promyshlennosti," in *Polnoe sobranie sochinenii v piatnadtsati tomakh* (Moscow: Gosudarstvennoe izdatel'stvo khudozhestvennoi literatury, 1953), 16:103 (emphasis added). In the original Russian, the measures Chernyshevsky gives are equal to 0.71 meter and 2.13 meters, respectively.

43. Nabokov's version, in his fictionalized biography of Chernyshevsky, is slightly different: "By lifting a corner of the green baize curtain the sentry could look through the peephole in the door at the prisoner." Vladimir Nabokov, *The Gift* (New York: Vintage International, 1991), 272.

44. Chernyshevskii, *Chto Delat'* 28.

45. Ibid., 89.

46. Ibid., 337. The delighted woman in black is a hidden reference to Chernyshevsky's real-life spouse, Olga Sokratovna.

47. Chernyshevskii, "Novosti literatury," 93. Later Chernyshevsky details how much glass has been used to create that impression: "The width of the Sydenham palace is almost equal to the length of our [St. Petersburg] Passage; the length is commensurate with this frightful [*strashnoi*] width. Thirty or forty Passages would barely add up to one Crystal Palace. . . . The glass used for its walls and roof could cover a space of 25 acres; if all these panes of glass were to be placed in a single row, the line would extend for 375 versts [roughly 563 miles]" (ibid.).

48. F. M. Dostoevskii, *Brat'ia Karamazovy*, in *Sobranie Sochinenii v Deviati Tomakh* (Moscow: Astrel', 2004), 266 and 484; Fedor Dostoevskii, *Besy* (St. Petersburg: Karavella, 1994), 308.

49. F. M. Dostoevskii, "Mal'chik u Khrista na elke," in *Dnevnik pisatelia za 1876 god, ianvar'-aprel', Polnoe sobranie sochinenii* (Moscow: Nauka, 1981), 23:15.

50. F. M. Dostoevskii, *Prestuplenie i nakazanie*, in *Polnoe Sobranie Sochinenii v Tridtsati Tomakh*, ed. V. G. Bazanov (Leningrad: Nauka, 1972), 7:63.

51. M. M. Bakhtin, "Forms of Time and Chronotope in the Novel," in *The Dialogic Imagination: Four Essays by M. M. Bakhtin*, ed. Michael Holquist, trans. Caryl Emerson and Michael Holquist (Austin: University of Texas Press, 1981), 248.

52. F. M. Dostoevskii, *Zapiski iz podpolia*, 177.

53. Georg Kohlmaier and Barna von Satory, *Houses of Glass: A Nineteenth-Century Building Type*, trans. John C. Harvey (Cambridge, Mass: MIT Press, 1986), 20.

CHAPTER FIVE

The chapter epigraph is quoted in Ulrich Conrads and Hans G. Sperlich, *The Architecture of Fantasy: Utopian Building and Planning in Modern Times*, trans. and ed. Christiane Crasemann Collins and George R. Collins (New York: Frederick A. Praeger, 1962), 133–34.

1. Daniel R. Brower, *The Russian City between Tradition and Modernity, 1850–1900* (Berkeley: University of California Press, 1990), 72.

2. Moreover, Armstrong argues that the structure, which contained "exotic trees, meandering pathways, shrubs, Greek sculpture, fish in crystal vases, and a grotto of looking glasses," influenced both the art of Charlotte Brontë and the architectural practice of Sydney Smirke, whose Pantheon arcade was built in London in 1832. Isobel Armstrong, *Victorian Glassworlds: Glass Culture and the Imagination, 1830–1880* (Oxford: Oxford University Press, 2008), 116, 140, 379n16.

3. Ibid., 170–71.

4. According to Anatole Kopp, "a dialectical conception of the role of the human environment" developed in the wake of the revolution: "a reflection of the new society, it was at the same time the mold in which that society was to be cast." *Town and Revolution: Soviet Architecture and City Planning 1917–1935*, trans. Thomas E. Burton (New York: George Braziller, 1970), 12.

5. "Steklo v sovremennoi arkhtitekture," *Sovremennaia arkhitektura* 3 (1926): 63.

6. Bletter, "Interpretation of the Glass Dream," 31. This article provides a detailed account of the evolution of the mystical associations surrounding glass.

7. Qtd. in John Milner, *Vladimir Tatlin and the Russian Avant-Garde* (New Haven, Conn.: Yale University Press, 1983), 34.

8. See Anatole Kopp, "Foreign Architects in the Soviet Union during the First Two Five Year Plans," in *Reshaping Russian Architecture: Western Architecture, Utopian Dreams*, ed. William Craft Brumfield (Cambridge, Eng.: Cambridge University Press, 1990), 233–34.

9. Nikolai Kachalov, introduction to Levinson et al., *Khudozhestvennoe steklo*, 10.

10. Hughes, *Shock of the New*, 178. Compare Kachalov's assumption that no one would break a window intentionally: "a pane of glass mounted in a window frame may last for dozens of years, *unless it is accidentally broken*" (Kachalov, *Steklo*, 13, emphasis added).

11. "Steklo v sovremennoi arkhitekture." The original text reads: "Вместо спящего, инертного, каменного массива-монумента—гибкий, динамический, напряжённый и разумный организм."

12. Ibid. This attack on the cloistered petit-bourgeois mentality of those who are hostile to glass architecture echoes the words of Behne, cited in the epigraph to this chapter.

13. N. F. Popov, "Novaia Moskva—ne muzei stariny," *Izvestiia* 267 (November 22, 1925); reprinted in K. N. Afanas'ev, ed., *Iz istorii sovetskoi arkhitektury, 1917–1925 gg*. (Moscow: Akademiia nauk SSSR, 1963), 50.

14. In fact, the attack on stone architecture is typical of the rhetoric among progressive architects of the time. See K. Selinskii, "Style and Steel" (1923): "Inflexible, restricted, and tortuous in its dynamic possibilities, stone is incapable of keeping up with the rapid pace of life." Selinskii goes on to suggest that the Palace of Labor be realized as a gigantic, rotating edifice, its various parts in perpetual motion, "a great building of glass and aluminum walls that can be easily disassembled." The latter details recall the Chernyshevskian Crystal Palace as well as its real-life prefabricated prototype of 1851. Qtd. in Conrads and Sperlich, *The Architecture of Fantasy*, 153–54.

15. El Lissitzky, "Suprematism in World Reconstruction," in *Russian Art of the Avant-Garde: Theory and Criticism 1902–1934*, ed. and trans. John Bowlt, rev. ed. (New York: Thames and Hudson, 1988), 155.

16. Ibid., 156 (punctuation omitted in the original).

17. A feature entitled "Why We Live Here," published in *Boston Magazine*, April 2002, placed "the reflection of Trinity Church on the Hancock Tower" as the third item on the list. Perhaps the attraction is the way in which the reflection of the venerable church in the sleek skyscraper visually seems to convey the harmony between historical epochs epitomized in the different architectural styles, to say nothing of the functions, of the two buildings in question.

18. El Lissitzky, "New Russian Art: A Lecture" (1922), in *El Lissitzky: Life-Letters-Texts* (Greenwich, Conn.: New York Graphic Society, 1968), 133.

19. L. Trotskii, *Literatura i revoliutsiia* (1923; Moscow: Izdatel'stvo politicheskoi literatury, 1991), 196.

20. Ibid., 197.

21. John Bowlt, "The Presence of Absence: The Aesthetic of Transparency in Russian Modernism," *The Structurist* 27–28 (1987–88): 15.

22. In his discussion of the Crystal Palace, Mikhail Iampolskii draws a parallel between the capacity of glass to become invisible, the way that it stimulates the imagination, and its aura of magic (*Nabliudatel'*, 121).

23. Qtd. in Milka Bliznakov, "The Realization of Utopia: Western Technology and Soviet Avant-Garde Architecture," in *Reshaping Russian Architecture*, ed. Brumfeld, 145 (emphasis in the original). Konstantin Tsiolkovsky's utopian novel *Beyond the Planet Earth*, published in 1920 and set in 2017, also

features glass houses filled with greenery that hover weightless in space. See Milner, *Vladimir Tatlin*, 178–79. Tsiolkovsky's cosmic, crystalline vision is very close to that of Scheerbart at the turn of the century.

24. "Voyage of the Red Star Pioneer Troop to Wonderland," in *Mass Culture in Soviet Russia: Tales, Poems, Songs, Movies, Plays and Folklore 1917–1953*, ed. James Von Geldern and Richard Stites (Bloomington: Indiana University Press, 1995), 103 (translation slightly revised). For the original, see I. N. Zhukov, *Puteshestvie zvena "Krasnoi zvezdy" v stranu chudes: Povest'* (Kharkov: Izdatel'stvo Vseukrainskogo obshch-va sodeistviia Iunomu Lenintsu, 1924), 50.

25. See Timothy Colton, *Moscow: Governing the Socialist Metropolis* (Cambridge, Mass.: Belknap Press, 1995), 265.

26. Yury Olesha, *No Day without a Line: From Notebooks by Yury Olesha*, ed., trans., and intro. Judson Rosengrant (Evanston, Ill.: Northwestern University Press, 1998), 99 (translation slightly revised). Original in Iurii Olesha, *Kniga Proshchaniia* (Moscow: Vagrius, 1999).

27. Bletter documents Scheerbart's influence on Gropius ("Interpretation of the Glass Dream," 37–38).

28. Paul Scheerbart, *Glass Architecture*, trans. James Palmes, ed. Dennis Sharp (New York: Praeger, 1972), 46.

29. Ibid., 50–51.

30. Ibid., 63. German architect Adolf Behne, a devotee of Scheerbart, was just as enthusiastic about the potential of glass architecture to bring about "a new culture" by transforming the individual, or more precisely, by transforming his vision: it entices "the contemplation of—not man and his accomplishments—but the infinite universe." Cited in Conrads and Sperlich, *The Architecture of Fantasy*, 134.

31. Scheerbart, *Glass Architecture*, 72.

32. We recall the religious function of glass in medieval Russia, in the form of ritual glass vessels and, most famously, the Kievan church mosaics.

33. Scheerbart, *Glass Architecture*, 72.

34. This date has been confirmed by Larissa Zhadova ("Tolpa prozrachno-chistykh sot," *Nauka i zhizn'* 8 [1976]: 104).

35. Velimir Khlebnikov, *Collected Works of Velimir Khlebnikov*, trans. Paul Schmidt, ed. Charlotte Douglas (Cambridge, Mass.: Harvard University Press, 1987), 1:347; Velimir Khlebnikov, *Tvoreniia*, ed. M. Ia. Poliakov (Moscow: Sovetskii pisatel', 1986), 595. (I use Schmidt's translation throughout, modified as needed.)

36. Khlebnikov, *Collected Works*, 3:73. The importance of the sense of sight for Khlebnikov is well documented; hence glass would appeal to him as the material that engages with the sense of sight more than any other, and a glass book would naturally suggest itself as that which is apprehended visually. See Robin Milner-Gulland, "Khlebnikov's Eye," in *Russian Literature, Modernism*

and the Visual Arts, ed. Catriona Kelly and Stephen Lovell (Cambridge, Eng.: Cambridge University Press, 2000), 211.

37. The honeycomb can be read as the communal house of worker bees: the worker bee was a popular utopian metaphor and model of the time—see, for example, Alexandra Kollontai's popular 1923 novel *The Love of Worker Bees*.

38. Khlebnikov, *Collected Works*, 1:350.

39. See the discussion of Khlebnikov and organic architecture in Julia Vaingurt, *Wonderlands of the Avant-Garde: Technology and the Arts in Russia of the 1920s* (Evanston, Ill.: Northwestern University Press, 2013).

40. That, as well as its prefabricated quality, strongly recalls Paxton's Crystal Palace of 1851, one of the sites where utopian architecture originated.

41. Khlebnikov, *Collected Works*, 1:351.

42. Khlebnikov, *Tvoreniia*, 119. The original is "и алошарая вершина / Светла венком стеклянной проседи."

43. The original has "ящик из гнутого стекла или походная каюта [. . .] стеклянный шатёр [. . .] стекло-хата [. . .] оболочка" (Khlebnikov, *Tvoreniia*, 350–51).

44. Ibid., 113–14.

45. This connection has been noted by Elizabeth Klosty Beaujour in "Architectual Discourse and Early Soviet Literature," *Journal of the History of Ideas* 44, no. 3 (July–September 1983): 484; and by Emma Widdis in *Visions of a New Land: Soviet Film from the Revolution to the Second World War* (New Haven, Conn.: Yale University Press, 2003), 51.

46. In 1927, Moisei Ginzburg—the editor of *Sovremennaia arkhitektura*—named "the cabins of a passenger ship, airplane or sleeping wagon" as prototypes for the new home. Cited in Papernyi, *Kul'tura "Dva,"* 61.

47. Mikhail Okhitrovich, "K probleme goroda," *Sovremennnaia arkhitektura* 4 (1929): 134.

48. Khlebnikov, *Collected Works*, 1:353–56.

49. Katerina Clark sheds light on Khlebnikov's use of "*griaznyi iashchik*": there was a discourse in early twentieth-century Russia directed against small, closed spaces, exemplified in the sardine tin that conceals a bomb in Bely's *Petersburg*. See *Petersburg, Crucible of Cultural Revolution* (Cambridge, Mass.: Harvard University Press, 1995).

50. Khlebnikov, *Collected Works*, 3:73 / *Tvoreniia*, 119.

51. Mumford, *Technics and Civilization*, 28.

52. Khlebnikov, *Collected Works*, 3:178–79 / *Tvoreniia*, 290.

53. Khlebnikov, *Collected Works*, 3:94.

54. On Khlebnikov's attempt to synthesize landscape and architecture, see Zhadova, "Tolpa prozrachno-chistykh sot," 107.

55. See Kohlmaier and von Satory, *Houses of Glass*, 20.

56. Khlebnikov, *Collected Works*, 1:397–98 / *Tvoreniia*, 566. Aside from

the overwhelming interest in glass they share, Iampolskii cites two other parallels between Scheerbart and Khlebnikov: the former's invention of a plantlike house in a work from 1910, and his enthusiasm for mobile cities (Iampolskii, *Nabliudatel'*, 147).

57. Gogol's novel *Taras Bulba* contains a reference to this kind of armor.

58. I use the term "anti-utopia" to refer to a text that questions the very concept of utopianism, as well as to a polemical response to an existing positive utopia; *We* fulfills both criteria. See the glossary in Schaer et al., eds., *Utopia*, 15.

59. Milner, *Vladimir Tatlin*, 243.

60. Ibid., 152–53.

61. Nikolai Punin, "Pamiatnik III Internatsionala," in *O Tatline: Arkhiv russkogo avangarda* (Moscow: Literaturno-khudozhestvennoe agenstvo "RA," 1994), 18. Subsequent citations of this source will be indicated by in-text page references.

62. A similar mindset was at work in the case of the unrealized design of the U.N. building. The glass of its walls was meant to signify the honesty of the human beings within and the transparency of the political system. See also Svetlana Boym, *The Future of Nostalgia* (New York: Basic Books, 2001), 216–17 on the false transparency of the Reichstag building redesigned in 1990.

63. Milner, *Vladimir Tatlin*, 151.

64. Il'ia Erenburg, *A vse-taki ona vertitsia* (Moscow: Gelikon, 1922), 19.

65. Konstantin Miklashevskii, *Gipertrofiia iskusstva* (Petrograd: Gosudarstvennaia tipografiia im. Evgenii Sokolovoi, 1924), 65.

66. Milner, *Vladimir Tatlin*, 160.

67. S. Frederick Starr has documented Mel'nikov's strategic use of glass in projects such as the Green City to expose the human body to the beneficent rays of the sun (*Melnikov: Solo Architect in a Mass Society* [Princeton, N.J.: Princeton University Press, 1978], 177 and 179). Khlebnikov names his utopia City of the Sun (*Solntsestan*), perhaps in reference to Campanella's utopia, which made a great impression on Lenin.

68. "Steklo v sovremennoi arkhitekture," 63.

69. This sun worship can be seen in Mel'nikov's design for his own house (1926–27), whose walls had over 200 hexagonal corbeled windows (around sixty of which were glassed-in) and was entirely fronted with glass. See Starr, *Melnikov*, 122–23.

70. Osip Mandelstam, *The Egyptian Stamp*, in *The Noise of Time: The Prose of Osip Mandelstam*, ed. and trans. Clarence Brown (New York: Penguin Books, 1993), 69 (translation slightly revised).

71. The Lubyanka had negative associations by the time that Mandelstam wrote this work; see Vitaly Shentalinsky, *Arrested Voices: Resurrecting the Disappeared Writers of the Soviet Regime*, trans. John Crowfoot (New York: Martin Kessler Books, 1993).

72. According to one Soviet source, 259 Russian glass factories were in operation on the eve of World War I. Many of the factories ceased to function during the war; at the time of the October Revolution, the number of working glass factories compared to 1913 was reduced by 34 percent, the number of workers by 32 percent, and the volume of production by 52 percent. After four years of war, the glass industry found itself at the level where it had been at the turn of the century. The nationalization of glass factories began in 1919. In 1921 glass production enterprises were put on a self-supporting basis, and territorial trusts were established. These NEP measures increased the quantity of production by 4,123 tons, or almost 40 percent in a year (Boldyrev, "Stekol'naia promyshlennost'," 222). New glass factories were built in the mid-1920s. With an increase in construction and the development of various branches of industry, the demand for all types of glass grew and mechanical methods of glass production were quickly adopted (ibid., 223).

73. "The Lights of Dagestan"—the first glass factory to be built in the U.S.S.R. after the Bolshevik Revolution—began to produce sheet glass by means of vertical extraction in 1926 (Boldyrev, 223). The Soviet Union invited foreign glassmaking specialists from Germany, Czechoslovakia, Belgium, and elsewhere "to instruct the mountaineers" in this unfamiliar method, using machines invented by the Belgian Emile Fourcauld. These machines were replaced by Soviet-made ones in 1937. S. B. Babakhanov, *Fakely "Ognei"* (Makhachkala: Dagestanskoe knizhnoe izdatel'stvo, 1991), 25.

74. "Steklo v sovremennoi arkhitekture," 63.

75. Boldyrev, "Stekol'naia promyshlennost'," 223.

76. Qtd. in Keith Bell, "Glass in Architecture," *The Structurist* 27–28 (1987–88): 73 (emphasis added).

77. Starr, *Melnikov*, 72.

78. Iampolskii documents how thinkers saw in the transparency of the Crystal Palace and similar glass structures a symbol of the dissolution of boundaries and the hope of social unity; this is relevant to the dream of harmony embodied in glass architecture, a dream shared by Khlebnikov and company (*Nabliudatel'*, 122–23).

79. See, for example, Gary Kern on the preservation of mandatory happiness in the One State: "So that this happiness not be threatened by freedom, all houses are made of glass. This facilitates the work of the 'Bureau of Guardians,' special agents who watch the citizens to ensure their uninterrupted tranquility." *Zamyatin's "We": A Collection of Critical Essays*, ed. Gary Kern (Ann Arbor, Mich.: Ardis, 1988), 11–12.

80. Evgenii Zamiatin, *My*, in *Izbrannoe* (Moscow: Pravda, 1989), 418. Subsequent citations of this source will be indicated by in-text page references.

81. S. A. Cowan, "The Crystalline Center of Zamyatin's *We*," *Extrapolation* 29, no. 2 (Summer 1988): 161.

82. Qtd. in Conrads and Sperlich, *The Architecture of Fantasy*, 134.

83. Thus, the glass *Integral* is constructed by glass cranes sliding along glass rails (361); even the people participating in the construction look to D as if they themselves were made of glass: their foreheads are "mirror-like, unclouded by the madness of thoughts."

84. William Hutchings compares the *Integral* to Tatlin's Tower on the basis of form and function in "Structure and Design in a Soviet Dystopia: H. G. Wells, Constructivism, and Yevgeny Zamyatin's *We*," *Journal of Modern Literature* 9, no. 1 (1981/1982): 98.

85. Alexei Tolstoi, *Aelita: Giperboloid inzhenera Garina* (Moscow: Izdatel'stvo "Pravda," 1986), 162.

86. In Mikhail Zoshchenko's story "Happiness" (1924), a glazier's only recollection of the titular emotion is connected with installing a new plate-glass window in a tavern; juxtaposed with the contemporary works by Zamyatin and Tolstoi (the former of which circulated widely in unofficial copies), this suggests that Zoshchenko is parodying an association between glass and happiness that other authors of the time present earnestly.

87. On the influence of Dostoevskian texts on *We*, see Robert Louis Jackson, *The Underground Man in Russian Literature* (The Hague: Mouton, 1958), 157; and Efraim Sicher, "By Underground to Crystal Palace: The Dystopian Eden," *Comparative Literature Studies* 22, no. 3 (Fall 1985): 383.

88. See Vladimir Mayakovsky, *The Bedbug and Selected Poetry*, trans. Max Hayward and George Reavey, ed. Patricia Blake (Bloomington: Indiana University Press, 1975), 278, 284, 288, and 291, respectively. For the original, see V. V. Maiakovskii, *Klop*, in *Sochineniia v dvukh tomakh*, vol. 2 (Moscow: Pravda, 1988), 568, 572, 575, and 576, respectively.

89. Such parallels include the "mirror-like foreheads" cited above; the implied analogy between the semispherical (*polushar*) glass dome of the auditorium and the spherical (*sharoobrasnykh*) shaven heads of the numbers within (Zamiatin, *My*, 317); and the way the "enemy of the state" seems to turn to glass when he is being put to death (337).

90. I am borrowing this term from Louis Althusser, who used it to refer to institutions in a capitalist society—educational systems, family, religion, the mass media—that keep its subjects under control, willingly participating in their subjugation. In contrast to the Repressive State Apparatuses such as the police and the army, the ISAs do their work through persuasion, not force. They are omnipresent, omnipotent, and carry on their work of indoctrination invisibly. See Althusser's essay "Ideology and Ideological State Apparatuses: Notes Toward an Investigation" in *Lenin and Philosophy*, trans. Ben Brewster (London: New Left Books, 1971).

91. See Zamyatin's 1921 essay "Paradise," which ends with a citation from a novel by H. G. Wells: "And the teacher of eternal questing, eternal rebellion, Satan, replied 'Yes, without me time and space would freeze into crystalline

perfection.'" *Soviet Heretic: Essays by Yevgeny Zamyatin*, ed. and trans. Mirra Ginsburg (Chicago: University of Chicago Press, 1970), 67.

92. See Christopher Collins, "Zamyatin's *We* as Myth," in *Zamyatin's "We": A Collection of Critical Essays*, ed. Gary Kern (Ann Arbor, Mich.: Ardis, 1988), 71.

93. The sensation, enabled by mirrors, of being at once "here" and "elsewhere" may be what Michel Foucault has in mind when he discusses mirrors in the context of what he calls the heterotopia. This is a real site in which "all the other real sites that can be found within the culture are simultaneously represented, contested, and inverted." See his essay "Of Other Spaces," *Diacritics* (Spring 1986): 24.

94. Scheerbart, *Glass Architecture*, 47–48.

95. Only in 1835 did Julius von Leibeg invent a process of backing mirror glass with silver instead of mercury. Jane Turner, ed., *Dictionary of Art* (New York: Grove's Dictionaries, 1996), 721.

96. Robert Russell, "The Modernist Tradition," in *Cambridge Companion to the Classic Russian Novel*, ed. Malcolm E. Jones and Robin Feuer Miller (New York: Cambridge University Press, 1998), 220.

97. The glass structures that order the One State can be seen as an Ideological State Apparatus of which D suddenly becomes aware: seeing it from an unfamiliar angle instantly renders it visible.

98. Trained as a naval engineer, Zamyatin received a commission in 1916 to supervise the construction of Russian icebreakers in Newcastle. Zamyatin spent a year and a half in England and returned to Russia in time to witness the October Revolution. See Alex M. Shane, *The Life and Works of Evgenij Zamjatin* (Berkeley: University of California Press, 1968), 12–13.

99. Evgenii Zamiatin, "O moikh zhenakh, o ledokolakh i o Rossii," *Mosty* 9 (1962): 21.

100. Ibid., 22–25.

101. Alan Myers, "Zamyatin in Newcastle," *Foundation* 59 (Autumn 1993): 76.

102. See also Russell on this point—D's "alter ego, the intuitive creative artist, senses the fragility underlying the massively solid exterior of the state" (*Zamyatin's "We,"* Kern, ed., 90). Beaujour discusses the ambiguity of glass in "Zamyatin's *We* and Modernist Architecture," *The Russian Review* 47, no. 1 (1988), 59–60.

103. According to the "glass crown" method, molten glass blown out into a bubble, then twirled on the end of the blowpipe over the artisan's head; glass disks spun out in this way were thicker in the middle than at the edge. Glaziers installed the thicker part of the windowpane at the bottom for stability. See Armstrong, *Victorian Glassworlds*, 39–41.

104. This use of glass imagery is developed in Zamyatin's "Story about the Main Thing" (1923).

105. Bowlt, "The Presence of Absence," 16.

106. Ibid., 17.

107. Douglas Fairbanks and Mary Pickford, enthralled by *The Battleship Potemkin*, visited Eisenstein in 1926 and invited him to Hollywood; he went there in 1930. His idea was rejected by the Hollywood producers, and even by close friends, as outlandish and unprofitable; he was persecuted in the United States as a suspected Bolshevik agent, only to meet even worse treatment back home. See Ronald Bergan, *Eisenstein: A Life in Conflict* (Woodstock, N.Y.: Overlook, 1999).

108. Bordwell, *The Cinema of Eisenstein*, 46.

109. Ibid., 195. The 28mm lens and other short-focus lenses allowed Eisenstein to create "dynamically deep images" (ibid., 46).

110. Nesbet uses Eisenstein's concept of plasmaticness, his term to designate a body's potential for metamorphosis, to analyze the dialogue between the *Ivan the Terrible* films and the animated work of Disney (*Savage Junctures*, 187–203).

111. Sergei Eisenstein, *Nonindifferent Nature*, trans. Herbert Marshall (Cambridge, Eng.: Cambridge University Press), 47. These essays, written mostly in 1945–47, provide insights into Eisenstein's thinking about lenses and optical effects.

112. Ibid., 48–49 (translation slightly revised).

113. Bergan, *Eisenstein: A Life in Conflict*, 122.

114. Oksana Bulgakowa, *Sergei Eisenstein: A Biography*, trans. Anne Dwyer (Berlin: Potemkin, 2001), 63; see also 115–16.

115. Naum Kleiman, " 'Stekliannyi dom' S. M. Eizenshteina: k istorii zamysla," *Iskusstvo kino* 3 (1979): 94, 100. This article features excerpts from Eisenstein's notebooks along with Kleiman's commentary.

116. Ibid., 110.

117. Cited in Bulgakowa, *Sergei Eisenstein: A Biography*, 48.

118. Ibid., 104. Mike Figgis's film *Time Code* (2000), set in Hollywood, features a screen divided into four sections, each showing a different story unfolding simultaneously; here this device is used for ironic juxtapositions and social critique as well.

119. Ivor G. S. Montague, *With Eisenstein in Hollywood* (New York: International, 1969), 103.

120. Kleiman, " 'Stekliannyi dom' S. M. Eizenshteina," 103. The punning original reads: " 'G.H.' для нас записать как ряд марксистских 'положений,' как монтаж формул. . . . Комедию положений сменяет—комедия 'положений.' "

121. I am grateful to Julia Vaingurt for bringing this poem to my attention. See her *Wonderlands of the Avant-Garde*, 174.

122. Kleiman, " 'Stekliannyi dom' S. M. Eizenshteina," 96. Subsequent citations of this source will be indicated by in-text page references.

123. Sergei Eisenstein, "Disnei," in *Problemy sinteza v khudozhestvennoi kul'ture*, ed. A. V. Prokhorov et al. (Moscow: Nauka, 1985), 221.

124. Ibid., 246.

125. As Bulgakowa argues, "*The Glass House* took vision as its theme—both the perfect vision of the medium and also the voyeurism of man" (*Sergei Eisenstein*, 116).

126. This interpretation of Eisenstein's use of the term "mystery play" belongs to Naum Kleiman ("'Stekliannyi dom' S. M. Eizenshteina," 113).

127. Qtd. in Bergan, *Eisenstein: A Life in Conflict*, 196.

128. Qtd. in Jay Leyda and Zina Voynow, *Eisenstein at Work* (New York: Pantheon, 1982), 37.

129. While Eisenstein was editing *October* in November 1927, Stalin paid a visit to his studio and, after watching several sequences, demanded the deletion of scenes involving Trotsky and those showing Lenin "in an unsatisfactory light." This was the first time that Eisenstein had to subject his art to drastic change on the direct order of the state. See Bergan, *Eisenstein: A Life in Conflict*, 134.

130. Bulgakowa, *Sergei Eisenstein*, 69.

131. Cited ibid., 190.

132. Sergei Eisenstein, *Selected Works*, vol. 2, *Towards a Theory of Montage*, ed. Michael Glenny and Richard Taylor, trans. Michael Glenny (London: BFI, 1991), 232.

133. For a detailed analysis of mirror imagery in *Strike*, see my article "No Mere Reflection: Mirrors as Windows on Russian Culture," *Studies in Twentieth- and Twenty-First Century Literature* 34, no. 2 (Summer 2010): 170–206.

134. Eisenstein, *Selected Works*, 2:232–33.

135. Ibid., 233.

136. Kleiman, "'Stekliannyi dom' S. M. Eizenshteina," 95.

137. Bordwell also notes this juxtaposition (*The Cinema of Eisenstein*, 82).

138. Such decanters, with four different chambers for four different wines, date back to the eighteenth century. The Museum of Applied and Folk Art (DPI) in Moscow has in its collection a similar object, made at the imperial glassworks: a late eighteenth-century carafe with four compartments, monogrammed, with gold design on clear glass with milky-white Venetian thread depicting musical instruments on the sides.

139. Bordwell, *The Cinema of Eisenstein*, 85.

140. Referring to the film's "Gods" sequence, Herbert Eagle characterizes this type of montage as a technique of "narration through *things*." Herbert Eagle, "Visual Patterning, Vertical Montage, and Ideological Protest: Eisenstein's Stylistic Legacy to East European Filmmakers," in *Eisenstein at 100: A Reconsideration*, ed. Al LaValley and Barry Scherr (New Brunswick, N.J.: Rutgers University Press, 2001), 177.

141. Cited in Nikita Lary, "Viktor Shklovsky: The Good and Awkward

Friend," in LaValley and Scherr, *Eisenstein at 100*, 124; original in "Konets barokko," *Literaturnaia gazeta* 32 (July 17, 1932).

142. Yury Tsivian, "Ivan the Terrible: Eisenstein's Rules of Reading," in La Valley and Scherr, *Eisenstein at 100*, 284.

143. Bordwell characterizes the conflict within *October* as framed in terms of stasis (that of statues and other still visual images) versus motion (*The Cinema of Eisenstein*, 93–94).

144. Already in *Strike* a similar effect can be seen in the repeated shots of lavish wineglasses; this glittering stemware is associated with the forces hostile to the strike.

145. Kleiman sees this building as standing in opposition to "the glass skyscraper of solitary souls (*odinochek*)" ("'Stekliannyi dom' S. M. Eizenshteina," 106).

146. Bulgakowa, *Sergei Eisenstein*, 68.

147. Sergei Eisenstein, *Selected Works*, vol. 4, *Beyond the Stars: The Memoirs*, ed. Richard Taylor, trans. William Powell (London: BFI, 1995), 138–39 (translation slightly revised); original cited in Viktor Shklovskii, *Eizenshtein* (Moscow: Iskusstvo, 1973), 62.

CHAPTER SIX

1. Popov, "Novaia Moskva—ne muzei stariny," 50.

2. Kopp, *Town and Revolution*, 192.

3. Blair A. Ruble, "Moscow's Revolutionary Architecture and Its Aftermath: A Critical Guide," in *Reshaping Russian Architecture*, ed. Brumfeld, 134.

4. In his 1923 book *Towards an Architecture*, Le Corbusier wrote: "a house is a machine for living in [*machine a habiter*]."

5. Cited in Jean-Louis Cohen, *Le Corbusier and the Mystique of the USSR: Theories and Projects for Moscow, 1928–1936* (Princeton, N.J.: Princeton University Press, 1992), 96.

6. S. N. Kozhin, "Oshibki zamysla," *Arkhitektura SSSR* 2, no. 12 (1934): 9 (emphasis added). See also D. Arkin, "Dom na ulitse Kirova," *Arkhitektura SSSR* 10 (1936): 34.

7. E. Kriger, qtd. in Papernyi, *Kul'tura "Dva,"* 161.

8. See M. Gor'kii, "Pozhary," in *Sobranie sochinenii v tridtsati tomakh* (Moscow: Gosudarstvennoe izdatel'stvo khudozhestvennoi literatury, 1951), 15:143–44. Gor'kii dates the story to 1922.

9. In 1783, the chemist and designer Aimé Argand was the first to encase the flame of a lamp in a glass cylinder. See Schivelbusch, *Disenchanted Night*, 12.

10. Although I consider the evolution of light imagery over several decades, my main goal is not to establish causality; I am primarily interested in tracing the

manifestations of the discourse concerning light in written and visual sources as well as exploring the creation of the light-producing objects that themselves generated such discourses. For a broader historical framework within which to view the evolution of light imagery discussed in this chapter, as well as a compelling approach to the interpretation of visual propaganda, see Victoria Bonnell, *The Iconography of Power: Soviet Political Posters under Lenin and Stalin* (Berkeley: University of California Press, 1997).

11. Wortman, *Scenarios of Power* 1:3.

12. For example, see James von Geldern, *Bolshevik Festivals, 1917–1920* (Berkeley: University of California Press, 1993); and Karen Petrone, *Life Has Become More Joyous, Comrades: Celebrations in the Time of Stalin* (Bloomington: University of Indiana Press, 2000). On the "performative culture" of the Stalin era, see Jeffrey Brooks, *Thank You, Comrade Stalin! Soviet Public Culture from Revolution to Cold War* (Princeton, N.J.: Princeton University Press, 2001).

13. Richard Stites, "The Origins of Soviet Ritual Style," in *Symbols of Power: The Esthetics of Political Legitimation in the Soviet Union and Eastern Europe*, ed. Claes Arvidsson and Lars Erik Blomquist (Stockholm: Almqvist & Wiksell International, 1987).

14. For an insightful discussion of the practical as well as the symbolic significance of the electrification campaign and the proliferation of "lampochki Il'icha," see Emma Widdis, *Visions of a New Land: Soviet Film from the Revolution to the Second World War* (New Haven, Conn.: Yale University Press, 2003), 22–27.

15. The Church of the Annunciation and the Church of the Savior in the Wood—the oldest church in Moscow—were destroyed in 1932 and 1933, respectively. Both were located in the Kremlin. The Cathedral of Christ the Savior, situated half a kilometer from the Kremlin, was destroyed in 1931. See Colton, *Moscow*, 260–62 and 268.

16. Constructivist architects drew an explicit connection between glass and good health in the article "Steklo v sovremennoi arkhitekture," *Sovremennaia arkhitektura* 3 (1926): 63.

17. See the essay "Lenin's Light Bulb" by Diane P. Koenker, as well as the accompanying photograph of a peasant woman looking on as electric light is installed in her hut, in Peter Fritzsche and Charles Stewart, eds., *Imagining the Twentieth Century* (Urbana: University of Illinois Press, 1997), 30. I should note that we are now seeing another wave of excitement around incandescent bulbs as they are poised to be swept aside by LED lighting. See Dan Koeppel, "Let There Be Light," *Wired* (September 2011): 110–19.

18. For a more detailed discussion of light imagery in the service of the young Soviet state, see my article "Light in Captivity: Spectacular Glass and Soviet Power in the 1920s and 1930s," *Slavic Review* 66, no. 1 (Spring 2007): 82–105.

19. "Over a bright and free world . . . the Red Army star shines with an international light. Its inextinguishable rays show scarlet through the fog, and the workers of the world walk toward it as pilgrims once did." See Ivan Esaulov, "Sotsrealizm i religioznoe soznanie," in *Sotsrealisticheskii kanon*, ed. Hans Günther and Evgeny Dobrenko (St. Petersburg: Akademicheskiĭ Proekt, 2000), 51.

20. The poster is reproduced in White, *The Bolshevik Poster*, 48 (plate 3.10). I am grateful to John Malmstad for bringing this poster to my attention.

21. See Olga Velikanova, *Making of an Idol: On Uses of Lenin* (Göttingen: Muster-Schmidt, 1996), 104.

22. Here I am following Nina Tumarkin's definition of the Lenin cult as the organized system of veneration around the leader. See Nina Tumarkin, *Lenin Lives! The Lenin Cult in Soviet Russia* (Cambridge, Mass.: Harvard University Press, 1983), 80–87.

23. Cited in Andrei Kotyrev, *Mavzolei V. I. Lenina: Proektirovanie i stroitel'stvo* (Moscow: Sovetskii khudozhnik, 1971), 18. The words of the Soviet state anthem (1944) continue the Lenin-as-light motif: "The sun of freedom shone to us through the storms, and great Lenin lit the way for us."

24. Indeed, the sun was a sacred symbol for the Russian peasantry. The popularity of the sun as a visual motif in Russian peasant art can help to explain why this association was propagated in images of Lenin meant to appeal to large sectors of the Russian population. On the centrality of the sun in peasant artwork, see Anthony Netting, "Images and Ideas in Russian Peasant Art," *Slavic Review* 35, no. 1 (March 1976): 53–54.

25. In 1875 the Russian inventor Pavel Yablochkov created the glass-encased arc light known as the "Yablochkov candle"; he patented it in Paris in the same year, and demonstrated his universal lighting system in England—at, among other venues, a sports stadium where fans watched the first soccer match played at night—and at the Universal Exhibition in Paris in 1878. Companies using the system were set up in France, England, and the United States. However, as Loren Graham recounts, Yablochkov was unable to duplicate his success when he returned to Russia, and "the major cities of the Russian Empire were eventually electrified by foreigners." See Loren Graham, "The Fits and Starts of Russian and Soviet Technology," in *Technology, Culture, and Development: The Experience of the Soviet Model*, ed. James P. Scanlan (Armonk, N.Y.: M. E. Sharpe, 1992). See also John A. Jakle, *City Lights: Illuminating the American Night* (Baltimore: Johns Hopkins University Press, 2001), 39–40; and the illustration in Maurice Déribéré, *Préhistoire et histoire de la lumière* (Paris: France-Empire, 1979), 257.

26. In his writings, Lenin argued that the wholesale electrification of Russia was the crucial step in creating an industrial base for the new socialist society, as well as in overhauling the agricultural system. See I. P. Verkhovtsev, ed., *Svet*

nad Rossiei: Ocherki po istorii elektrifikatsii SSSR (Moscow: Gosudarstvennoe izdatel'stvo politicheskoi literatury, 1960), 6–7.

27. Stites, *Revolutionary Dreams*, 48–49.

28. Jean Starobinski, *1789: The Emblems of Reason*, trans. Barbara Bray (Cambridge, Mass.: MIT Press, 1988), 58. Martin Jay discusses the "solar myth" of the French revolution in *Downcast Eyes: The Denigration of Vision in Twentieth-Century French Thought* (Berkeley: University of California Press, 1993), 94.

29. Verkhovtsev, ed., *Svet nad Rossiei*, 310. On November 14, 1955, the front page of *Leningradskaia pravda* reported that the village of Kashino was celebrating the thirty-fifth anniversary of Lenin's visit and referred to Kashino as "the birthplace of 'Lenin's little lamp.'" "Tam, gde vpervye zazhglas' 'lampochka Il'icha,'" *Leningradskaia pravda*, November 14, 1955. See also V. Iu. Steklov, *V. I. Lenin i elektrifikatsiia* (Moscow: Nauka, 1975), 226–29.

30. As Mumford observes: "The glass hothouse . . . lengthened the growing period of Northern Europe, increased, so to say, the climatic range of a region, and utilized solar energy which would otherwise have been wasted . . . Even more important for industry, glass lengthened the span of the working day in cold or in inclement weather, particularly in the northern regions" (*Technics and Civilization*, 125).

31. M. Isakovskii, "Vdol' derevni," in *Poet sovetskaia strana*, comp. I. A. Shvedov (Moscow: Moskovskii rabochii, 1962), 97. Isakovskii's frequent collaborator V. Zakharov set the poem to music. I am grateful to Valery and Larisa Bekman for bringing this song to my attention.

32. Quoted in Pavel Belitskii, "Poet, vernuvshii pesniu: K 100-letiiu Mikhaila Isakovskogo," *Nezavisimaia gazeta* no. 8, January 19, 2000.

33. GUM is the State Department Store (Gosudarstvennyi Univermag). The original text reads: "Дайте солнце ночью! Где найдёшь его? Покупай в ГУМе—ослепительно и дёшево." The poster is reproduced in Selim O. Khan-Magomedov, *Rodchenko: The Complete Work*, intro. and ed. Vieri Quilici (Cambridge, Mass.: MIT Press, 1987), 149.

34. Quoted in Frank J. Miller, *Folklore for Stalin: Russian Folklore and Pseudofolklore of the Stalin Era* (Armonk, N.Y.: M. E. Sharpe, 1990), 164. I am grateful to Polina Rikoun for this reference.

35. See Bonnell, *The Iconography of Power*, 120.

36. Stalin came to appropriate the luminous aspect (among others) of the Lenin cult. Starting in the late 1920s, literature and particularly folklore praised Stalin in metaphorical language that invoked light or the sun. See Jan Plamper, "The Spatial Poetics of the Personality Cult: Circles around Stalin," in *The Landscape of Stalinism: The Art and Ideology of Soviet Space*, ed. Evgeny Dobrenko and Eric Naiman (Seattle: University of Washington Press, 2003), 25–27.

37. The fact that the smaller, darker profile of Stalin is placed inside the larger, lighter profile of Lenin may have been an additional cause for concern.

38. Alexander Zakharov, "Mass Celebrations in a Totalitarian System," in *Tekstura: Russian Essays on Visual Culture*, ed. and trans. Alla Efimova and Lev Manovich (Chicago: University of Chicago Press, 1993), 210.

39. "'Lenin's little lamp' is a phrase that has spread throughout the country and has become an expression of the people's gratitude to their great leader for his tireless energy in reconstructing the entire national economy on the basis of electrification and for his concern for the people's well-being." Verkhovtsev, *Svet nad Rossiei*, 310.

40. Mikhail Zoshchenko, "Elektrifikatsiia," in *Uvazhaemye grazhdane*, ed. M. Z. Dolinskii (Moscow: Knizhnaia palata, 1991), 221; originally published in *Krasnyi voron*, no. 17 (1924).

41. The landlady cuts the wires only in her own room and insists on living in darkness and filth "as before"; in case any ambiguity remains, a character not present in the first version calls her a "degenerate petite bourgeois." Mikhail Zoshchenko, "Bednost'," in *Rasskazy, fel'etony, povesti* (Moscow: Gosudarstvennoe izdatel'stvo khudozhestvennoi literatury, 1958), 29.

42. Gaston Bachelard, *La flamme d'une chandelle* (Paris, 1961) 3; cited in Schivelbusch, *Disenchanted Night*, 29.

43. See Mikhail Zoshchenko, "Malen'kaia khitrost'," in *Povesti i rasskazy* (New York: Izdatel'stvo imeni Chekhova, 1952), 319–20.

44. *Moskovskii bolshevik*, April 9, 1948, cited in Verkhovtsev, ed., *Svet nad Rossiei*, 311.

45. In a still later edition (1965) it received the neutral title "Lenin's Little Lamp." These dates are cited in Thomas Seifrid, *Andrei Platonov: Uncertainties of Spirit* (Cambridge, Eng.: Cambridge University Press, 1992).

46. Andrei Platonov, "O potukhshei lampochke Il'icha," in *Sobranie sochinenii v piati tomakh* (Moscow: Informpechat', 1998), 1:327. Subsequent references are in the text.

47. Reproduced in B. S. Butnik-Siverskii, *Sovetskii plakat epokhi grazhdanskoi voiny, 1918–1921* (Moscow: Izdatel'stvo Vsesoiuznoi knizhnoi palaty, 1960), 685.

48. For broader discussions of light and optical imagery in Olesha, see Elizabeth Klosty Beaujour, *The Invisible Land: A Study of the Artistic Imagination of Iurii Olesha* (New York: Columbia University Press, 1970); Marietta Chudakova, *Masterstvo Iuriia Oleshi* (Moscow: Nauka, 1972); Kazimiera Ingdahl, *The Artist and the Creative Act: A Study of Jurij Oleša's Novel "Zavist'"* (Stockholm: University of Stockholm Press, 1984); and Nils Ake Nilsson, "Through the Wrong End of Binoculars: An Introduction to Jurij Olesha," *Scando-Slavica* 11 (1965): 40–68.

49. Yury Olesha, *Envy*, in *The Portable Twentieth-Century Russian Reader*,

ed. Clarence Brown (New York: Viking,, 1985), 251. For the original, see Iu. K. Olesha, "Zavist'," in *Ni dnia bez strochki*, 4. Subsequent references to this source will be in the text.

50. The notion of Kavalerov's conflict with the "men of action" is developed by Janet G. Tucker in *Revolution Betrayed: Jurij Olesa's "Envy"* (Columbus, Ohio: Slavica, 1996).

51. Not only is this a central image in *Envy*, but the image also appears literally at the center of the book—Olesha places it roughly halfway through the novel.

52. Olesha, *Envy*, 326. This translation has been revised. For the original, see Olesha, *Zavist'*, 64.

53. During the interrogation sequence, Ivan uses such phrases as "peaceful revolt," "peaceful demonstration of feelings," and, in a draft, "shock troop of feelings." As Ingdahl points out, such expressions "parody the code of the Revolution." Ingdahl, *Artist and the Creative Act*, 84. This suggests that there are other potentially parodic moments in the interrogation sequence.

54. Writing of his visit to Moscow during the period of the NEP, Walter Benjamin mentions the hourly power outages and the flickering light of Soviet lamps. See Benjamin, "Moscow," in *Reflections: Essays, Aphorisms, Autobiographical Writings*, trans. Edmund Jephcott (New York: Schocken, 1978), 110.

55. Velikanova's statistics illustrate the remarkable growth of the Lenin cult in publishing in the years when Olesha was working on the novel, especially 1924–25 (*Making of an Idol*, 156–57).

56. As Eliot Borenstein argues, Olesha "not only understood his culture's code, but offered the novel as a complex parody of it." See "Defying Interpretation: Allegory and Ideology in Jurij Oleša's *Envy*," *Russian Literature* 49 (2001): 25.

57. In this novel structured by oppositions, the burned-out bulb appears as a counter-image to the hundred-watt bulb, a garish emblem of the technological and aesthetic triumph of the new world that illuminates Andrei and his cronies as they feast on his brand-new sausage. Olesha, *Zavist'*, 23.

58. The street mirror appears at the end of part 1. Ivan's lightbulb is just as central an image—it appears on the other side of the looking glass, at the beginning of part 2.

59. Olesha, *Zavist*, 49.

60. The revitalization of the surrounding world—everything "repeats itself with all the three-dimensionality and brilliancy conveyed only via the wrong end of the binoculars"—also suggests stepping back in time: the street mirror as fountain of youth.

61. Other mirror imagery in Olesha's novel is distressing with respect to Kavalerov and other representatives of the old world, with one exception: the widow's bed with mirrored arcs in the headboard and footboard. As it is being

transported to her home, the arcs reflect the blue sky and resemble beautiful blue eyes opening and closing (Zavist', 75)—a lovely, tranquil image (Nabokov paid tribute to it in *The Gift*); here the bed-mirror also functions as a *street mirror* since it is reflecting the dynamic outside world.

62. Edison took out the first patent for a working lightbulb in 1879. Other inventors, such as Sir Joseph William Swan, came up with similar devices, but Edison was the one to elaborate an entire infrastructure of power lines and other equipment to make electrical lighting practical. Thus he is generally recognized as the inventor who brought the lightbulb into being.

63. Cited in Igor Sukhikh, "Ostaetsia tol'ko metafora . . . 1927: 'Zavist' Iurii Oleshi," *Zvezda* 10 (2002): 224 (emphasis added).

64. The final light source in Olesha's novel—wielded by the widow Propokovich—is a wood splinter (*luchina*), a traditional torch for peasant huts that the electric bulb was meant to drive out; hence the agitprop slogan: "We used to have the splinter and the candle, but now we'll have Lenin's lamp" (Была лучина и свеча, а теперь будет лампа Ильича). Cited in V. M. Mokienko, *Tolkovyi slovar' iazyka Sovdepii* (St. Petersburg: Folio-press, 1998), 307.

65. Iurii Olesha, "Zagovor chuvstv," in *P'esy: Stat'i o teatre i dramaturgii* (Moscow: Iskusstvo, 1968), 83.

66. Olesha, "Avtor o svoei p'ese," in *P'esy*, 261.

67. M. A. Topolin, *Kremlevskie zvezdy* (Moscow: Moskovskii rabochii, 1975), 40.

68. Ibid., 42.

69. The following account is based on coverage in *Pravda*, October 10, 11, 18, 19, 23, 24, 25, 26, 27, and 28, 1935; and Topolin, *Kremlevskie zvezdy*, 16–22.

70. The red star became the official emblem of the Red Army in April 1918 and was made into a badge to be worn on the breast; in July of that year, the new constitution incorporated the red star into the state coat of arms, and by the end of the year the star was made part of the Soviet flag. See Stites, "Origins of Soviet Ritual Style"; and Maria Gough, "Switched On: Notes on Radio, Automata, and the Bright Red Star," in *Building the Collective: Soviet Graphic Design 1917–1937*, ed. Leah Dickerman (New York: Princeton Architectural Press, 1996), 40. On the red star as symbol, see V. V. Pokhlebkin, *Slovar' mezhdunarodnoi simvoliki i emblematiki* (Moscow, 1994), 209–11.

71. In July 1935, Stalin publicized his Plan for the Reconstruction of Moscow. The decree to make the first set of stars was issued just a few months later. See the remarkable album with commentary by Viktor Shklovskii, *Moskva rekonstruiruetsia: Al'bom diagram, toposkhem i fotografii po rekonstruktsii gor. Moskvy* (Moscow: In-t izobrazitel'noii statistiki sov. stroitel'stva i khoziiaistva TSUNKhU gosplana SSSR, 1938).

72. Topolin, *Kremlevskie zvezdy*, 18.

73. The stars measured 16 feet across and weighed an average of 3,300 pounds. A photograph in *Pravda*, October 12, 1935, p. 6, shows a worker dwarfed by one of the stars.

74. The remaining three stars were raised over the next three days.

75. Topolin, *Kremlevskie zvezdy*, 23.

76. The Mechanical Engineering Research Institute in Moscow was given two months to manufacture five new stars of a "size and shape in accordance with [the wishes of] the commandant's office in the Kremlin." V. N. Iashanova, "Kremlevskie zvezdy 1937 g.," *Otechestvennye arkhivy*, no. 4 (1997): 77. The Konstantinovskii glass factory in Donbass was charged with making the special ruby-red glass for the stars, and more than a dozen other organizations took part in their creation. See Topolin, *Kremlevskie zvezdy*, 28.

77. The information in this paragraph is from *Pravda*, September 29–30 and October 4, 5, 9, 16, and 23, 1937; and Topolin, *Kremlevskie zvezdy*, 23–33.

78. The stars were red on the outside and white on the inside; without the white glass, the red glass would have appeared black in the daytime.

79. Brooks points out the prevalence of the "cleansing" metaphor in official discourse at the height of the Great Purge (*Thank You, Comrade Stalin!*, 142–43). The purges provide an important context in which to view the Kremlin stars. In 1937 Soviet citizens were commanded to look *up*, to marvel at the exploits of Soviet aviators and dirigible pilots, rather than look *around* to see what was happening. In fact, the back page of *Pravda* on October 4, 1937 features an article with the headline "Stars on the Kremlin Towers" next to a photograph of the dirigible SSSR-6 and its pilot.

80. The interior of each tower had to be rebuilt to make room for this equipment, and the rickety old *shater* roof of the Nikolskaya tower was replaced with a new, metal one. *Pravda*, September 29, 1937, 3.

81. The remaining stars were raised on October 4, 9, 14, and 23, 1937. A typical headline announced: "Ruby Stars Blaze over the Kremlin." *Pravda*, October 5, 1937.

82. Three years later, Viktor Govorkov created a poster, "Stalin in the Kremlin Cares about Every One of Us," depicting the leader surrounded by light sources—flanked by his ornate table lamp on one side and a bright Kremlin star on the other—and appearing in association with them as another source of light.

83. The description in the epigraph to this chapter is typical.

84. Arnold Whittick, *Symbols, Signs and Their Meaning and Uses in Design*, 2nd ed. (London: Leonard Hill, 1971), 132–33, cited in Christel Lane, *The Rites of Rulers: Ritual in Industrial Society—The Soviet Case* (Cambridge, Eng.: Cambridge University Press, 1981), 199.

85. Lane describes a "lit-up globe rotating in the sky with Lenin's name above it" used at a political demonstration, and comments: "The propensity to

project lit-up objects or names into the sky must be seen as an effort to achieve permanence, to become like one of the timeless stars of the sky" (*The Rites of Rulers*, 199–200).

86. In her long poem *Requiem* (1935–40), Anna Akhmatova makes her own use of the Bible, associating the Kremlin star with the star Wormwood from the Book of Revelations. It now presages, not the coming of a messiah, but the apocalypse. See Anna Akhmatova, *Sochineniia*, 2nd ed. (Munich: Mezhdunarodnoe literaturnoe sodruzhestvo, 1967), 1:363 and 365.

87. "Всё ярче и краше / сверкает она." A. Kovalenkov, "Zvezda," *Pravda*, October 2, 1937.

88. The English text is cited from the King James Version; the Russian is from the Synodal version. The word *goret'* can mean both to burn like a fire and to blaze like a light.

89. "The Star" was the first of numerous songs and poems that presented the Kremlin stars as visible from anywhere on the globe. For details, see my "Light in Captivity."

90. The fact that this letter comes from abroad also underscores the idea that the Soviets have the support of socialist brethren around the world.

91. "Nam svetiat zvezdy Kremlia," *Pravda*, November 6, 1937. On the metaphor of the "path" in the 1920s and 1930s, see Brooks, *Thank You, Comrade Stalin!*, 136.

92. A poem by Aleksandr Zharov that appeared in *Pravda* on September 15, 1937, two weeks before the announcement of the new glass stars, ends with the lines "Guided by our stars, people everywhere now seek the road to joy and happiness."

93. Vladimir Murav'ev, comp., *S zemli do zvezd vstaet Moskva: Moskva v sovetskoi poezii* (Moscow: Moskovskii rabochii, 1989), 164.

94. "Tvortsy kremlevskogo sozvezdiia," in *Na krasnoi ploshchadi u mavzoleia: Sbornik*, ed. M. N. Alekseev et al. (Moscow: Sovetskaia Rossiia, 1972), 80. The article reports that on the factory's hundred-year anniversary, one of the old master glassworkers was asked to fill out a questionnaire; in reply to a question about the "path" that he had traveled in his career, he answered, "From church icon-lamps to the Kremlin stars" (ibid).

95. One such illumination, featuring an allegorical scene that celebrated Russia's military might, is described in chapter 2 above; the image is reproduced in Asharina, "Russkoe khudozhestvennoe steklo," 86. In 1918, the Red Army distributed leaflets to explain the symbolic meaning of its new emblem, the red star. See Tumarkin, *Lenin Lives!*, 70–72.

96. See her essay "Sotsrealism i sacralizatsiia prostranstva" in *Sotsrealisticheskii kanon*, ed. Hans Gunther and Evgeny Dobrenko (St. Petersburg: Akademicheskii proekt, 2000).

97. Cited in Greg Castillo, "Stalinist Modern: Constructivism and the Soviet

Company Town," in *Architectures of Russian Identity: 1500 to the Present*, ed. James Cracraft and Daniel B. Rowland (Ithaca, N.Y.: Cornell University Press, 2003), 138.

98. See Hugh Hudson, Jr., *Blueprints and Blood: The Stalinization of Soviet Architecture, 1917–1937* (Princeton, N.J.: Princeton University Press, 1994).

99. I am grateful to David Brandenberger for suggesting this idea to me.

100. Papernyi analyzes the spires atop the Palace of Soviets and its surrogates as an embodiment of the hierarchical nature of Stalinist culture (*Kul'tura "Dva,"* 125–26).

101. Qtd. in Alexei Tarkhanov and Sergei Kavtaradze, *Architecture of the Stalin Era* (New York: Rizzoli International, 1992), 132.

102. See Papernyi, *Kul'tura "Dva,"* 126; and Tarkhanov and Kavtaradze, *Architecture of the Stalin Era*, 141.

103. See Beaujour, "Architectual Discourse and Early Soviet Literature," 494.

104. Bowlt, "The Presence of Absence," 21–22.

105. Construction on the MGU building began in 1949 and concluded in 1953. It remained the tallest building in Europe until 1988.

106. The builders of MGU turned to glass when seeking an economical alternative to covering the spire with gold. A special golden-yellow glass was manufactured (the color resulted from the addition of carbon to the molten glass). Pulverized aluminum was applied to the reverse side of the glass. Rectangular plates of the glass were then affixed to the metal spire. (Levinson et al., *Khudozhestvennoe steklo*, 167).

107. Dmitrii Semenov, "Pervyi sovetskii neboskreb," *Moskovskaia Pravda*, May 18, 1991, 3.

108. Papernyi documents: "As every Muscovite knew, centers of anti-aircraft defense were located inside [the Moscow high-rises]. These . . . 'monuments of contemporary architecture' were also pedestals, but not for the figure of the leader, as in the case of the Palace of Soviets, but for the all-seeing eye of defense" (*Kul'tura "Dva,"* 310). The Kremlin stars, as emblems of the Red Army, would also serve as perpetual reminders of war, the empire thus always in a state of martial readiness, even in peacetime.

109. Dmitrii Semenov, "Etazhi so znakom minus," *Moskovskaia Pravda*, October 12, 1991, 1.

110. Ibid.

111. Boris Iofan's original 1948 design for the MGU featured, in place of a spire, the figure of Lenin "with disproportionately long legs (so that he would look normal from the ground), arms tensed, purposefully striding off somewhere," as Semenov discovered when poring through the archives in 1991. Thus MGU would inherit the look of the Palace of Soviets, which Iofan likewise designed to be crowned with a gigantic figure of Lenin, as seen in a photograph of an architectural model of MGU from 1949 (Semenov, "Etazhi so znakom," 3).

112. Just before the 1980 Olympics, the university made an attempt to spruce up the spire, but the results were less than stellar. The MGU administration hired freelance steeplejacks to attach new orange glass to the top of the spire. Unfortunately, the new glass panes soon fell out as well (Semenov, "Pervyi sovetskii neboskreb," 3).

113. G. V. Pototskaia, *Kontrol' produktsii na zavodakh tekhnicheskogo stekla* (Moscow: Promstroiizdat, 1953), 11.

114. Two decades later a book on Soviet construction materials made the hyperbolic claim that Soviet scientists had invented a glass whose durability exceeded that of steel. A. S. Boldyrev, ed., "Stekol'naia promyshlennost'," in *Promyshlennost' stroitel'nykh materialov SSSR 1917–1967* (Moscow: Izdatel'stvo literatury po stroitel'stvu, 1967), 245.

115. The references, all from 2005, are from the *New York Times*, October 5 (Poltavchenko, Mikhalkov, Novodvorskaia, Orlova) and *ANSA News*, October 12 (Ziuganov).

116. Starr, *Melnikov*, 81.

117. Nina Tumarkin, *Lenin Lives!*, 179.

118. Boris Malkiel', "To, o chem nikogda ne zabyt'," *Pravda*, January 27, 1924, 3.

119. For discussions of possible conceptual sources for the Lenin mausoleum, see Alexander A. Panchenko, "The Cult of Lenin and 'Soviet Folklore,'" *FOLKLORICA: Journal of the Slavic and East European Folklore Association* 10, no. 1 (2005): 28–29; and Stites, *Revolutionary Dreams*, 120.

120. Tumarkin, *Lenin Lives!*, 186.

121. Cited ibid., 173.

122. Cited in Zbarskii, *Mavzolei Lenina* (Leningrad: Gosudarstvennoe izdatel'stvo politicheskoi literatury, 1946), 22. For a challenge to the Soviet historiography, see Velikanova (*Making of an Idol*, 58 and 67), who argues that the decision to embalm and display Lenin had been made before any "proposals 'from below.'"

123. Zbarskii, *Mavzolei Lenina*, 25.

124. Ibid., 46.

125. In the days following Lenin's death, the Burial Commission debated methods of preserving his body. For details, see my essay "From Lenin's Tomb to Avtovo Station: Illusion and Spectacle in Soviet Subterranean Space," in *Rites of Place: Public Commemoration in Russia and Eastern Europe*, ed. Julie Buckler and Emily Johnson (Evanston, Ill.: Northwestern University Press), 2013.

126. Cited by Walter Duranty, "Lenin Is Lifelike as He Lies in Tomb," *New York Times*, August 4, 1924, 1.

127. These ideas appear in Tumarkin, *Lenin Lives!*; and Panchenko, "The Cult of Lenin," respectively.

128. Duranty, "Lenin Is Lifelike."

129. Qtd. in Iurii Koginov, *Almaznaia gran': Dokumental'naia povest'* (Moscow: Profizdat, 1977), 149. Lenin's exclamation in the original reads as follows: "Ого, вот бы нытиков эстетов сюда, полюбоваться этими чудесными вещицами!"

130. Katerina Clark, "Sotsrealism i sacralizatsiia prostranstva," 126.

131. Nikolai Bukharin, "Tovarishch," *Pravda*, January 24, 1924, 1.

132. In his poem "Vladimir Il'ich" (1920), Mayakovsky praises Lenin as "the brains" behind the Revolution: "The wail of the war was building when Lenin's gigantic head appeared, towering over the world." The poem ends with the prescient image of the sky strewn with red stars, although here it is still just a metaphor: "the sky of the immeasurable Workers' and Peasants' Party is covered with five-pointed stars."

133. Starr, *Melnikov*, 81.

134. S. O. Khan-Magomedov, *Mavzolei Lenina: Istoriia sozdaniia i arkhitektura* (Moscow: Prosveshchenie, 1972), 57. The sarcophagus ended up as a simpler cone-shaped pyramid.

135. Starr, *Melnikov*, 249.

136. Ibid., 202.

137. Kotyrev, *Mavzolei V. I. Lenina*, 137–38.

138. A. Abramov, *Mavzolei Lenina* (Moscow: Moskovskii rabochii, 1963), 50.

139. Andrei Voznesenskii, "Lonzhiumo," in *Lenin v sovetskoi poezii*, ed. P. B. Val'be (Leningrad: Sovetskii pisatel', 1970), 665. The poem originally appeared in *Pravda*, October 13, 1963.

140. Abramov, *Mavzolei Lenina*, 60.

141. See I. B. Zbarskii, "Ot Rossii do Rossii," in *Pod "kryshei" mavzoleia*, comp. E. E. Zaitseva (Tver': Polina, 1998), 236.

142. Another example of behind-the-scenes glass in the mausoleum are the banners decorating the walls, made of the blood-red glass known as purpurine, whose closely guarded recipe was invented by a jeweler in the employ of Carl Faberge, an artisan named Petukhov. See Henry Charles Bainbridge, *Peter Carl Faberge: His Life and Work* (New York: B. T. Batsford, 1949), 54.

143. See ""Protestuia ot imeni millionov trudiashchikhsia SSSR, krest'ianin Nikitin vystrelil v sarkofag s telom Lenina, a zatem ubil sebia," *Fakty i kommentarii*, October 22, 1999, http://www.facts.kiev.ua/oct99/2210/10.htm.

144. Kotyrev, *Mavzolei V. I. Lenina*, 137–38.

145. Zbarskii, *Mavzolei Lenina*, 46.

146. Another potential inspiration for Lenin's glass coffin can be found in a 1910 dystopian novel by H. G. Wells (who was widely read in Russia), *When the Sleeper Awakes*, which features a protagonist who falls into a trance; as he lies for centuries inside "a case of thin glass," politically motivated myths arise that designate him a savior who will liberate the people upon awakening. See Wells, *When the Sleeper Awakes: A Critical Text of the 1899 New York and London*

First Edition, ed. Leon Stover (Jefferson, N.C.: McFarland, 2000), 78. Zamyatin, who greatly admired Wells, would have taken note of the glass dome that covers the future city in this novel.

147. Reports from the OKARTU (Okrug Artillery School) (undated), cited in Velikanova, *Making of an Idol*, 97n17.

148. Starr, *Melnikov*, 81.

149. Ibid., 249. In the Grimms' "Glass Coffin" tale, the sleeping beauty lies in a glass coffin *and* in a subterranean setting. Her rescuer steps on a magical stone that transports him underground, to a spacious hall, where he finds "a maiden of the greatest beauty" lying as if asleep in a glass chest. "Her eyes were closely shut, but the brightness of her complexion . . . left no doubt that she was alive." According to Panchenko ("The Cult of Lenin," 27) the tale of "Sleeping Beauty" was "hugely popular in nineteenth- and twentieth-century Russian culture thanks to Pushkin's verse rendering, the translation of Perrault's fairy tales, [and] Tchaikovsky's ballet."

150. "Земная лежит оболочка, / Как в сказке, / В стеклянном гробу."

151. See Vitaly Komar and Alexander Melamid, "We Remember, or So It Seems," in *Monumental Propaganda*, ed. Dore Ashton (New York: Independent Curators International, 1995), 45–47.

152. In this connection, see Panchenko ("The Cult of Lenin," 29): "It is possible that the rhetoric of Lenin, which had already taken shape by the mid-1920s and presented the leader as an immortal and omnipresent being . . . did not seem, to many people, consonant with the material presence of the 'eternally alive' leader's mummified corpse on display in a glass coffin."

153. Olesha, *Zavist'*, 21. Mikhail Vaiskopf also sees this glass cube as a "veiled, but still easily reconstructed motif of the mausoleum" (although he does not discuss the glass sarcophagus itself). See "Andrei Babichev i ego proobraz v 'Zavisti' Iuriia Oleshi," *Izvestiia Akademii Nauk, Seriia Literatury i Iazyka* 53, no. 5 (1994): 73.

154. *Novyi mir*, no. 11, 1925, cited in Panchenko, "The Cult of Lenin," 24.

155. Ibid. 32. Panchenko suggests that the plot of "Sly Lenin" may have been "based upon rumors actually circulating among the peasants immediately after Lenin's death." A rural correspondent reported that "there exists a legend among the peasants . . . that Lenin is alive and walking the earth incognito, observing the work of Soviet authorities" ("The Cult of Lenin," 27). The important thing is this image/myth was put into popular circulation even if it came from above, not from below.

156. Tumarkin, *Lenin Lives!*, 198.

157. I. B. Zbarsky and Samuel Hutchinson, *Lenin's Embalmers*, trans. Barbara Bray (London: Harvill, 1999), 93–94.

158. I. B. Zbarskii, "'Zhizn'' mumii i sud'ba cheloveka: Iz vospominanii khranitelia tela Lenina," *Otechestvennaia istoriia* 5 (1993): 160.

159. This information comes from a memorandum marked "Secret" from the U.S.S.R. Minister of Health S. Kurashov to the Central Committee of the Communist Party, dated July 16, 1960. Reproduced in *Neizvestnaia Rossiia XX vek*, ed. V. A. Kozlov, vol. 4 (Moscow: Istoricheskoe nasledie, 1993), 465.

160. See I. B. Zbarskii, "Ot Rossii do Rossii," in *Pod "kryshei" mavzoleia*, comp. E. E. Zaitseva (Tver': Polina, 1998), 268–69; and Zbarsky and Hutchinson, *Lenin's Embalmers*.

161. Schivelbusch, *Disenchanted Night*, 98.

162. This claim also appears in travel guides from more recent times: see Pavel Kann, *Leningrad: A Guide* (Moscow: Planeta, 1990), 10.

163. Levinson et al., *Khudozhestvennoe steklo*, 138–39.

164. The information about the columns is from A. M. Baskakov, ed., *Metropoliten Leningrada-Peterburga: Stranitsy istorii* (St. Petersburg: Ivan Fedorov, 1995), 164. The station also contains a monumental mosaic of the very kind that Lomonosov, living in the same city, sought to make nearly 200 years earlier.

165. A book issued on the forty-year anniversary of the Leningrad metro claims: "When you are inside the metro station, you do not feel that you are deep underground" thanks to the ample electric light (Baskakov, *Metropoliten Leningrada-Peterburga*, 193).

166. Karen Kettering, "An Introduction to the Design of the Moscow Metro in the Stalin Period: 'The Happiness of Life Underground,'" *Studies in the Decorative Arts* 7, no. 2 (Spring/Summer 2000): 8–9.

167. Ibid.

168. Kettering writes with regard to the "*zhizneradost'*" that these subterranean spaces were meant to generate: "If such a sensation of joy could be created underground, the Metro interior would be yet another site demonstrating the widely propagandized ability of Soviet citizens to overcome and transform any natural force, be it darkness, damp, cold, or frozen earth" ("Introduction to the Design," 8).

169. Catherine Cooke, "Beauty as a Route to the 'Radiant Future': Responses of Soviet Architecture," *Journal of Design History* 10, no. 2 (1997): 147. An explicit association between brightness/light and glass can be seen in Platonov's story "Doubting Makar" (1929). Makar comes upon a construction site for an "eternal" building of the future; a worker tells him that it is made of "iron, concrete, steel, and bright glass [*svetloe steklo*]."

170. Cited in Schivelbusch, *Disenchanted Night*, 98.

171. I am grateful to Julie Buckler for this idea. A letter to the editor of *Leningradskaia Pravda* from November 15, under the title "One of the Greatest Monuments of the Epoch" characterized the "station-palaces" as a Soviet answer to the tsarist legacy: "In the days of the celebration [of the anniversary of the October Revolution] I examined the beautiful station-palaces along with thousands of my fellow Leningraders . . . In Leningrad there are many architectural

monuments. Most of them were created by the Russian architects of the past. The metro is one of the greatest monuments of our epoch."

172. This claim is echoed in A. M. Sokolov, *Stantsii Leningradskogo metro* (Leningrad: Gosudarstvennoe izdatel'stvo literatury po stroitel'stvu i arkhitekture, 1957), 24: "The necessary composition of glass was obtained with the help of specialists who ardently responded to the call of the metro builders. This glass is more durable than marble."

173. Andrew Jenks, "A Metro on the Mount: The Underground as a Church of Soviet Civilization," *Technology and Culture* 41, no. 4 (2000): 713.

174. Kachalov, *Steklo*, 358.

175. "During World War II, the front border of the defense of the besieged city was close to the current site of the Avtovo station. In the central hall of this station is a beautiful glass mosaic panel titled 'The Motherland,' and the façade of the vestibule features group bas-reliefs devoted to the theme of the war." Baskakov, *Metropoliten Leningrada-Peterburga*, 164.

176. See Susan Reid, "Destalinization and Taste, 1953–1963," *Journal of Design History* 10, no. 2 (1997): 177; and Cooke, "Beauty as a Route," 138.

177. Sokolov uses the same rhetoric of palaces and light in his discussion of the metro (*Stantsii Leningradskogo metro*, 20).

178. E. Simakova and V. Bobarykina, letter to *Leningradskaia Pravda*, November 15, 1955 (emphasis added). References to fairy tales, miracles, and magic were prevalent in the official rhetoric of the early Soviet period. A classic example is the song "Ever Higher," which opens with the line: "We are born to make fairy tales come true." Such rhetoric was meant to convey the idea that the Soviets had transformed humdrum life into a wondrous fairy tale. (In fact, the escalator in the metro was dubbed *lesenka-chudesenka*, "the magic staircase," a term that is still in use today.)

179. On the "obsession with palaces that came to dominate Soviet aesthetics," see Beaujour, "Architectual Discourse and Early Soviet Literature"; Beaujour cites a 1922 speech by Kirov that looks ahead to the construction of an "enchanted palace of workers and peasants" that will persuade observers in other lands "that we are here to stay" (488).

180. Cited in Baskakov, *Metropoliten Leningrada-Peterburga*, 22.

181. Another Leningrad station is praised for lighting that "creates the illusion of a fresh, brisk morning." A similarly laudatory reference to illusion can be found in a 1935 memoir of a Moscow metro builder: "The Komsomol station, with its luxuriant detail, took the passenger 'into a world of illusion and call[ed] forth feelings of being in a theater lobby"; cited in Jenks, "A Metro on the Mount," 713n37.

182. According to Kann, the design solution was found "with the aid of optical researchers . . . : facets on the inner surface of the glass slabs were cut at an angle of 80°. As a result the light reflected by the facets does not reach the con-

crete shafts [and] all the columns seem to be glass monoliths." The same team of artists created a gigantic crystal vase that was given to Stalin for his seventieth birthday in 1949; they speak with pride of successfully disguising the vase's metal skeleton through a combination of strategic faceting and well-placed mirrors (*Leningrad: A Guide*, 34–38, 42).

183. In this connection, see the discussion of the "'Socialist Realist' 'reality' within which Soviet citizens were supposed to have dwelled" by Thomas Seifrid, "'Illusion' and Its Workings in Modern Russian Culture," *Slavic and East European Journal* 45, no. 2 (Summer 2001): 211. Seifrid posits that modern Russian culture is characterized by illusion-making, the substitution of illusion for reality, as well as a tradition of reflecting on this process.

184. I am grateful to Julia Vaingurt for this insight.

185. Jane Friedman argues that the Moscow metro not only transported passengers in a literal sense but also provided "imagined and ideological transport." See her article "Soviet Mastery of the Skies at the Mayakovsky Metro Station" in *Studies in the Decorative Arts* 7, no. 2 (Spring/Summer 2000): 48.

186. Khan-Magomedov, *Mavzolei Lenina: Istoriia sozdaniia*, 117.

187. Sokolov, *Stantsii Leningradskogo metro*, 25.

188. Metro architect Alexei Dushkin makes an argument about the power of architecture to convey messages that is particularly applicable to the subterranean spaces under discussion: "Architectural works exert a continuous ideological influence that is not weakened by the passage of time. On the contrary, historical events accumulate in the architectural monument, supplementing and enriching its essential meaning." Cited at http://www.metro.ru/library/architecture/81/.

CONCLUSION

The first chapter epigraph is taken from Epstein, *Cries in the New Wilderness*, 147.

The second chapter epigraph is taken from Kachalov, *Steklo*, 441.

1. В стеклянные дворцы на курьих ножках /Я даже тенью лёгкой не войду.

2. Peter Steiner, "Poem as Manifesto: Mandelstam's 'Notre-Dame,'" *Russian Literature* 5 (1977): 242.

3. Osip Mandel'shtam, *Izbrannoe* (Rostov-on-Don: Feniks, 1995), 87. The original reads "Зажглось каюты толстое стекло." Subsequent references to this edition will be indicated by in-text citations.

4. Le Corbusier's building was called a "hut on chicken legs" because of its unprecedented construction: the entire house was raised on concrete pillars (pilotis)—hence the impression of "legs." See Vladimir Paperny, "Movement—Immobility," *Tekstura: Russian Essays*, 64–65.

5. Nadezhda Ia. Mandelstam, *Kniga tret'ia* (Paris: YMCA, 1987), 166. Mandelstam's poem "Today one can make decals [Segodnia mozhno sniat' dekal'komani] . . ." depicts a sports festival in the lines directly preceding the reference to the Tsentrosiuiuz building: "Never will I march in step with the youth / On lined stadiums."

6. See Paperny, "Movement—Immobility," 64–65.

7. The poem, "Sleep Defends My Don Drowsiness [Oboroniaet son moiu donskuiu son']," is from the Voronezh cycle, as is "Stanzas."

8. See Gregory Friedin, "Mandel'shtam's Ode to Stalin: History and Myth," *Russian Review* 41, no. 2 (October 1982): 409.

9. Kiril Taranovsky points out that the line "Рабу не быть рабом, рабе не быть рабой" (slaves shall be slaves no more), a quotation from the *Internationale*, "contains an onomatopoeia of the Kremlin chimes (*bu—by—bom //b'e—by—boi*)." See his *Essays on Mandel'štam*, Harvard Slavic Studies 6 (Cambridge, Mass: Harvard University Press, 1976), 131.

10. Velimir Khlebnikov, *Zangezi*, in *Sobranie sochinenii* (Munich: W. Fink, 1968), 2:324. I am grateful to Alfred Sproede for bringing this passage to my attention.

11. "Blue Fetters" ("*Sinie okovy*"), another long poem from the same year, has a variation on this theme: "The log cabin of events sometimes has a window cut through it—the pensive *and yet* of glasswork": "В избе бревенчатой событий / Порой прорублено окно / Стеклянных дел задумчивое *но*." Abstract "events" are imagined as a concrete "log cabin" whose window stands for hesitation and doubt—the glass expanse becomes a lexical utterance, the word *но*, signifying "but" or "yet."

12. Although Mandelstam did slight the Futurists and their "word as such" in his Acmeist manifesto, he greatly admired Khlebnikov as an artist. Mandelstam praises Khlebnikov's innovative use of language in such essays as "Notes about Poetry" (1923, reworked 1928) and "Storm and Stress" (1923). See *Osip Mandelstam: Selected Essays*, trans. Sidney Monas (Austin: University of Texas Press, 1977), 82 and 152, respectively.

13. Clare Cavanagh analyzes the imagery of sacred architecture in the work of both poets in "Modernist Church-Building: Pound, Khlebnikov, Mandelstam," *Paideuma: A Journal Devoted to Ezra Pound Scholarship* 28, no. 2–3 (Fall-Winter 1999): 149–72. For more on their relationship, see G. G. Amelin and V. Ia. Morderer, *Miry i stolknoveniia Osipa Mandel'shtama* (Moscow: Iazyki russkoi kul'tury, 2000). The authors document that Mandelstam challenged Khlebnikov to a duel in 1913 for reading anti-Semitic verse at the Stray Dog cabaret. Subsequently the poets made peace with one another; http://magazines.russ.ru/novyi_mi/filos/amelin/m04.htm.

14. Дано мне тело—что мне делать с ним, / Таким единым и таким моим? // За радость тихую дышать и жить / Кого, скажите, мне благодарить? // Я и

садовник, я же и цветок / В темнице мира я не одинок. / На стёкла вечности уже легло / Моё дыхание, моё тепло. // Запечатлеестя не нём узор, / Неузнаваемый с недавних пор. // Пускай мгновения стекает муть— / Узора милого не зачеркнуть.

15. Osip Mandelstam, "About the Nature of the Word," in *Selected Essays*, 75.

16. The original Russian text reads as follows: ""Эллинизм— . . . это домашняя утварь, посуда, всё окружение *тела*; эллинизм—это *тепло* очага, ощущаемое, как священное . . . очеловечение окружаещего мира, согревание его *тончайшим телеологическим теплом*." Osip Mandelstam, "O prirode slova," in *Sobranie sochinenii v chetyrekh tomakh* (Moscow: Art-Biznes Tsentr, 1993), 1:227 (emphasis added).

17. "Рисунок, вычерченный метко,—/Когда его художник милый /Выводит на стеклянной тверди." Clarence Brown points out that both this poem and "A body has been given to me" involve a "pattern traced on glass" in his study *Mandelstam* (Cambridge, Eng.: Cambridge University Press, 1973), 169.

18. Epstein, *Cries in the New Wilderness*, 147.

19. According to Brown, in the latter half of the 1920s Mandelstam "lived mostly by translations" (*Mandelstam*, 121).

20. Не искушай чужих наречий, но постарайся их забыть: /Ведь всё равно ты не сумеешь стекло зубами укусить!

21. Note also the recurrence of "moving lips" in his verse as a figure for poetry and its survival; see Jane Gary Harris, *Osip Mandelstam*, Twayne's World Author Series 799 (Boston: Twayne, 1988), 103.

22. On Mandelstam's problematic relationship toward language and the notion of tongue-tiedness in his work, see Cavanagh, *Modernist Creation of Tradition*.

23. Freidin writes, "Mandelstam constructed the [Ode to Stalin] at least in part, out of contemporary official rhetoric" (Mandel'shtam's *Ode to Stalin*: History and Myth," *Russian Review* 41, no. 2 [October 1982]: 412).

24. See Steiner, "Poem as Manifesto," 251; and E. Kantor, "V tolpokrylatom vozdukhe kartin: Iskusstvo i tvorchestvo O. E. Mandel'shtama," *Literaturnoe obozrenie* 1 (1991): 65.

25. O. I. Voronova, *Vera Ignat'evna Mukhina* (Moscow: Iskusstvo, 1976), 164. The original reads: "Не было человека, который не погладил бы его руками. Нравилось."

26. Maria Zavialova, personal correspondence, May 29, 2009.

27. Hughes, *Shock of the New*, 175–76.

28. Robert Sowers, *The Language of Stained Glass* (Forest Grove: Timber, 1981), 40.

29. Ingdahl sees the visual presentation of events in *Envy* in terms of "a kind of double exposure reminiscent of film techniques in which the protagonist

perceives what is happening before his eyes as both a common observer and as an artist" (*The Artist and the Creative Act*, 31).

30. This idea was championed by ideologues such as Bukharin (in 1917) as well as avant-garde artists such as Sergei Tret'iakov (who stated that the Futurists sought to "re-forge" mankind). See also Olesha's story "Human Material" (1929).

31. Rolf Hellebust analyzes Ostrovsky's novel within the context of a larger study of metal imagery in Soviet art and political discourse, with special emphasis on how the New Soviet Man came to be imagined in terms of the human body's metallization, in *Flesh to Metal: Soviet Literature and the Alchemy of Revolution* (Ithaca, N.Y.: Cornell University Press, 2003). This stimulating work, along with Kiaer's *Imagine No Possessions*, are two hopeful signs that scholars are increasingly turning their attention to the material world, and furthermore, showing how Russia is a crucial place to look for insights and revelations into the relationship between persons and things.

32. See Iurii Koginov, *Almaznaia gran': Dokumental'naia povest'* (Moscow: Profizdat, 1977), 75, 188.

33. Cited in Iampol'skii, *Nabliudatel'*, 134n56.

34. See Carla Gottlieb, *The Window in Art: From the Window of God to the Vanity of Man; A Survey of Window Symbolism in Western Painting* (New York: Abaris, 1981), 135.

Works Cited

Abramov, A. *Mavzolei Lenina*. Moscow: Moskovskii rabochii, 1963.

Afanas'ev, K. N., ed. *Iz istorii sovetskoi arkhitektury. 1917–1925 gg.: Dokumenty i materialy*. Moscow: Akademiia Nauk SSSR, 1963.

Akhmatova, Anna. *Sochineniia*. 2nd ed. Vol. 1. Munich: Mezhdunarodnoe literaturnoe sodruzhestvo, 1967.

Alekseev, M. N., et al., eds. *Na krasnoi ploshchadi u mavzoleia: Sbornik*. Moscow: Sovetskaia Rossiia, 1972.

Althusser, Louis. "Ideology and Ideological State Apparatuses: Notes toward an Investigation." In *Lenin and Philosophy*, translated by Ben Brewster. London: New Left Books, 1971.

Amelin, G. G., and V. Ia. Morderer. *Miry i stolknoveniia Osipa Mandel'shtama*. Moscow: Iazyki russkoi kul'tury, 2000.

Anderes, Fred, and Ann Agranoff. *Ice Palaces*. New York: Abbeville, 1983.

Andrews, Edna. "Seeing Is Believing: Visual Categories in the Russian Lexicon." In *Meaning as Explanation: Advances in Linguistic Sign Theory*, edited by Ellen Contini-Morava and Barbara Sussman Goldberg. Berlin: Mouton, 1995.

Anisimov, N. G. *Ogni nad Volgoi: Ocherk istorii Vasil'evskogo steklozavoda "Pobeda Truda."* Kazan: Tatknigoizdat, 1967.

Arkin, D. "Dom na ulitse Kirova." *Arkhitektura SSSR* 10 (1936): 34–35.

Armstrong, Isobel. "Technology and Text: Glass Consciousness and Nineteenth-Century Culture." In *Culture, Landscape and Environment: The Linacre Lectures 1997*, edited by Kate Flint and Howard Morphy. Oxford: Oxford University Press, 2000.

———. "Transparency: Towards a Poetics of Glass in the Nineteenth Century." In *Cultural Babbage: Technology, Time and Invention*, edited by Francis Spufford and Jenny Uglow. London: Faber and Faber, 1996.

———. *Victorian Glassworlds: Glass Culture and the Imagination, 1830–1880*. Oxford University Press, 2008.

Arvidsson, Claes, and Lars Erik Blomqvist, eds., *Symbols of Power: The Esthetics of Political Legitimation in the Soviet Union and Eastern Europe*. Stockholm: Almqvist & Wiksell International, 1987.

Asharina, N. A. "Kubki s emblematami." *Nauka i zhizn'* 6 (1972): 69–71.

———. "'Shutikhi' sela Izmailova." *Nauka i zhizn'* 11 (1973): 151–53.

———. "Russkie zavody khudozhestvennogo stekla XVII–XVIIIvv." In *Iz istorii russkoi keramiki i stekla XVII–XIX vekov: Sbornik trudov*, edited by N. A. Asharina. Moscow: Gosudarstvennyi ordena Lenina Istoricheskii muzei, 1986.

———. "Russkoe khudozhestvennoe steklo." In *Na rubezhe dvukh vekov: Iz istorii preobrazovanii Petrovskogo vremeni*, edited by L. G. Beskrovnyi. Moscow: Sovetskaia Rossiia, 1978.

Asharina, N. A., Tamara Malinina, and Liudmila Kazakova. *Russian Glass of the 17th–20th Centuries*. Corning, N.Y.: Corning Museum of Glass, 1990.

Babakhanov, S. B. *Fakely "Ognei."* Makhachkala: Dagestanskoe knizhnoe izdatel'stvo, 1991.

Babel', I. "Moi pervyi gus'." In *Odesskie Rasskazy: Konarmiia*. Moscow: Izvestiia, 1994.

Baehr, Stephen Lessing. *The Paradise Myth in Eighteenth-Century Russia: Utopian Patterns in Early Secular Russian Literature and Culture*. Stanford, Calif.: Stanford University Press, 1991.

Baiburova, P. "Russkii usadebnyi dom serediny XVIII veka kak element razvlekatel'noi kul'tury barokko." In *U istokov rezvlekatel'noi kul'tury Rossii novogo vremeni, XVIII–XIX veka*, edited by E. V. Dukov. Moscow: Gosudarstvennyi in-t iskusstvoznaniia, 1996.

Bainbridge, Henry Charles. *Peter Carl Faberge: His Life and Work*. New York: B. T. Batsford, 1949.

Bakhtin, M. M. "Forms of Time and Chronotope in the Novel." In *The Dialogic Imagination: Four Essays by M. M. Bakhtin*, edited by Michael Holquist, translated by Caryl Emerson and Michael Holquist. Austin: University of Texas Press, 1981.

Baranov, P., comp. *Opis' imennym vysochaishim ukazam tsaria-imperatora Petra Velikago 1704–1725*. St. Petersburg, 1872.

Barkhatova, E. V., ed. *Iz istorii russkogo plakata: "Okna" ROSTA i Glavolit prosveta 1919–1922: Katalog vystavki*. St. Petersburg: Rossiiskaia natsional'naia biblioteka, 2000.

Barthes, Roland. *Mythologies*. Translated by Annette Lavers. London: Paladin, 1972.

Baskakov, A. M., ed., *Metropoliten Leningrada-Peterburga: Stranitsy istorii*. St. Petersburg: Ivan Fedorov, 1995.

Batanova, Ekaterina I., and N. Voronov. *Sovetskoe khudozhestvennoe steklo*. Moscow: Iskusstvo, 1964.

Baudrillard, Jean. *The System of Objects*. Translated by James Benedict. London: Verso, 1996.

Beaujour, Elizabeth Klosty. "Architectual Discourse and Early Soviet Literature." *Journal of the History of Ideas* 44, no. 3 (July–September 1983): 477–95.

———. *The Invisible Land: A Study of the Artistic Imagination of Iurii Olesha*. New York: Columbia University Press, 1970.

———. "Zamyatin's *We* and Modernist Architecture." *The Russian Review* 47, no. 1 (1988): 49–60.

Belitskii, Pavel. "Poet, vernuvshii pesniu: K 100-letiiu Mikhaila Isakovskogo." *Nezavisimaia gazeta*. January 19, 2000, http://www.ng.ru/2000-01-19.

Bell, Keith. "Glass in Architecture." *The Structurist* 27–28 (1987–88): 73–79.

Benjamin, Walter. "Moscow." In *Reflections: Essays, Aphorisms, Autobiographical Writings*, translated by Edmund Jephcott. New York: Schocken, 1978.

———. "Paris, the Capital of the Nineteenth Century." In *Reflections: Essays, Aphorisms, Autobiographical Writings*, translated by Edmund Jephcott. New York: Schocken, 1978.

Bennett, Jane. *Vibrant Matter: A Political Ecology of Things*. Durham, N.C.: Duke University Press, 2010.

Beretta, Marco. *When Glass Matters: Studies in the History of Science and Art from Graeco-Roman Antiquity to Early Modern Era*. Florence: Leo S. Olschki, 2004.

Bergan, Ronald. *Eisenstein: A Life in Conflict*. Woodstock, N.Y.: Overlook, 1999.

Berger, John. *Ways of Seeing*. New York: Penguin, 1990 (reprint from 1972).

Berkov, P. N., ed. *Russkaia komediia i komicheskaia opera XVIII veka*. Moscow: Iskusstvo, 1950.

Bezborodov, M. A. "Issledovatel'skaia rabota Lomonosova po tsvetnym steklam." *Nauka* 1 (1947): 74–84.

———. *M. V. Lomonosov—Osnovopolozhnik nauchnogo steklodeliia*. Moscow: Gosudarstvennoe izdatel'svo literatury po stroitel'nym materialam, 1956.

Bletter, Rosemarie Haag. "The Interpretation of the Glass Dream—Expressionist Architecture and the History of the Crystal Metaphor." *Journal of the Society of Architectural Historians* 49 (March 1981): 20–43.

Bliznakov, Milka. "The Realization of Utopia: Western Technology and Soviet Avant-Garde Architecture." In *Reshaping Russian Architecture: Western Architecture, Utopian Dreams*, edited by William Craft Brumfield. Cambridge, Eng.: Cambridge University Press, 1990.

Boldyrev, A. N. "Khrustal'nyi tron." *Zvezda* 5–6 (1945): 153–55.

Boldyrev, A. S., ed. "Stekol'naia promyshlennost'." In *Promyshlennost' stroitel'nykh materialov SSSR 1917–1967*. Moscow: Izdatel'stvo literatury po stroitel'stvu, 1967.

Bol'sheva, K. A. "K istorii Mal'tsevskogo stekol'nogo proizvodstva." In *Izobrazitel'noe iskusstvo*. Gosududarstvennaia akademiia iskusstvoznaniia. Leningrad: Akademiia, 1927.

Bonnell, Victoria E. *Iconography of Power: Soviet Political Posters under Lenin and Stalin*. Berkeley: University of California Press, 1997.

Boorstin, Daniel J. *The Discoverers*. New York: Random, 1983.

Bordwell, David. *The Cinema of Eisenstein*. Cambridge, Mass.: Harvard University Press, 1993.

Borenstein, Eliot. "Defying Interpretation: Allegory and Ideology in Jurij Oleša's *Envy*." *Russian Literature* 49 (2001): 25–42.

Bowlt, John. "The Presence of Absence: The Aesthetic of Transparency in Russian Modernism." *The Structurist* 27–28 (1987–88): 15–22.

Boym, Svetlana. *The Future of Nostalgia*. New York: Basic, 2001.

Brewer, Ebenezer Cobham. *Brewer's Dictionary of Phrase and Fable*. 14th ed. New York: HarperCollins, 1989.

Brooks, Jeffrey. *Thank You, Comrade Stalin! Soviet Public Culture from Revolution to Cold War*. Princeton, N.J.: Princeton University Press, 2001.

Brower, Daniel R. *The Russian City between Tradition and Modernity, 1850–1900*. Berkeley: University of California Press, 1990.

Brown, Clarence. *Mandelstam*. Cambridge, Eng.: Cambridge University Press, 1973.

Brumfield, William Craft. *A History of Russian Architecture*. Cambridge, Eng.: Cambridge University Press, 1993.

Bukharin, Nikolai. "Tovarishch." *Pravda*, January 24, 1924, 1.

Bulgakowa, Oksana. *Sergei Eisenstein: A Biography*. Translated by Anne Dwyer. Berlin: Potemkin, 2001.

Bulgarin, Faddei. "Plausible Fantasies, or A Journey to the 29th Century." In *Pre-Revolutionary Russian Science Fiction: An Anthology*, edited and translated by Leland Fetzer. Ann Arbor, Mich.: Ardis, 1982.

Butler, William E. "On the Formation of a Russian Legal Consciousness: The Zertsalo." In *Russia and the Law of Nations in Historical Perspective: Collected Essays*. London: Wildy, Simmonds and Hill, 2009.

Butnik-Siverskii, B. S. *Sovetskii plakat epokhi grazhdanskoi voiny 1918–1921*. Moscow: Izdatel'stvo Vsesoiuznoi knizhnoi palaty, 1960.

Castillo, Greg. "Stalinist Modern: Constructivism and the Soviet Company Town." In *Architectures of Russian Identity: 1500 to the Present*, edited by James Cracraft and Daniel B. Rowland. Ithaca, N.Y.: Cornell University Press, 2003.

Cavanagh, Clare. "Modernist Church-Building: Pound, Khlebnikov, Mandelstam." *Paideuma: A Journal Devoted to Ezra Pound Scholarship* 28, no. 2–3 (Fall-Winter 1999): 149–72.

———. *Osip Mandelstam and the Modernist Creation of Tradition*. Princeton, N.J.: Princeton University Press, 1995.

Chadaga, Julia Bekman. "Light in Captivity: Spectacular Glass and Soviet Power in the 1920s and 1930s." *Slavic Review* 66, no. 1 (Spring 2007): 82–105.

———. "Mirror Writing: The Literary Traces of the Zertsalo." *The Russian Review* 61 (January 2002): 73–93.

———. "No Mere Reflection: Mirrors as Windows on Russian Culture." *Stud-*

ies in Twentieth- and Twenty-First Century Literature 34, no. 2 (Summer 2010): 170–206.

Chernov, Andrei. "Tak vot gde tailas' Rossiia moia. . . ." *Ogonek* 29 (July 1998): 50–55.

Chernyshevskii, N. G. *Chto delat'? Iz rasskazov o novykh liudiakh*. Edited by T. I. Ornatskaia and S. A. Reiser. Leningrad: Nauka, 1975.

———. "Novosti literatury, iskusstv, nauk i promyshlennosti." In *Polnoe sobranie sochinenii v piatnadtsati tomakh*. Vol. 16. Moscow: Gosudarstvennoe izdatel'stvo khudozhestvennoi literatury, 1953.

Chistiakov, A. S. *Istoriia Petra Velikogo*. Moscow: Buklet, 1992.

Chudakova, Marietta. *Masterstvo Iuriia Oleshi*. Moscow: Nauka, 1972.

Clark, Katerina. *Petersburg, Crucible of Cultural Revolution*. Cambridge, Mass.: Harvard University Press, 1995.

———. "Sotsrealism i sacralizatsiia prostranstva." In *Sotsrealisticheskii kanon*, edited by Hans Gunther and Evgeny Dobrenko. St. Petersburg: Akademicheskii proekt, 2000.

Cohen, Jean-Louis. *Le Corbusier and the Mystique of the USSR: Theories and Projects for Moscow, 1928–1936*. Princeton, N.J.: Princeton University Press, 1992.

Collins, Christopher. "Zamyatin's *We* as Myth." In *Zamyatin's "We": A Collection of Critical Essays*, edited by Gary Kern. Ann Arbor, Mich.: Ardis, 1988.

Colton, Timothy J. *Moscow: Governing the Socialist Metropolis*. Cambridge, Mass.: Belknap Press of Harvard University Press, 1995.

Conrads, Ulrich, and Hans G. Sperlich. *The Architecture of Fantasy: Utopian Building and Planning in Modern Times*. Translated and edited by Christiane Crasemann Collins and George R. Collins. New York: Frederick A. Praeger, 1962.

Cooke, Catherine. "Beauty as a Route to the 'Radiant Future': Responses of Soviet Architecture." *Journal of Design History* 10, no. 2 (1997): 137–60.

Corson, Richard. *Fashions in Eyeglasses*. 2nd rev. ed. London: Peter Owen, 1980.

Costlow, Jane T. *Worlds within Worlds: The Novels of Ivan Turgenev*. Princeton, N.J.: Princeton University Press, 1990.

Cowan, S. A. "The Crystalline Center of Zamyatin's *We*." *Extrapolation* 29, no. 2 (Summer 1988): 160–78.

Cracraft, James. *The Petrine Revolution in Russian Architecture*. Chicago: University of Chicago Press, 1988.

———. *The Petrine Revolution in Russian Imagery*. Chicago: University of Chicago Press, 1997.

Danilevskii, V. V., and N. P. Tikhonov. "Restavratsiia mozaiki Lomonosova 'Poltavskaia bataliia.'" *Problemy istoriii dokapitalisticheskikh obshchestv* 9 (1935): 170–91.

de la Shepard, I. "V Rossii." In *Russkii byt vo vospominaniiakh sovremennikov: XVIII vek*, edited by A. V. Butorov. Moscow: AST, 2012.

Déribéré, Maurice. *Préhistoire et histoire de la lumière*. Paris: France-Empire, 1979.

Derzhavin, G. R. *Sochineniia Derzhavina s ob"iasnitel'nymi primechaniiami I. A. Grota*. 2nd ed. 7 vols. St. Petersburg: Izdatel'stvo Imperatorskoi Akademii nauk, 1868–78.

Dodsley, Robert. *The Toy-Shop*. Augustan Reprint Society. Los Angeles: William Andrews Clark Memorial Library, University of California, 1983.

Dolgikh, E. V. *Russkoe steklo XVIII veka: Sobranie Gosudarstvennogo muzeia keramiki i "Usad'ba Kuskovo XVIII veka."* Moscow: Iskusstvo, 1985.

Dolgorukaia, Natal'ia Borisovna. *The Memoirs of Princess Natal'ja Borisovna Dolgorukaja*. Edited and translated by Charles E. Townsend. Columbus, Ohio: Slavica, 1977.

Dostoevskii, F. M. *Besy*. St. Petersburg: Karavella, 1994.

———. *Brat'ia Karamazovy*. Vol. 7 of *Sobranie Sochinenii v Deviati Tomakh*. Moscow: Astrel', 2004.

———. "Mal'chik u Khrista na elke." 1876. In *Dnevnik pisatelia za 1876 god. Ianvar'-aprel'*. Vol. 23 of *Polnoe sobranie sochinenii*. Moscow: Nauka, 1981.

———. *Prestuplenie i nakazanie*. Vol. 7 of *Polnoe sobranie sochinenii v tridtsati tomakh*. Edited by V. G. Bazanov. Leningrad: Nauka, 1972.

———. *Zapiski iz mertvogo doma*. Vol. 4 of *Polnoe sobranie sochinenii v tridtsati tomakh*. Edited by V. G. Bazanov. Leningrad: Nauka, 1972.

———. *Zapiski iz podpolia*. Vol. 5 of *Polnoe sobranie sochinenii v tridtsati tomakh*. Edited by V. G. Bazanov. Leningrad: Nauka, 1972.

Dostoevsky, Fyodor. *Notes from Underground*. Translated by Richard Pevear and Larissa Volokhonsky. New York: Vintage Classics, 1993.

Dukov, E. V., ed. *U istokov razvlekatel'noi kul'tury Rossii novogo vremeni, XVIII–XIX veka*. Moscow: Gosudarstvennyi in-t iskusstvoznaniia, 1996.

Dul'kina, T. I., and N. A. Asharina. *Russkaia keramika i steklo 18–19 vekov: Sobranie gosudarstvennogo istoricheskogo muzeia*. Moscow: Izobrazitel'noe iskusstvo, 1978.

Duranty, Walter. "Lenin Is Lifelike as He Lies in Tomb." *New York Times*, August 4, 1924, 1.

Eagle, Herbert. "Visual Patterning, Vertical Montage, and Ideological Protest: Eisenstein's Stylistic Legacy to East European Filmmakers." In *Eisenstein at 100: A Reconsideration*, edited by Al LaValley and Barry Scherr. New Brunswick, N.J.: Rutgers University Press, 2001.

Eaton, Ruth. "Architecture and Urbanism: The Faces of Utopia." In *Utopia: The Search for the Ideal Society in the Western World*, edited by Roland Schaer, Gregory Claeys, and Lyman Tower Sargent. New York: New York Public Library, 2000.

Efimov, A. I. *M. V. Lomonosov i russkii iazyk*. Moscow: Izdatel'stvo Moskovskogo universiteta, 1961.

Eisenstein, Sergei. *Beyond the Stars: The Memoirs*. Vol. 4 of *Selected Works*. Edited by Richard Taylor, translated by William Powell. London: BFI, 1995.

———. "Disnei." In *Problemy sinteza v khudozhestvennoi kul'ture*, edited by A. V. Prokhorov et al. Moscow: Nauka, 1985.

———. *Nonindifferent Nature*. Translated by Herbert Marshall. Cambridge, Eng.: Cambridge University Press, 1987.

———. *Towards a Theory of Montage*. Vol. 2 of *Selected Works*. Edited by Michael Glenny and Richard Taylor. Translated by Michael Glenny. London: BFI, 1991.

Ellis, William S. *Glass: From the First Mirror to Fiber Optics, the Story of the Substance That Changed the World*. New York: Avon, 1998.

Epstein, Mikhail. *Cries in the New Wilderness: From the Files of the Moscow Institute of Atheism*. Translated and introduction by Eve Adler. Philadelphia: Paul Dry, 2002.

———. "The Stature of Things in Russian Thought." http://www.russ.ru/antolog/intelnet/sympo_epstein_things.html.

———. "Thing and Word: On the Lyrical Museum." In *After the Future: The Paradoxes of Postmodernism and Contemporary Russian Culture*. Translated by Anesa Miller-Pogacar. Amherst: University of Massachusetts Press, 1995.

Erenburg, Il'ia. *A vse-taki ona vertitsia*. Moscow: Gelikon, 1922.

Erofeev, Aleksei. "Chto otkryvaetsia v Evropu?" *Smena—Informatsionnaia gazeta*, April 6, 2002. http://www.smena.ru/arc/22654-log.html.

Esaulov, Ivan. "Sotsrealizm i religioznoe soznanie." In *Sotsrealisticheskii kanon*, edited by Hans Gunther and Evgeny Dobrenko. St. Petersburg: Akademicheskii proekt, 2000.

Fauvel, Maryse. "From Iron to Glass: Transparency and Pluralism." *Studies in Twentieth-Century Literature* 20, no. 2 (Summer 1996): 337–49.

Fitzpatrick, Sheila. *Tear Off the Masks! Identity and Imposture in Twentieth-Century Russia*. Princeton, N.J.: Princeton University Press, 2005.

Foucault, Michel. *Discipline and Punish: The Birth of the Prison*. Translated by Alan Sheridan. New York: Penguin, 1977.

———. "Of Other Spaces." *Diacritics* (Spring 1986): 22–27.

Fourier, Charles. *Design for Utopia: Selected Writings of Charles Fourier*. Translated by Julia Franklin. New York: Schocken Books, 1971.

Frazier, Ian. "On the Prison Highway." *The New Yorker*, August 30, 2010.

Freidin, Gregory. "Mandel'shtam's *Ode to Stalin*: History and Myth." *Russian Review* 41, no. 2 (October 1982): 400–426.

Friedman, Jane. "Soviet Mastery of the Skies at the Mayakovsky Metro Station." *Studies in the Decorative Arts* 7, no. 2 (Spring/Summer 2000): 48–64.

Fritzsche, Peter, and Charles Stewart, eds. *Imagining the Twentieth Century*. Urbana: University of Illinois Press, 1997.

Frolova, Elena. "Ne ochen' prozrachnaia istoriia." *Material* 2 (2002). http://www.okna.spb.ru/okna/articles/?inset=glass_about3.phtml.

Gladkov, Fedor. *Tsement*. Moscow: n.p., 1927.

Gogol, Nikolai. *Dead Souls*. Translated and annotated by Richard Pevear and Larissa Volokhonsky. New York: Vintage, 1996.

———. "The Tale of How Ivan Ivanovich Quarreled with Ivan Nikiforovich." Vol. 2 of *The Complete Tales of Nikolai Gogol*, edited by Leonard J. Kent. Chicago: University of Chicago Press, 1985.

Gogol', N. V. *Mertvye dushi*. Vol. 5 of *Sobranie sochinenii v shesti tomakh*. Moscow: Gosudarstvennoe izdatel'stvo khudozhestvennoi literatury, 1953.

———. "Povest' o tom, kak possorilsia Ivan Ivanovich s Ivanom Nikiforovichem." Vol. 2 of *Sobranie khudozhestvennykh proizvedenii v piati tomakh*. Moscow: Izdatel'stvo Akademii Nauk SSSR, 1951.

———. *Shinel'*. Vol. 3 of *Sobranie sochinenii*. Moscow: Gosudarstvennoe izdatel'stvo khudozhestvennoi literatury, 1959.

———. *Taras Bul'ba*. Moscow: Akademiia nauk SSSR, 1963.

Goldberg, Benjamin. *The Mirror and Man*. Charlottesville: University Press of Virginia, 1985.

Gor'kii, M. "Pozhary." Vol. 15 of *Sobranie sochinenii v tridtsati tomakh*. Moscow: Gosudarstvennoe izdatel'stvo khudozhestvennoi literatury, 1951.

Gottlieb, Carla. *The Window in Art: From the Window of God to the Vanity of Man: A Survey of Window Symbolism in Western Painting*. New York: Abaris, 1981.

Gough, Maria. "Switched On: Notes on Radio, Automata, and the Bright Red Star." In *Building the Collective: Soviet Graphic Design 1917–1937*, edited by Leah Dickerman. New York: Princeton Architectural Press, 1996.

Grabes, Herbert. *The Mutable Glass: Mirror-Imagery in Titles and Texts of the Middle Ages and English Renaissance*. Translated by Gordon Collier. Cambridge, Eng.: Cambridge University Press, 1982.

Graham, Loren. "The Fits and Starts of Russian and Soviet Technology." In *Technology, Culture, and Development: The Experience of the Soviet Model*, edited by James P. Scanlan. Armonk, N.Y.: M. E. Sharpe, 1992.

Grohmann, Will. *Wassily Kandinsky: Life and Work*. Translated by Norbert Guterman. New York: Abrams, 1958.

Gurikov, Vladimir. "Obrabotka i shlifovka linz v epokhu Petra I." http:/www.optika.ru/pressa/history/5-2001/index.php.

Hammarberg, Gitta. "Eighteenth Century Narrative Variations on 'Frol Skobeev.'" *Slavic Review* 46, no. 3/4 (Autumn-Winter 1987): 529–39.

Harris, Jane Gary. *Osip Mandelstam*. Twayne's World Author Series 799. Boston: Twayne, 1988.

Hellebust, Rolf. *Flesh to Metal: Soviet Literature and the Alchemy of Revolution*. Ithaca, N.Y.: Cornell University Press, 2003.

Hellie, Richard. *The Economy and Material Culture of Russia, 1600–1725*. Chicago: University of Chicago Press, 1999.

Hudson, Hugh, Jr. *Blueprints and Blood: The Stalinization of Soviet Architecture, 1917–1937*. Princeton, N.J.: Princeton University Press, 1994.

Hughes, Lindsey. *Russia in the Age of Peter the Great*. New Haven, Conn.: Yale University Press, 1998.

Hughes, Robert. *The Shock of the New: Art and the Century of Change*. Rev. ed. New York: Knopf, 1991.

Hutchings, William. "Structure and Design in a Soviet Dystopia: H. G. Wells, Constructivism, and Yevgeny Zamyatin's *We*." *Journal of Modern Literature* 9, no. 1 (1981/1982): 81–102.

Iampolskii, Mikhail. "Le cinéma de l'architecture utopique." *Iris* (1991): 39–46.

———. *Nabliudatel': Ocherki istorii videniia*. Moscow: Ad Marginem, 2000.

Iashanova, V. N. "Kremlevskie zvezdy 1937 g." *Otechestvennye arkhivy*, no. 4 (1997): 77.

Ilardi, Vincent. *Renaissance Vision from Spectacles to Telescopes*. Philadelphia: American Philosophical Society, 2007.

Ingdahl, Kazimiera. *The Artist and the Creative Act: A Study of Jurij Oleša's Novel Zavist'*. Stockholm: University of Stockholm Press, 1984.

Isakovskii, M. "Vdol' derevni." In *Poet sovetskaia strana*, compiled by I. A. Shvedov. Moscow: Moskovskii rabochii, 1962.

Iurchuk, K. I. *Votchinnye manufaktury v stekol'noj promyshlennosti Rossii v kontse XVIII-pervoi polovine XIX veka: K probleme genezisa kapitalizma*. Voronezh: Izdatel'stvo Voronezhskogo universiteta, 1988.

Jackson, Robert Louis. *Dostoevsky's Underground Man in Russian Literature*. The Hague: Mouton, 1958.

Jakle, John A. *City Lights: Illuminating the American Night*. Baltimore: Johns Hopkins University Press, 2001.

Jay, Martin. *Downcast Eyes: The Denigration of Vision in Twentieth-Century French Thought*. Berkeley: University of California Press, 1993.

Jenks, Andrew. "A Metro on the Mount: The Underground as a Church of Soviet Civilization." *Technology and Culture* 41, no. 4 (2000): 697–724.

Kachalov, Nikolai. *Steklo*. Moscow: Izdatel'stvo Akademii Nauk SSSR, 1959.

Kamenskii, V. V. *Zhizn' s Maiakovskim*. Munich: Wilhelm Fink Verlag, 1974.

Kann, Pavel. *Leningrad: A Guide*. Moscow: Planeta, 1990.

Kantor, E. "V tolpokrylatom vozdukhe kartin: Iskusstvo i tvorchestvo O. E. Mandel'shtama." *Literaturnoe obozrenie* 1 (1991): 59–68.

Kapnist, V. V. *Iabeda*. Vol. 1 of *Sobranie sochinenii v dvukh tomakh*, edited by D. S. Babkin. Moscow: Izdatel'stvo Akademii nauk SSSR, 1960.

Karamzin, N. M. "Moia ispoved'." Vol. 1 of *Sochineniia v dvukh tomakh*, edited by G. P. Makogonenko. Leningrad: Khudozhestvennaia literatura, 1984.

Kelly, Catriona. "Territories of the Eye: The Russian Peep Show (Raek) and Pre-

Revolutionary Visual Culture." *Journal of Popular Culture* 31, no. 4 (1998): 49–74.

Kelly, Laurence. *Diplomacy and Murder in Tehran: Alexander Griboyedov and Imperial Russia's Mission to the Shah of Persia*. London: I. B. Tauris, 2002.

Kern, Gary, ed. *Zamyatin's "We": A Collection of Critical Essays*. Ann Arbor, Mich.: Ardis, 1988.

Kettering, Karen. "An Introduction to the Design of the Moscow Metro in the Stalin Period: 'The Happiness of Life Underground.'" *Studies in the Decorative Arts* 7, no. 2 (Spring/Summer 2000): 2–20.

Khan-Magomedov, S. O. *Mavzolei Lenina: Istoriia sozdaniia i arkhitektura*. Moscow: Prosveshchenie, 1972.

———. *Rodchenko: The Complete Work*. Edited by Vieri Quilici. Cambridge, Mass.: MIT Press, 1987.

Khlebnikov, Velimir. *Collected Works of Velimir Khlebnikov*. Translated by Paul Schmidt. Edited by Charlotte Douglas. 4 vols. Cambridge, Mass.: Harvard University Press, 1987–97.

———. *Tvoreniia*. Edited by M. Ia. Poliakov. Moscow: Sovetskii pisatel', 1986.

———. *Zangezi*. Vol. 2 of *Sobranie sochinenii*. Munich: W. Fink, 1968.

Kiaer, Christina. *Imagine No Possessions: The Socialist Objects of Russian Constructivism*. Cambridge, Mass: MIT Press, 2005.

Kivelson, Valerie A., and Joan Neuberger, eds. *Picturing Russia: Explorations in Visual Culture*. New Haven, Conn.: Yale University Press, 2010.

Kleiman, Naum. "'Stekliannyi dom' S. M. Eizenshteina: k istorii zamysla." *Iskusstvo kino* 3 (1979): 94–113.

Kochetkova, Natal'ia. "Zhal', chto ego bol'she net s nami." *Izvestiia*, July 18, 2009.

Koepnick, Lutz. *Framing Attention: Windows on Modern German Culture*. Baltimore: Johns Hopkins University Press, 2007.

Koeppel, Dan. "Let There Be Light." *Wired* (September 2011): 110–19.

Koginov, Iurii. *Almaznaia gran': dokumental'naia povest'*. Moscow: Profizdat, 1977.

Kohl, Johann Georg. *Russia and the Russians in 1842*. Vol. 1. 1842. Reprinted by Cleveland: Micro Photo Div., Bell & Howell, 1965.

Kohlmaier, Georg, and Barna von Satory. *Houses of Glass: A Nineteenth-Century Building Type*. Translated by John C. Harvey. Cambridge, Mass.: MIT Press, 1986.

Komar, Vitaly, and Alexander Melamid. "We Remember, or So It Seems." In *Monumental Propaganda*, edited by Dore Ashton. New York: Independent Curators International, 1995.

Kopp, Anatole. "Foreign Architects in the Soviet Union during the First Two Five Year Plans." In *Reshaping Russian Architecture: Western Architecture, Utopian Dreams*, edited by William Craft Brumfield. Cambridge, Eng.: Cambridge University Press, 1990.

———. *Town and Revolution: Soviet Architecture and City Planning 1917–1935*. Translated by Thomas E. Burton. New York: George Braziller, 1970.

Kopytoff, Igor. "The Cultural Biography of Things." In *The Social Life of Things: Commodities in Cultural Perspective*, edited by Arjun Appadurai. Cambridge, Eng.: Cambridge University Press, 1986.

Korolenko, V. G. "Istoriia moego sovremennika." Vol. 5 of *Sobranie sochinenii v 10-i tomakh*. Moscow: Gosudarstvennoe Izdatel'stvo khudozhestvennoi literatury, 1954.

Kotyrev, Andrei. *Mavzolei V. I. Lenina: proektirovanie i stroitel'stvo*. Moscow: Sovetskii khudozhnik, 1971.

Kozhin, S. N. "Oshibki zamysla." *Arkhitektura SSSR* 2, no. 12 (1934): 9.

Kraft, G. W. *Podlinnoe i obstoiatel'noe opisanie postroennogo v Sankt-Peterburge, v Genvare 1740 goda, ledianogo doma*. St. Petersburg: Imperatorskaia Akademiia nauk, 1741.

Krasheninnikov, V. V., ed. *S. I. Mal'tsov i istoriia razvitiia Mal'tsovskogo promyshlennogo raiona*. Briansk: Grani, 1994.

Krylov, I. A. *P'esy*. Vol. 1 of *Polnoe sobranie sochinenii v dvukh tomakh*. Moscow: Iskusstvo, 1944.

Kurashov, S. Secret memorandum to the Central Committee of the Communist Party. July 16, 1960. Reprinted in *Neizvestnaia Rossiia XX vek*, edited by V. A. Kozlov. Vol 4. Moscow: Istoricheskoe nasledie, 1993.

Lane, Christel. *The Rites of Rulers: Ritual in Industrial Society—The Soviet Case*. Cambridge, Eng.: Cambridge University Press, 1981.

Lary, Nikita. "Viktor Shklovsky: The Good and Awkward Friend." In *Eisenstein at 100: A Reconsideration*, edited by Al LaValley and Barry Scherr. New Brunswick, N.J.: Rutgers University Press, 2001.

Lazhechnikov, I. I. *Ledianoi dom*. Moscow: Izdatel'stvo "Sovetskaia Rossiia," 1977.

Lebedev, V. I., comp. *Reformy Petra I: Sbornik dokumentov*. Moscow: Gosudarstvennoe sotsial'no-ekonomicheskoe izdatel'stvo, 1937.

Lebedeva, O. B. *Russkaia vysokaia komediia XVIII veka: Genezis i poetika zhanra*. Tomsk: Izdatel'stvo Tomskogo universiteta, 1996.

Leonov, A. I., ed. *Russkoe dekorativnoe iskusstvo: 18-i vek*. Vol. 2. Moscow: Izdatel'stvo Akademii Khudozhestv, 1963.

Levinson, E. A., et al. *Khudozhestvennoe steklo i ego primemenie v arkhitekture*. Leningrad: Gosudarstvennoe izdatel'stvo literatury po stroitel'stvu i arkhitekture, 1953.

Levitt, Marcus C. *The Visual Dominant in Eighteenth-Century Russia*. DeKalb: Northern Illinois University Press, 2011.

Leyda, Jay, and Zina Voynow. *Eisenstein at Work*. New York: Pantheon, 1982.

Lissitzky, El. "New Russian Art: A Lecture" (1922). In *El Lissitzky: Life, Letters, Texts*. Greenwich, Conn.: New York Graphic Society: 1968.

———. "Suprematism in World Reconstruction." In *Russian Art of the Avant-*

Garde: Theory and Criticism 1902–1934, edited and translated by John Bowlt. Rev. ed. New York: Thames and Hudson, 1988.

Lodder, Christina. *Russian Constructivism*. New Haven, Conn.: Yale University Press, 1983.

Lomonosov, M. V. "Pis'mo o pol'ze stekla." In *Stikhotvoreniia*. Biblioteka poeta, Malaia Seriia. 3rd ed. Edited by A. Morozov. Leningrad: Sovetskii pisatel', 1954.

———. *Polnoe sobranie sochinenii*. Vol. 8. Moscow: Akademiia nauk SSSR, 1959.

Lotman, Iu. M. *Besedy o russkoi kul'ture: byt i traditsii russkogo dvorianstva XVIII–nachalo XIX veka*. St. Petersburg: Iskusstvo-SPB, 1994.

———. Commentaries to A. S. Pushkin, *Evgenii Onegin*. Moscow: Atrium, 1991.

———. "The Poetics of Everyday Behavior in Russian Eighteenth-Century Culture." In *The Semiotics of Russian Culture*, ed. Ann Shukman. Ann Arbor, Mich.: Michigan Slavic Contributions, 1984.

Lotman, Jurij M., and B. A. Uspenskij. "Echoes of the Notion 'Moscow as the Third Rome' in Peter the Great's Ideology." In *The Semiotics of Russian Culture*, edited by Ann Shukman. Michigan Slavic Contributions 11. Ann Arbor: University of Michigan, 1984.

Lukin, V. I. *Shchepetil'nik: Russkaia komediia i komicheskaia opera XVIII veka*. Edited by P. N. Berkov. Moscow: Iskusstvo, 1950.

Luppov, S. P. *Istoriia stroitel'stva Peterburga v pervoi chetverti XVIII veka*. Moscow: Izdatel'stvo Akademii nauk SSSR, 1957.

Macfarlane, Alan, and Gerry Martin. *Glass: A World History*. Chicago: University of Chicago Press, 2002.

Maiakovskii, V. V. *Klop*. Vol. 2 of *Sochineniia v dvukh tomakh*. Moscow: Pravda, 1988.

Makarov, V. K. *Khudozhestvennoe nasledie M. V. Lomonosova: Mozaiki*. Moscow: Izdatel'stvo Akademii nauk SSSR, 1950.

Malkiel', Boris. "To, o chem nikogda ne zabyt'." *Pravda*, January 27, 1924.

Mandelker, Amy. *Framing Anna Karenina: Tolstoy, the Woman Question, and the Victorian Novel*. Columbus: Ohio State University Press, 1993.

Mandelstam, Nadezhda Ia. *Kniga tret'ia*. Paris: YMCA, 1987.

Mandel'shtam, Osip. *Izbrannoe*. Rostov-on-Don: Feniks, 1995.

Mandelstam, Osip. "About the Nature of the Word." In *Osip Mandelstam: Selected Essays*, translated by Sidney Monas. Austin: University of Texas Press, 1977.

———. *The Egyptian Stamp*. In *The Noise of Time: The Prose of Osip Mandelstam*, edited and translated by Clarence Brown. New York: Penguin, 1993.

———. "O prirode slova." Vol. 1 of *Sobranie sochinenii v chetyrekh tomakh*. Moscow: Art-Biznes Tsentr, 1993.

Man'kov, A. G., ed. *Zakonodatel'stvo perioda stanovleniia absoliutizma: Rossiiskoe zakonodatel'stvo X–XX vekov v deviati tomakh*. Moscow: Iuridicheskaia literatura, 1986.

Marly, Pierre. "Spectacles Through the Ages, from the *Clouants* of the 13th Century to the Modern Day." In *Spectacles & Spyglasses*, translated by Barry Tulett. Liguge, Poitiers: Editions Hoebeke, 1988.

Matsai, A. *"Iabeda" V. V. Kapnista*. Kiev: Izdatel'stvo Kievskogo gosudarstvennogo universiteta im. T. Shevchenko, 1958.

Mauss, Marcel. *The Gift: Forms and Functions of Exchange in Archaic Societies*. Translated by Ian Cunnison. New York: Norton, 1967.

Mayakovsky, Vladimir. *The Bedbug and Selected Poetry*. Translated by Max Hayward and George Reavey. Edited by Patricia Blake. Bloomington: Indiana University Press, 1975.

McLean, Hugh. "The Adventures of an English Comedy in Eighteenth-Century Russia: Dodsley's *Toy Shop* and Lukin's *Ščepetil'nik*." In *American Contributions to the Fifth International Congress of Slavists, Sofia, September 1963*. The Hague: Mouton, 1963.

Mel'gunova-Stepanova, P. E. *Russkii byt vo vospominaniiakh sovremennikov: XVIII vek: Sbornik otryvkov iz zapisok, vospominanii i pisem*. Moscow: Zadruga, 1914.

Meneley, Anne. "Oleo-Signs and Quali-Signs: The Qualities of Olive Oil." *Ethnos* 73, no. 3 (September 2008): 303–26.

Miklashevskii, Konstantin. *Gipertrofiia iskusstva*. Petrograd: Gosudarstvennaia tipografiia im. Evgenii Sokolovoi, 1924.

Miller, Daniel. "Artefacts and the Meaning of Things." In *Companion Encyclopedia of Anthropology*, edited by Tim Ingold. London: Routledge, 1994.

Miller, Frank J. *Folklore for Stalin: Russian Folklore and Pseudofolklore of the Stalin Era*. Armonk, N.J.: M. E. Sharpe, 1990.

Milner, John. *Vladimir Tatlin and the Russian Avant-Garde*. New Haven, Conn.: Yale University Press, 1983.

Milner-Gulland, Robin. "Khlebnikov's Eye." In *Russian Literature: Modernism and the Visual Arts*, edited by Catriona Kelly and Stephen Lovell. Cambridge, Eng.: Cambridge University Press, 2000.

Mokienko, V. M. *Tolkovyi slovar' iazyka Sovdepii*. St. Petersburg: Folio-press, 1998.

Montague, Ivor Goldsmidt Samuel. *With Eisenstein in Hollywood*. New York: International, 1969.

Moreno, Shonquis. "Through the Looking Glass." In *Forefront: The Culture of Shop Window Design*. Amsterdam: Birkhäuser, 2005.

Morozov, Aleksandr. Commentary to "Pis'mo o pol'ze stekla" by M. V. Lomonosov. In *Polnoe sobranie sochinenii*, vol. 8. Moscow: Akademiia nauk SSSR, 1959.

———. "Lomonosov i barokko." *Russkaia literatura* 2 (1965): 70–96.

Mumford, Lewis. *Technics and Civilization*. New York: Harcourt, Brace, 1934.

Muntian, T. N. "Izdeliia Nikol'sko-Bakhmetevskogo stekol'nogo zavoda v sobranii muzeev Kremlia." In *Dekorativnoe i prikladnoe iskusstvo: materialy i issledovaniia*, edited by Aida Nasibova. Moscow: Moskovskii Kreml', 1993.

Murav'ev, Vladimir, comp. *S zemli do zvezd vstaet Moskva: Moskva v sovetskoi poezii*. Moscow: Moskovskii rabochii, 1989.

Myers, Alan. "Zamyatin in Newcastle." *Foundation* 59 (Fall 1993): 70–78.

Nabokov, Vladimir. *The Gift*. New York: Vintage International, 1991.

Nesbet, Anne. *Savage Junctures: Sergei Eisenstein and the Shape of Thinking*. London: I. B. Tauris, 2003.

Netting, Anthony. "Images and Ideas in Russian Peasant Art." *Slavic Review* 35, no. 1 (1976): 48–68.

Nilsson, Nils Ake. "Through the Wrong End of Binoculars: An Introduction to Jurij Olesha." *Scando-Slavica* 11 (1965): 40–68.

Noonan, Thomas, et al. "The Development and Diffusion of Glassmaking in Pre-Mongol Russia." In *The Prehistory and History of Glassmaking Technology*, edited by Patrick McGray. Westerville, Ohio: American Ceramic Society, 1998.

Novak, Anna. "Ice Palace Unveiled in St. Petersburg." RIA Novosti, February 8, 2006.

Odoevskii, V. F. "The Year 4338. Letters from Petersburg." In *Pre-Revolutionary Russian Science Fiction: An Anthology*, edited and translated by Leland Fetzer. Ann Arbor, Mich.: Ardis, 1982.

———. *4338-I god: Peterburgskie pis'ma*. Edited by Orest Tsekhovitser. Moscow: Izdatel'stvo "Ogonek," 1926.

Okhitrovich, Mikhail. "K probleme goroda." *Sovremennnaia arkhitektura* 4 (1929): 130–34.

"Okno." In *Entsiklopedicheskii slovar'*, vol. 21a, edited by I. E. Andreevskii. 43 vols. St. Petersburg: F. A. Brokgauz and I. A. Efron, 1897.

Olesha, Iurii. "Avtor o svoei p'ese." In *P'esy: Stat'i o teatre i dramaturgii*. Moscow: Iskusstvo, 1968.

———. *Kniga Proshchaniia*. Moscow: Vagrius, 1999.

———. *Zagovor chuvstv*, in *P'esy: Stat'i o teatre i dramaturgii*. Moscow: Iskusstvo, 1968.

———. *Zavist'*, in *Ni dnia bez strochki*. Minsk: Izdatel'stvo BGU im. V. I. Lenina, 1982.

Olesha, Yury. *Envy*. In *The Portable Twentieth-Century Russian Reader*. Edited by Clarence Brown. New York: Viking, 1985.

———. *No Day without a Line: From Notebooks by Yury Olesha*. Edited and translated by Judson Rosengrant. Evanston, Ill.: Northwestern University Press, 1998.

Onufrieva, R. I., and E. V. Gil', eds. *Ermitazh: Istoriia i arkhitektura zdanii*. Leningrad: Avrora, 1974.

Oreshnikov, A. "Aptekarskaia posuda vremeni Petra Velikago." *Starye gody* (February 1908): 87–91.

Ortega y Gasset, José. "The Dehumanization of Art." In *The Dehumanization of Art, and Other Writings on Art and Culture*. Garden City, N.Y., Doubleday, 1956.

Outka, Elizabeth. *Consuming Traditions: Modernity, Modernism, and the Commodified Authentic*. New York: Oxford University Press, 2009.

Panchenko, Alexander A. "The Cult of Lenin and 'Soviet Folklore.'" *FOLKLORICA: Journal of the Slavic and East European Folklore Association* 10, no. 1 (2005).

Paperno, Irina. *Chernyshevsky and the Age of Realism: A Study in the Semiotics of Behavior*. Stanford, Calif.: Stanford University Press, 1988.

Paperny, Vladimir. "Movement—Immobility." In *Tekstura: Russian Essays on Visual Culture*, edited and translated by Alla Efimova and Lev Manovich. Chicago: University of Chicago Press, 1993.

Papernyi, Vladimir. *Kul'tura "Dva."* Ann Arbor, Mich.: Ardis, 1985.

Parfenov, V. *Biulleten' "Steklo mira"* 3 (2001). http://www.akma.spb.ru/html/articles/gplant.htm.

Paustovskii, Konstantin. "Stekol'nyi master." Vol. 6 of *Sobranie sochinenii v vos'mi tomakh*. Moscow: Khudozhestvennaia literatura, 1969.

Peterson, Claes. *Peter the Great's Administrative and Judicial Reforms: Swedish Antecedents and the Process of Reception*. Stockholm: Bloms Boktryckeri AB, 1979.

Petrone, Karen. *Life Has Become More Joyous, Comrades: Celebrations in the Time of Stalin*. Bloomington: University of Indiana Press, 2000.

Plamper, Jan. "The Spatial Poetics of the Personality Cult: Circles around Stalin." In *The Landscape of Stalinism: The Art and Ideology of Soviet Space*, edited by Evgeny Dobrenko and Eric Naiman. Seattle: University of Washington Press, 2003.

Platonov, Andrei. "O potukhshei lampochke Il'icha." Vol. 1 of *Sobranie sochinenii v piati tomakh*. Moscow: Informpechat', 1998.

Plavil'shchikov, P. A. *Sochineniia*. St. Petersburg, 1816.

Pokhlebkin, V. V. *Chai i vodka v istorii Rossii*. Krasnoiarsk: Krasnoiarskoe knizhnoe izdatel'stvo, 1995.

———. *Slovar' mezhdunarodnoi simvoliki i emblematiki*. Moscow: Mezhdunarodnye otnosheniia, 1994.

Poltoratskii, Viktor. *Gnezdo khrustal'nogo gusia: Rasskaz o proshlom, nastoiashchem i budushchem rossiiskogo steklograda, o zamechatel'nykh masterakh i khudozhnikakh russkogo khrustalia*. Moscow: Sovetskaia Rossiia, 1959.

Popov, N. F. "Novaia Moskva—ne muzei stariny." *Izvestiia*, November 22, 1925.

"Posol'stvo poruchika Noskova v Persiiu s khrustal'noi krovat'iu." *Istoricheskii Vestnik* 30 (November 1887): 425–40.

Pototskaia, G. V. *Kontrol' produktsii na zavodakh tekhnicheskogo stekla*. Moscow: Promstroiizdat, 1953.

Printseva, G. A. *Pamiatniki russkoi kul'tury vremeni M. V. Lomonosova v Gosudarstvennom Ermitazhe*. Leningrad: Izdatel'stvo Gosudarstvennogo Ermitazha, 1961.

Prokof'ev, Evgenii P. *Russkii khrustal': Gusevskii khrustal'nyi zavod*. Leningrad: Khudozhnik RSFSR, 1970.

"Protestuia ot imeni millionov trudiashchikhsia SSSR, krest'ianin Nikitin vystrelil v sarkofag s telom Lenina, a zatem ubil sebia." *Fakty i kommentarii*, October 22, 1999. http://www.facts.kiev.ua/oct99/2210/10.htm.

Prown, Jules David. "The Truth of Material Culture: History or Fiction?" In *History through Things: Essays on Material Culture*, edited by Steven Lubar and W. David Kingery. Washington, D.C.: Smithsonian Institution, 1993.

Punin, Nikolai. "Pamiatnik III Internatsionala." In *O Tatline: Arkhiv russkogo avangarda*. Moscow: Literaturno-khudozhestvennoe agenstvo "RA," 1994.

Pushkin, A. S. "Pikovaia dama." In *Stikhotvoreniia, Poemy, Proza*. Moscow: Panorama, 1995.

Pyliaev, M. I. *Zabytoe proshloe okrestnostei Peterburga*. St. Petersburg: Izdatel'stvo A. S. Suvorina, 1889.

Reid, Susan. "Destalinization and Taste, 1953–1963." *Journal of Design History* 10, no. 2 (1997): 177–201.

Rets, Kirill. "Teatral'nye binokli i lornety." http://goodcoins.narod.ru/antic/raznoe/teatral.htm.

Revzin, Grigorii. "Khram kuptsa-spasitelia." *Kommersant"-Vlast'*, March 27, 2001. http://archi.ru/press/revzin/vlast2703.htm.

Riasanovsky, Nicholas V. *A History of Russia*. 5th ed. New York: Oxford University Press, 1993.

Richards, Thomas. *The Commodity Culture of Victorian England: Advertising and Spectacle 1851–1914*. Stanford, Calif.: Stanford University Press, 1990.

Rivosh, Ia. N. *Vremia i veshchi: Ocherki po istorii material'noi kul'tury v Rossii nachala XX veka*. Moscow: Iskusstvo, 1990.

Rosen, E. "The Invention of Eyeglasses." *Journal of the History of Medicine and Allied Sciences* 11, no. 1 and 2 (1956): 13–46, 183–218.

Rosen, Nathan. "The Magic Cards in *The Queen of Spades*." *SEEJ* 19, no. 3 (Autumn 1975): 268.

Röthel, Hans Konrad. Introduction to *Vasily Kandinsky: Painting on Glass (Hinterglasmalerei): Anniversary Exhibition*. Solomon R. Guggenheim Museum. New York: S. R. Guggenheim Foundation, 1966.

Ruane, Christine. *The Empire's New Clothes: A History of the Russian Fashion Industry, 1700–1917*. New Haven, Conn.: Yale University Press, 2009.

Ruble, Blair A. "Moscow's Revolutionary Architecture and Its Aftermath: A Critical Guide." In *Reshaping Russian Architecture: Western Technology, Utopian Dreams*, edited by William Craft Brumfield. Washington, D.C.: Woodrow Wilson International Center for Scholars, 1990.

Ruskin, John. *Seven Lamps of Architcture*. London: J. M. Dent, 1928.

Russell, Robert. "The Modernist Tradition." In *Cambridge Companion to the Classic Russian Novel*, edited by Malcolm E. Jones and Robin Feuer Miller. New York: Cambridge University Press, 1998.

———. *Zamyatin's "We."* London: Bristol Classical, 2000.

Schaer, Roland, Gregory Claeys, and Lyman Tower Sargent, eds. *Utopia: The Search for the Ideal Society in the Western World*. New York: New York Public Library, 2000.

Schaffer, Paul. "A Survey of Trends in the Russian Decorative Arts in the First Half of the Nineteenth Century." In *Art and Culture in Nineteenth-Century Russia*, edited by T. G. Stavrou. Bloomington: Indiana University Press, 1983.

Scheerbart, Paul. *Glass Architecture*. Translated by James Palmes. Edited by Dennis Sharp. New York: Praeger, 1972.

Schivelbusch, Wolfgang. *Disenchanted Night: The Industrialization of Light in the Nineteenth Century*. Translated by Angela Davies. Berkeley: University of California Press, 1988.

Sears, Robert. *An Illustrated Description of the Russian Empire*. New York: R. Sears, 1855.

Sedov, Vladimir. "Koshmar shuta." www.projectclassica.ru.

Seifrid, Thomas. *Andrei Platonov: Uncertainties of Spirit*. Cambridge, Eng.: Cambridge University Press, 1992.

———. "'Illusion' and Its Workings in Modern Russian Culture." *Slavic and East European Journal* 45, no. 2 (Summer 2001): 205–15.

Semenov, Dmitrii. "Etazhi so znakom minus." *Moskovskaia Pravda*, October 12, 1991, 1–3.

———. "Pervyi sovetskii neboskreb." *Moskovskaia Pravda*, May 18, 1991, 3.

Shane, Alex M. *The Life and Works of Evgenij Zamjatin*. Berkeley: University of California Press, 1968.

Shangina, I. I. *Russkii traditsionnyi byt: Entsiklopedicheskii slovar'*. St. Petersburg: Azbuka-klassika, 2003.

Shentalinsky, Vitaly. *Arrested Voices: Resurrecting the Disappeared Writers of the Soviet Regime*. Translated by John Crowfoot. New York: Martin Kessler Books, 1993.

Shklovskii, Viktor. *Eizenshtein*. Moscow: Iskusstvo, 1973.

———. "Konets barokko." *Literaturnaia gazeta*, July 17, 1932.

Shvedov, I. A., comp. *Poet sovetskaia strana*. Moscow: Moskovskii rabochii, 1962.

Sicher, Efraim. "By Underground to Crystal Palace: The Dystopian Eden." *Comparative Literature Studies* 22, no. 3 (Fall 1985): 377–93.

Simpson, John, and Jennifer Speake, comp. *Oxford Concise Dictionary of Proverbs*, 3rd ed. New York: Oxford University Press, 1998.

Skrine, Peter N. *The Baroque: Literature and Culture in Seventeenth-Century Europe*. London: Methuen, 1978.

Snoek, G. J. *Medieval Piety from Relics to the Eucharist: A Process of Mutual Interaction*. Leiden: E. J. Brill, 1995.

Sokolov, A. M. *Stantsii Leningradskogo metro*. Leningrad: Gosudarstvennoe izdatel'stvo literatury po stroitel'stvu i arkhitekture, 1957.

Solov'ev, S. M. *Istoriia Rossii s drevneishikh vremen*. Book 14 of vol. 27–28. Moscow: Mysl', 1965.

———. *Istoriia Rossii s drevneishikh vremen v piatnadtsati knigakh*. Book 8. Moscow: Izdatel'stvo Sotsial'no-ekonomicheskoi literatury, 1962.

Sowers, Robert. *The Language of Stained Glass*. Forest Grove: Timber, 1981.

Starobinski, Jean. *1789: The Emblems of Reason*. Translated by Barbara Bray. Cambridge, Mass.: MIT Press, 1988.

Starr, S. Frederick. *Melnikov: Solo Architect in a Mass Society*. Princeton, N.J.: Princeton University Press, 1978.

Stearns, Peter N. *Consumerism in World History*. London: Routledge, 2001.

Steiner, Peter. "Poem as Manifesto: Mandelstam's 'Notre-Dame.'" *Russian Literature* 5 (1977): 239–56.

"Steklo v sovremennoi arkhitekture." *Sovremennaia arkhtitektura* 3 (1926): 63.

Steklov, V. Iu. *V. I. Lenin i elektrifikatsiia*. Moscow: Nauka, 1975.

Stites, Richard. "The Origins of Soviet Ritual Style." In *Symbols of Power: The Esthetics of Political Legitimation in the Soviet Union and Eastern Europe*, ed. Claes Arvidsson and Lars Erik Blomqvist. Stockholm: Almqvist & Wiksell International, 1987.

———. *Revolutionary Dreams: Utopian Vision and Experimental Life in the Russian Revolution*. New York: Oxford University Press, 1989.

Sukhikh, Igor. "Ostaetsia tol'ko metafora . . . 1927: 'Zavist' Iurii Oleshi." *Zvezda* 10 (2002). http://magazines.russ.ru/zvezda/2002/10/suh.html.

Syromiatnikov, B. I., ed. *Zakonodatel'nye akty Petra I*. Vol. 1. Moscow: Izdatel'stvo akademii nauk Soiuza SSR, 1945.

Sytova, Alla, comp. *The Lubok: Russian Folk Pictures, 17th to 19th Century*. Translated by Alex Miller. Leningrad: Avrora, 1984.

Taranovsky, Kiril. *Essays on Mandel'štam*. Harvard Slavic Studies 6. Cambridge, Mass: Harvard University Press, 1976.

Targoff, Ramie. *John Donne, Body and Soul*. Chicago: University of Chicago Press, 2008.

Tarkhanov, Alexei, and Sergei Kavtaradze. *Architecture of the Stalin Era*. New York: Rizzoli International, 1992.

Tolstoi, Alexei. *Aelita: Giperboloid inzhenera Garina*. Moscow: Izdatel'stvo "Pravda," 1986.

Tolstoi, L. N. *Anna Karenina*. Vol. 8 of *Sobranie Sochinenii v 14-i tomakh*. Edited by K. M. Malyshev. Moscow: Gosudarstvennoe izdatel'stvo khudozhestvennoi literatury, 1952.

Tolstoy, Leo. *Anna Karenina*. Translated by Louise and Aylmer Maude, revised by George Gibian. Norton Critical Edition. 2nd ed. New York: Norton, 1970.

Tomkins, Calvin. *Duchamp: A Biography*. New York: H. Holt, 1998.

Topolin, M. A. *Kremlevskie zvezdy*. Moscow: Moskovskii rabochii, 1975.

Torti, Anna. *The Glass of Form: Mirroring Structures from Chaucer to Skelton*. Cambridge, Eng.: D. S. Brewer, 1991.

Trotskii, L. *Literatura i revoliutsiia*. 1923. Moscow: Izdatel'stvo politicheskoi literatury, 1991.

Tseitlin, M. A. "Kazennye (imperatorskie) 'stekliannyi' i 'zerkal'nyi' zavody v S.-Peterburge." In *Sbornik nauchnykh trudov Leningradskogo finansovo-ekonomicheskogo instituta*. Leningrad: Institut, 1948.

Tsivian, Yury. "Ivan the Terrible: Eisenstein's Rules of Reading." In *Eisenstein at 100: A Reconsideration*, edited by Al LaValley and Barry Scherr. New Brunswick, N.J.: Rutgers University Press, 2001.

Tucker, Janet G. *Revolution Betrayed: Jurij Oleša's "Envy."* Columbus, Ohio: Slavica, 1996.

Tumarkin, Nina. *Lenin Lives! The Lenin Cult in Soviet Russia*. Cambridge, Mass.: Harvard University Press, 1983.

Turgenev, I. S. *Ottsy i deti*. Vol. 8 of *Polnoe sobranie sochinenii i pisem v dvadtsati vos'mi tomakh*. Moscow: Nauka, 1964,

Turner, Jane, ed. *Dictionary of Art*. New York: Grove's Dictionaries, 1996.

Vaingurt, Julia. *Wonderlands of the Avant-Garde: Technology and the Arts in Russia of the 1920s*. Evanston, Ill.: Northwestern University Press, 2013.

Vaiskopf, Mikhail. "Andrei Babichev i ego proobraz v 'Zavisti' Iuriia Oleshi." *Izvestiia Akademii Nauk, Seriia Literatury i Iazyka* 53, no. 5 (1994): 69–76.

Val'be, P. B., ed. *Lenin v sovetskoi poezii*. Leningrad: Sovetskii pisatel', 1970.

Velikanova, Olga. *Making of an Idol: On Uses of Lenin*. Gottingen: Münster-Schmidt Verlag, 1996.

Verkhovtsev, I. P., ed. *Svet nad Rossiei: Ocherki po istorii elektrifikatsii SSSR*. Moscow: Gosudarstvennoe izdatel'stvo politicheskoi literatury, 1960.

Volkhovskoi, M. G., comp. *Domashnii byt russkikh tsarei v XVI-XVII vv. po Zabelinu, Kliuchevskomu, Karnovichu i drugim*. 1904. Moscow: Panorama, 1992.

Volobaeva, T. V. "Vitrazh v russkoi kul'ture: Sankt-Peterburg i ego pamiatniki." Dissertation, St. Petersburg State University, 1999. http://www.nature.ru/db/msg.html?mid=1156475&uri=general.htm.

von Geldern, James. *Bolshevik Festivals, 1917–1920*. Berkeley: University of California Press, 1993.

Voronov, N. V., and M. M. Dubova. *Nevskii khrustal': Ocherki osnovnykh etapov razvitiia*. Leningrad: Khudozhnik RSFSR, 1984.

Voronova, O. I. *Vera Ignat'evna Mukhina*. Moscow: Iskusstvo, 1976.

Voznesenskii, Andrei. "Lonzhiumo." In *Lenin v sovetskoi poezii*, edited by P. B. Val'be. Leningrad: Sovetskii pisatel', 1970.

Wells, H. G. *When the Sleeper Awakes: A Critical Text of the 1899 New York and London First Edition*. Edited by Leon Stover. Jefferson, N.C.: McFarland, 2000.

Werness, Hope B. *The Symbolism of Mirrors in Art from Ancient Times to the Present*. Lewiston, N.Y.: Edwin Mellen, 1999.

White, Stephen. *The Bolshevik Poster*. New Haven, Conn.: Yale University Press, 1988.

Whittick, Arnold. *Symbols, Signs and Their Meaning and Uses in Design*. 2nd ed. London: Leonard Hill, 1971.

Widdis, Emma. *Visions of a New Land: Soviet Film from the Revolution to the Second World War*. New Haven, Conn.: Yale University Press, 2003.

Wimsatt, James. *Allegory and Mirror: Tradition and Structure in Middle English Literature*. New York: Pegasus, 1970.

Wortman, Richard S. *The Development of a Russian Legal Consciousness*. Chicago: University of Chicago Press, 1976.

———. *Scenarios of Power: Myth and Ceremony in Russian Monarchy*. Vol. 1. Princeton, N.J.: Princeton University Press, 1995.

Zabelin, I. E. *Domashnii byt russkikh tsarei v XVI i XVII stoletiiakh*. Book 1. Moscow: Kniga, 1990.

Zakharov, Alexander. "Mass Celebrations in a Totalitarian System." In *Tekstura: Russian Essays on Visual Culture*, edited and translated by Alla Efimova and Lev Manovich. Chicago: University of Chicago Press, 1993

Zamiatin, Evgenii. *My*, in *Izbrannoe*. Moscow: Pravda, 1989.

———. "O moikh zhenakh, o ledokolakh i o Rossii." *Mosty* 9 (1962): 21–25.

Zamyatin, Yevgeny. "Paradise." In *Soviet Heretic: Essays by Yevgeny Zamyatin*, edited and translated by Mirra Ginsburg. Chicago: University of Chicago Press, 1970.

Zbarskii, B. I. *Mavzolei Lenina*. Leningrad: Gosudarstvennoe izdatel'stvo politicheskoi literatury, 1946.

Zbarskii, I. B. "Ot Rossii do Rossii." In *Pod "kryshei" mavzoleia*, compiled by E. E. Zaitseva. Tver': Polina, 1998.

———. "'Zhizn'' mumii i sud'ba cheloveka: Iz vospominanii khranitelia tela Lenina." *Otechestvennaia istoriia* 5 (1993): 158–64.

Zbarsky, I. B., and Samuel Hutchinson. *Lenin's Embalmers*. Translated by Barbara Bray. London: Harvill, 1999.

Zhadova, Larissa. "Tolpa prozrachno-chistykh sot." *Nauka i zhizn'* 8 (1976): 102–7.

Zhivov, V. M. "Istoriia russkogo prava kak lingvo-semioticheskaia problema." In *Semiotics and the History of Culture: In Honor of Jurij Lotman; Studies in Russian*, edited by Morris Halle et al. Columbus, Ohio: Slavica, 1988.

Zhivov, V. M., and B. A. Uspenskii. "Tsar' i bog: Semioticheskie aspekty sakralizatsii monarkha v Rossii." In *Iazyki kul'tury i problemy perevodimosti*, edited by B. A. Uspenskii. Moscow: Nauka, 1987.

Zholkovsky, Alexander. "'Window' in the Poetic World of Boris Pasternak." In *Themes and Texts: Toward a Poetics of Expressiveness*. Ithaca, N.Y.: Cornell University Press, 1984.

Zhukov, Innokenty. "Voyage of the Red Star Pioneer Troop to Wonderland." In *Mass Culture in Soviet Russia: Tales, Poems, Songs, Movies, Plays and Folklore 1917–1953*, edited and translated by James Von Geldern and Richard Stites. Bloomington: Indiana University Press, 1995.

Zhukov, I. N. *Puteshestvie zvena "Krasnoi zvezdy" v stranu chudes: Povest*. Khar'kov: Izdatel'stvo Vseukrainskogo obshch-va sodeistviia Iunomu Lenintsu, 1924.

Ziolkowski, Theodore. *Disenchanted Images: A Literary Iconology*. Princeton, N.J.: Princeton University Press, 1977.

Zoshchenko, Mikhail. "Bednost'." In *Rasskazy, Fel'etony, Povesti*. Moscow: Gosudarstvennoe izdatel'stvo khudozhestvennoi literatury, 1958.

———. "Elektrifikatsiia." In *Uvazhaemye grazhdane*, edited by M. Z. Dolinskii. Moscow: Knizhnaia palata, 1991.

———. "Malen'kaia khitrost'." In *Povesti i rasskazy*. New York: Izdatel'stvo im. Chekhova, 1952.

Index

Page numbers in **bold** refer to illustrations.